THE LUNG
NORMAL AND DISEASED

THE LUNG
NORMAL AND DISEASED

Michael E. Whitcomb, M.D.

Professor of Medicine and Director, Pulmonary Disease Division,
The Ohio State University College of Medicine,
Columbus, Ohio

with 152 illustrations

The C. V. Mosby Company

ST. LOUIS • TORONTO • LONDON   1982

MOSBY

A TRADITION OF PUBLISHING EXCELLENCE

Editor: John Lotz
Assistant editor: Anne Gunter
Manuscript editor: Jean Kennedy
Design: Susan Trail
Production: Margaret B. Bridenbaugh

Printed in the United States of America

The C.V. Mosby Company
11830 Westline Industrial Drive, St. Louis, Missouri 63141

Library of Congress Cataloging in Publication Data

Whitcomb, Michael E.
    The lung, normal and diseased.

    Includes index.
    1. Lungs—Diseases. 2. Lungs. I. Title.
[DNLM: 1. Lung. 2. Lung diseases. 3. Respiratory
insufficiency.   WF 600 W581L]
RC756.W48   616.2'407   81-16816
ISBN 0-8016-5421-1   AACR2

C/D/D 9 8 7 6 5 4 3 2 1   01/C/043

PREFACE

The Lung: Normal and Diseased has been written specifically for students interested in the normal and diseased lung. The organization of the text incorporates concepts used in teaching an introductory course in clinical pulmonary medicine to medical students at The Ohio State University College of Medicine. Traditionally, medical students are taught the structure and function of the normal and diseased lung and the clinical manifestations of the various lung diseases in separate courses (anatomy, histology, physiology, pathology, and pulmonary medicine). Several years ago, the introductory clinical pulmonary disease course at Ohio State was reorganized based on the premise that students are able to understand the clinical features of the various lung diseases better if they first understand the basic structure-function relationships of the normal and diseased lung. The course is organized in such a way that discussion revolves around the three major structural components of the lung—the airways, alveoli, and pulmonary vasculature. The normal structure and function of each component is first reviewed, then the impact of disease on the normal structure-function relationships is discussed. Finally, the clinical, roentgenographic, and physiologic manifestations of the diseases principally affecting each component are described. The diseases are not discussed in great detail, but enough information is provided so that the students can make the association between clinical manifestations common to a number of diseases that primarily affect the same structural component of the lung and basic structure-function relationships. The clinical manifestations of the various lung diseases should be learned in far greater detail during the student's clinical rotations.

Unfortunately, no single text covers all of this information in a way that is appropriate for students and in a size they find practical. *The Lung: Normal and Diseased* was written to fill this need and to help students expand their knowledge of lung diseases throughout the clinical portion of the curriculum. This text is divided into five major sections. The first three sections cover, respectively, the airways, gas-exchanging parenchyma (alveoli), and the pulmonary vasculature. The initial chapters in each section discuss the normal and abnormal structure-function relationships of the component of the lung under consideration and then describe the diseases that most appropriately fit into each section. Most diseases fit easily into this classification system. However, this approach does result in some departures from tradition. For example, emphysema is discussed in the section on alveolar wall diseases. In a more traditional physiologic classification scheme, emphysema is usually discussed along with certain airway diseases as an "obstructive lung disease." However, emphysema is truly a disease of the alveolar wall. In my experience, students are better able to understand and learn the clinical features of this disease when it is presented in this context, rather than associating it with asthma, chronic bronchitis, or other airways diseases.

Sections four and five cover the topics of respiratory failure and pulmonary infections. The initial chapters in both sections describe functions of the whole lung (gas exchange and ventilation and the pulmonary defense mechanisms) that are relevant to the clinical entities discussed in subsequent chapters. This is appropriate, since respiratory failure and pulmonary infection are, in a sense, simply pathophysiologic states resulting from altered ventilation and gas exchange or altered pulmonary defenses regardless of the specific causes of the lung disease.

As with any organizational scheme, the approach used in this text has some unavoidable inconsistencies. However, I believe that the organization of the text allows students to learn the clinical features of lung disease within a conceptual framework which allows them to actually *understand* the disease process far better than if diseases are presented in a more traditional physiologic or roentgenographic classification system. Although these classification systems serve a useful purpose for individuals with substantial knowledge of lung diseases, I believe that students approaching clinical pulmonary medicine for the first time are able to understand the subject better when the diseases are presented in a system based on the structure-function relationships of individual components of the lung or the lung as a whole.

Michael E. Whitcomb

CONTENTS

Section one

THE AIRWAYS

Chapter 1

NORMAL STRUCTURE
AND FUNCTION

STRUCTURE

The tracheobronchial tree, or airways, consists of a series of branching tubes whose main function is to conduct gases into and out of the lung. In addition to serving as conducting tubes, the airways also provide certain defense mechanisms that protect both the airway mucosa and the alveolar surface from a multitude of environmental noxious agents. These functions should be kept in mind when considering the varied structure of the airways at different points along the tracheobronchial tree.

Sequential division of the airways results in approximately twenty-two to twenty-five generations of airways. The combined cross-sectional area of two subdivisions of a parent trunk is always greater than the area of the parent airway. As a result, the total cross-sectional area of the airways increases substantially with each succeeding generation (Table 1). The importance of the increase in determining certain characteristics of flow in the airways will be discussed later.

The trachea and main stem bronchi are mediastinal structures that lie outside the confines of the lung. The remaining subdivisions of the tracheobronchial tree are intrapulmonary structures. The first fourteen intrapulmonary generations lie within the supporting interstitial connective tissue of the lung and are not in intimate contact with gas-exchanging parenchynal tissue. The remaining airways are closely surrounded by lung parenchyma. The terminal bronchioles, approximately the sixteenth generation, are the last airways to have a continuous mucosal lining. At least three generations of respiratory bronchioles lie beyond the terminal bronchioles. The respiratory bronchioles have a discontinuous mucosal lining with alveoli intermittently protruding directly from the wall of the airway. Beyond the respiratory bronchioles are a variable number of alveolar ducts whose walls are completely lined with alveoli. The alveolar ducts terminate in alveolar sacs (Fig. 1-1).

When viewed tangentially, the wall of an airway can be divided into mucosal and submucosal layers. The components of these layers vary markedly at different points along the tracheobronchial tree. The varying histologic features of the airways have functional significance and will be considered in some detail.

TABLE 1
Dimensions of the tracheobronchial tree and lung parenchyma at different levels

Structure	Number	Total cross-sectional area
Trachea	1	5 cm^2
Subsegmental bronchi	38	66 cm^2
Terminal bronchioles	4×10^4	116 cm^2
Terminal respiratory bronchioles	6×10^5	1000 cm^2
Alveoli	300×10^6	70 m^2

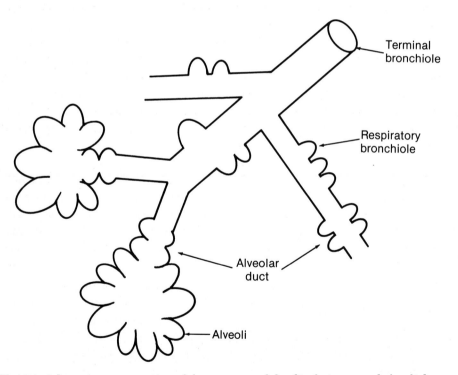

Fig. 1-1. Schematic representation of the structure of the distal airways and alveoli demonstrating the presence of respiratory epithelium (alveolar sacs) in respiratory bronchioles and alveolar ducts.

Mucosa

The mucosa consists of the epithelium, a basement membrane, and the lamina propria. The cells of the epithelium are attached to the basement membrane. The lamina propria lies below the basement membrane and contains lymphocytes, plasma cells, occasional polymorphonuclear leukocytes, and numerous mast cells. An elastic tissue layer forms the boundary of the lamina propria.

A number of different cell types have been identified in the epithelium at some point along the tracheobronchial tree. The functional significance of some of these cells is unknown, and they will not be discussed in any detail. The large airways are lined by a pseudostratified columnar epithelium (Fig 1-2), which consists predominantly of *ciliated cells* and *goblet cells* (Fig. 1-3). Approximately five ciliated cells exist for every goblet cell. The main purpose of the ciliated cells is to propel airway secretions toward the larynx, whereas the goblet cells are actively involved in the synthesis and secretion of mucus (Fig. 1-4). *Nonciliated serous cells* also appear to be distinct cells of the epithelium. The exact function of these cells is unknown, but they may be involved in synthesis of a protein necessary for the transport of a specific immunoglobulin (IgA) onto the airway surface. All these cells are attached to the underlying basement membrane by fine, cytoplasmic foot processes.

Basal, or *germinal cells*, and *intermediate cells* are scattered along the basement membrane. These cells do not reach the surface of the airway and are thus responsible for the pseudostratified appearance of the bronchial epithelium. These cells appear to be precursors of the ciliated and goblet cells. *Argyrophilic cells* (Kulchitsky cells) have also been identified within the basal cell layer. These cells contain neurosecretory granules and appear to have the potential to synthesize a number of bioactive polypeptides. Their significance in the normal lung is unknown, but they are extremely important in certain airway diseases.

The columnar epithelium gradually becomes cuboidal in distal airways. Goblet cells are not present in small bronchioles, whereas *Clara cells* first appear in these airways (Fig. 1-5). Although their exact function has yet to be elucidated, Clara cells are rich in secretory granules and are probably the source of at least one component of the fluid lining the smallest airways. These airways do not have

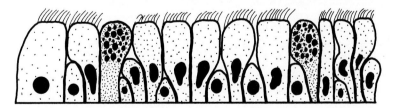

Fig. 1-2. Schematic representation of the pseudostratified columnar epithelium lining the large airways.

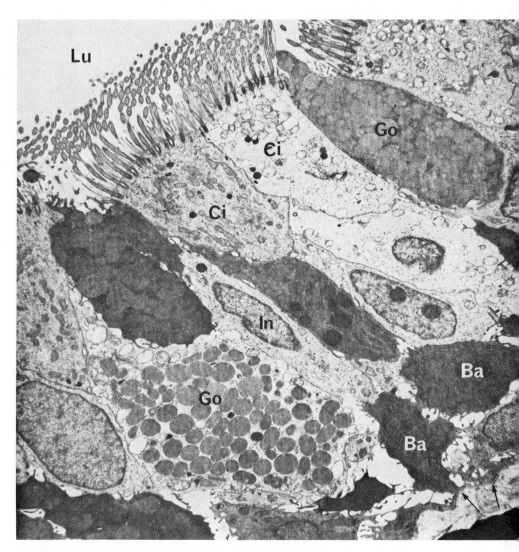

Fig. 1-3. Ultrastructure of the bronchial mucosa. Ciliated (*Ci*), goblet (*Go*), intermediate (*In*), and basal (*Ba*) cells are present. The secretory granules in the goblet cells are abundant. *Lu*, Lumen of the bronchus.

From Breeze, R.G., and Wheeldon, E.B.: REB: the cells of the pulmonary airways, Am. Rev. Respir. Dis. **116:**705, 1977.

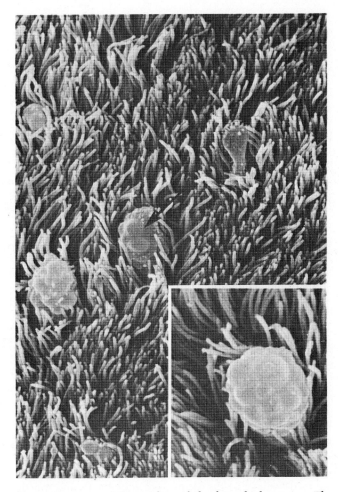

Fig. 1-4. Scanning microscopy of the surface of the bronchial mucosa. The secretions of goblet cells are interspersed in the microvilli of the ciliated cells. The insert shows in greater detail a single goblet cell discharging its secretion.

From Breeze, R.G., and Wheeldon, E.B.: REB: the cells of the pulmonary airways, Am. Rev. Respir. Dis. **116**:705, 1977.

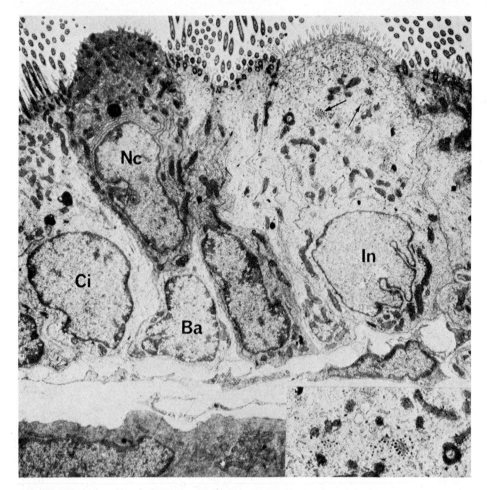

Fig. 1-5. Ultrastructure of the bronchiolar mucosa demonstrating a nonciliated (*Nc*), bronchiolar secretory cell (Clara cell). Ciliated (*Ci*), basal (*Ba*), and intermediate (*In*) cells are also depicted.

From Breeze R.G., and Wheeldon, E.B.: REB: the cells of the pulmonary airways, Am. Rev. Respir. Dis. **116**:705, 1977.

a mucous lining layer reflecting the absence of goblet cells and mucous glands. The cilia of the ciliated cells in these airways are bathed, however, in a watery, protein-rich layer that appears to have surface active properties. Although the source of the various constituents of this fluid is not agreed upon totally, it is agreed that Clara cells are probably important in its production.

Lymphoid nodules are important components of the lamina propria at some sites along the tracheobronchial tree (Fig. 1-6). At these sites the epithelium overlying the nodules is modified and consists of flattened, nonciliated cells resembling lymphoepithelium in other areas of the body (Fig. 1-7). This bronchus-associated

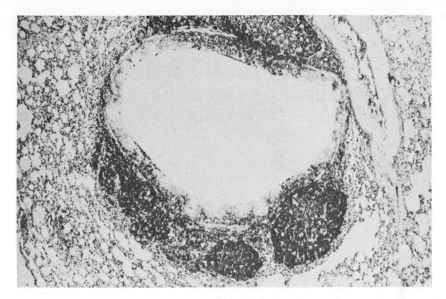

Fig. 1-6. Transverse section of a bronchus demonstrating the presence of bronchus-associated lymphatic tissue (*BALT*).

From Kirkpatrick, C.H., and Reynolds, H.Y.: Immunologic and infectious reaction in the lung, New York, 1976, Marcel Dekker, Inc.

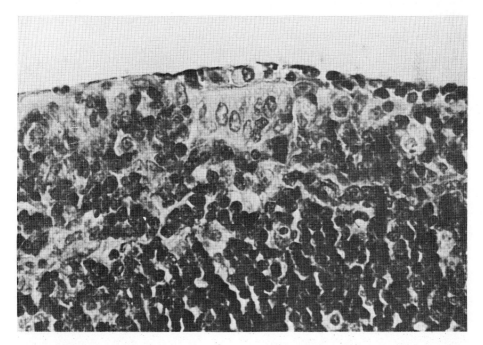

Fig. 1-7. High-power view demonstrating the epithelium overlying the bronchus-associated lymphatic tissue (*BALT*).

From Kirkpatrick, C.H., and Reynolds, H.Y.: Immunologic and infectious reaction in the lung, New York, 1976, Marcel Dekker, Inc.

lymphoid tissue is thought to be analogous to the Peyer patches of the intestine. This tissue is probably important in a variety of immune responses occurring in the lungs and may be particularly important in localizing cells committed to the production of immunoglobulin A (IgA).

Submucosa

Mucous glands, smooth muscle, and cartilaginous plates are the principal components of the submucosa. The submucosal glands contain both serous and mucous cells. Secretions from these cells empty into secretory tubules and then pass into collecting ducts. These ducts are directly contiguous with ciliated ducts whose epithelium is continuous with the lining of the airway. As the airways progress through succeeding generations, the number of complex mucous glands diminish, ultimately disappearing in bronchi less than 2 mm in diameter.

Smooth muscle forms a discontinuous layer in the innermost portion of the submucosa. The muscle bundles spiral in both directions around the airway. Additional muscle fibers insert into the cartilage plates that lie outside the connective tissue plane containing the bronchial mucous glands. In the trachea and main stem bronchi, the cartilage plates are incomplete rings that fail to meet posteriorly. In lobar and segmental bronchi the cartilage rings are complete. In more distal bronchi, cartilage plates are present but do not form rings. The more distal airways that do not contain cartilage are termed "bronchioles." Fine muscle bundles of elastic fibers lie beneath the epithelial surface of these airways.

Alveolar ducts form the final conducting airways. The walls of these ducts are

TABLE 2
Distinguishing features of airways

Airway	Mucosa	Submucosal glands	Cartilage
Trachea	Pseudostratified columnar epithelium, goblet and ciliated cells	Present	Incomplete rings
Bronchi	Pseudostratified columnar epithelium, goblet and ciliated cells	Present	Complete rings, individual plates distally
Bronchioles	Cuboidal epithelium, Clara cells, no goblet cells	Absent	Absent
Respiratory bronchioles	Discontinuous cuboidal epithelium	Absent	Absent
Alveolar ducts	Alveolar epithelium	Absent	Absent

completely lined by alveoli. Within the walls of the ducts fine muscle fibers form a geodesic network that surrounds each alveolar opening in a sphincter-like arrangement. Alveolar ducts terminate in four or occasionally fewer alveolar sacs. The major distinguishing features of the airways at various sites along the tracheobronchial tree are outlined in Table 2.

FUNCTION
Airway defense mechanisms

The exposure of the lung to our environment exceeds that of any other organ of the body except perhaps the skin. Approximately 6000 L of air reach the surface of the alveoli each day. The airways play an important role in protecting the alveolar membrane from noxious elements in the ambient air. The frequent occurrence of lung diseases caused by airborne agents reflects the fact that this defense system is imperfect. Nonetheless, if one simply inspects the air over any industrial city or in the environments in which humans must reside (e.g., cigarrette smoke–filled rooms, mines, factories,), the remarkable efficiency of the airway defense mechanisms is apparent. Following are the airway defense mechanisms:

Nonimmunologic
    reflexes
        cough
        sneeze
    mucociliary function
Immunologic
    humoral factors
        secretory IgA (other immunoglobulins)
        properdin system
    cellular factors
        bronchus-associated lymphocytes
        macrophages

Nasal function

Before considering the specific defense mechanism of the airways, it is important to recognize that the nose and upper respiratory tract perform the important function of adjusting the temperature and humidity of inhaled air. Temperature adjustment begins as soon as inspired air enters the nose. Even when breathing very warm or very cool air, the temperature will reach 28° to 37° C (82.4° to 98.6° F) in the nasopharynx. Further adjustment of air to body temperature is completed before the air reaches the alveoli. The addition of water vapor parallels the temperature adjustment. If the temperature and humidity of inhaled air were not adjusted, cold, unhumidified air would reach the vast surface of the alveolar-capillary membrane. Under these circumstances, it is likely that substantial fluid would be lost from the body, and maintenance of the core body temperature would be extremely difficult.

The structure of the nose provides maximum contact between inspired air and the nasal mucosa. The nasal submucosa contains a rich capillary bed that is under automatic control and very adaptable to changing ambient conditions. The shape and size of the nasal passage may be altered by engorgement of erectile vessels. In addition, changes in capillary bed blood flow and mucosal interstitial fluid may result in increased water at the mucosal surface.

The adjustments in the temperature and humidity of inspired air are extremely important in protecting the distal airways and alveoli against injury. Bypassing these nasal defenses results in metaplasia of the epithelial lining cells of the large airways. As a result, ciliary function in these airways is lost. Thus the whole airway defense system is somewhat dependent on this important function of the nose.

Cough

A number of reflexes involving the respiratory tract are designed to protect the lungs from a variety of insults. Rhinorrhea, sneezing, coughing, laryngeal closure, and bronchial constriction may occur on exposure to noxious substances. Of these various reflexes, cough is of greatest importance as an airway defense mechanism. It clears the airways of excess secretions or foreign materials. Since cough is a common symptom of respiratory disease, it is important to be aware of the physiology of this reflex event.

Cough occurs in response to stimulation of afferent fibers belonging to both the glossopharyngeal and vagus nerves. The sensory endings of the fibers are located in the pharynx, larynx, trachea, and bronchi. Other cough-producing afferent impulses may arise from the esophagus, pleural surface, and external auditory canal. In addition to particulates, noxious gases, and accumulated secretions, cough may be stimulated by cold or hot air.

A cough usually begins with a brief, rapid inspiration that is greater than the normal inspiratory volume. This is followed by closure of the glottis for a brief period during which both the thoracic and abdominal wall muscles contract in an attempt at a forced expiratory effort. Since the glottis is closed, the expiratory muscle activity increases intrathoracic pressure to maximum levels, reaching 100 torr or greater. The glottis then suddenly opens, and expiratory flow accelerates. The presence of a large pressure differential between the alveoli and the atmosphere when the glottis opens and the transient narrowing of the airways produces exceedingly high flow rates within the trachea and airways. Flow may exceed 12 L/second at the mouth within 30 to 50 msec. This expiratory effort is accompanied by a characteristic explosive sound. The vibrations generated by this sound may play a role in suspending secretions in the rapidly moving air column.

A cough produces sufficiently rapid airflow for clearance of foreign material or secretions that are located in the larger airways. In the bronchioles and alveoli, flow is too feeble to effect significant clearance. Foreign material in these regions must be transported to the larger bronchi by ciliary action before cough has an effect on their clearance.

Mucociliary system

Particulate material constitutes the major airborne threat to the lungs. The size of particles dictates how the material is handled by the various respiratory defense mechanisms. The largest particles in the environment, those greater than 10 μm in diameter, are usually trapped in the nose and upper respiratory tract and do not make their way into the lung to confront the airway defense mechanisms. In the nose, long hairs, known as vibrissae, filter out these particles. Turbulence and inertial impaction brought about by the angles that inhaled air must traverse through the nose cause the larger particles escaping the vibrissae to be entrapped in mucus lining the nasal cavities. Similarly, very small particles, those less than 0.3 μm in diameter, do not challenge the lung's defense mechanisms. These particles generally remain suspended in inhaled gas and are simply exhaled back into the environment. Slightly larger particles, 0.5 to 3 μm in diameter, may escape the airway defense mechanisms and be inhaled into the alveoli. These particles, however, may sediment in the alveolus where they are subject to the defense mechanisms of the alveolar membrane (see Chapter 26).

Particles between 2 and 10 μm in diameter constitute the greatest challenge to the airway defense mechanisms. The geometry of airway branching and the mucociliary transport system combine to trap and remove these particles before they reach the alveolus. Since air velocity drops rapidly at points of bifurcation of the airways, both vertical impaction and sedimentation may contribute to the deposition of these particles on the surface of the airway at these points. The particles land on the mucous blanket that coats the surface of the airways. This mucous blanket is constantly propelled toward the mouth by the cilia of the ciliated mucosal cells at an approximate velocity of 10 to 20 mm/minute. Each ciliated cell has approximately 200 cilia that beat up to 1000 times/minute. The cilia in one field beat in one direction while those of adjacent fields beat in slightly different directions.

The mucous blanket consists of two layers. A serous, watery sol layer is in direct contact with the epithelium and bathes the cilia. The cilia beat within this layer but reach up to penetrate and propel the upper zone of mucus toward the mouth (Fig. 1-8). The upper gel layer has a high viscosity and is stickier than the sol layer. The gel layer is occasionally continuous but usually exists as small clumps or streams of mucus. Particles are entrapped in the gel layer and propelled toward the mouth with it. The sources of the various components of the mucous blanket have not been completely identified, but mucous glands and goblet cells contribute

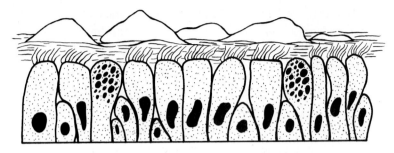

Fig. 1-8. Schematic representation of the mucociliary blanket. The cilia of the mucosal cells beat within a continuous sol layer and the upper gel layer exists in clumps.

to the composition of the mucous layer. Approximately 95% of the mucous blanket is water. Distinct glycoproteins are the most prominent constituent of mucus. These glycoproteins are dispersed as a continuous mesh of fibers within the gel phase. A number of other proteins are found in the sol phase. IgA and lysozyme are the most prominent components of this phase. A number of serum proteins are also found in the sol phase.

Immunologic defense

The airways also contribute to the immunologic defense against inhaled pathogenic microorganisms. Local antibody production by plasma cells in the airway wall is at least one of the mechanisms by which this is accomplished. Immunoglobulin G (IgG) is the major immunoglobulin class in serum and is of major importance in the host's systemic response to bacterial infection. Although IgG is also present in airway secretions, the concentration of IgA in airway secretions is approximately five times greater than that of IgG. In this respect, airway secretions are similar to other body secretions.

The molecular structure of IgA in bronchial secretions (secretory IgA) differs from that of circulating IgA. Secretory IgA is composed of two IgA molecules linked by a "J" chain and attached to a unique "secretory piece." IgA is synthesized as a dimer by plasma cells in the lamina propria of the airway wall. The secretory piece is synthesized by the serous epithelial cells and apparently added to the IgA dimer within the cell. The exact function of the secretory piece is unknown. However, it may play a role not only in facilitating the transport of IgA to the surface of the airway but also in protecting the IgA molecule from proteolysis within the lumen (Fig. 1-9).

The exact function of secretory IgA is not known. It has been suggested that this antibody plays a major role in protection against viral infection. However, the mechanism by which this might occur is unclear. Activation of complement and opsonization, a process that promotes ingestion by phagocytic cells, are both im-

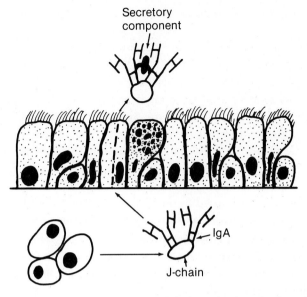

Fig. 1-9. Synthesis of secretory immunoglobulin A (IgA) in the bronchial wall.

portant antibacterial defense mechanisms. IgA does not activate complement by the classic pathway and does not opsonize bacteria for phagocytosis. Thus its role in defense against bacterial infection is even less clear. However, IgA might contribute to the protection against bacteria by other mechanisms. IgA may prevent absorption or attachment of bacteria to specific epithelial cell receptors thus preventing tissue invasion. In addition, it appears that bacteria coated with secretory IgA may be lysed by activation of complement through the properdin pathway.

It also appears that other constituents of the fluid layer lining the airways may have antibacterial properties. This is an area of active investigation, and it is too early to draw conclusions about the importance of these substances for defense of the lung against pathogenic bacteria.

Ventilation

The role of the airways as conducting tubes for the movement of air into and out of the lung is crucial for normal lung function. Diseases of the airways that alter normal gas flow have a profound effect on gas exchange by the lung. Thus it is important to understand the physiology of gas movement in the airways.

To begin, it must be clearly understood that the forces required for the movement of gas within the airways are generated independently of the airways themselves. Since the characteristics of flow within the airways are determined by the relationship between the pressure generating flow and resistance within the airways, it is important first to understand the mechanism by which the driving pressure is generated. Air moves into and out of the lung whenever respiratory muscle activity or recoil forces of the lung and chest wall result in alveolar pressures that are either lower than or greater than atmospheric pressure. Since the pressure at the mouth is always atmospheric, generation of alveolar pressures that are other than atmospheric produces a pressure gradient across the airways. When alveolar pressure falls below atmospheric pressure, the pressure gradient dictates that air flows into the lungs and the lungs inflate. When alveolar pressure is greater than atmospheric pressure, the pressure gradient dictates that flow be mouthward and the lungs must deflate. Changes in alveolar pressure are primarily generated by inspiratory and expiratory muscle activity.

The muscles ordinarily used in quiet breathing (tidal ventilation) are the diaphragm and external intercostal muscles. As these muscles contract, they enlarge the thoracic cavity, thus decreasing intrapleural pressure. The fall in intrapleural pressure similarly produces a fall in alveolar pressure that promotes the flow of gas into the lung and inflation of the lung. The rate of flow and the volume of gas entering the lung will obviously vary with the rapidity and amount of inspiratory force generated by inspiratory muscle activity.

Traditionally, little emphasis has been placed on the characteristics of gas flow during inspiration. It is important to recognize, however, that normal inspiratory airflow is essential for the normal distribution of ventilation throughout the lung. However, since the distribution of ventilation is also affected by the mechanical properties of the alveoli, abnormalities in the distribution of ventilation cannot necessarily be attributed to abnormalities in the mechanical properties of the airways. Thus interest has primarily focused on the dynamics of flow during expiration, since these events are almost totally determined by the mechanical properties of the airways. Consequently, the physiology of expiratory airflow must be discussed in some detail.

During normal tidal ventilation, expiration occurs passively. The force that is responsible for expiration is actually generated during the active inspiratory effort. Inflation of the lung during inspiration imparts potential energy to the elastic tissue of the lung. Therefore, when the inspiratory muscles are relaxed, the lung will recoil inward as a result of this elastic force. The static recoil pressure can be determined for any lung volume by inflating or deflating the lung to a measured volume and, after allowing a few seconds for the lung to come to rest, measuring the intrapleural pressure required to hold the lung at that volume. The static recoil pressure of the lung (Pst [l]) is defined as the alveolar pressure (Palv) minus the pleural pressure (Ppl). Since under a condition of no flow Palv is atmospheric, the Pst (l) is equal to Ppl. When the muscle force maintaining intrapleural pressure is relaxed, this pressure is transmitted to the alveolus and promotes expiratory flow (Fig. 1-10). Expiration continues passively until the inward Pst (l) is balanced by the outward recoil pressure of the chest wall. At this point Palv will equal atmo-

Fig. 1-10. Intrathoracic pressures after modest inspiratory effort. Pleural pressure (*Ppl*) is held at -15 cm H_2O by active inspiratory muscle effort. With the glottis open, pressure in the alveolus equilibrates with atmospheric pressure, which is considered to be zero for reference purposes. Under this circumstance the static recoil pressure (*Pst*) of the lung is 15 cm H_2O. If the inspiratory muscles are relaxed and no active expiratory muscle effort is made, the only pressure on the alveolus generating expiratory airflow will be the Pst of the lung.

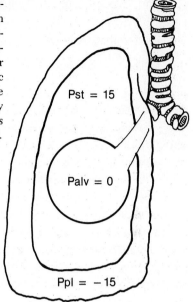

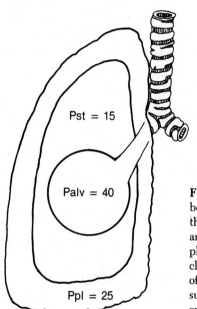

Fig. 1-11. Intrathoracic pressure relationships at the beginning of an active expiratory effort. In contrast to the situation depicted in Fig. 1-10, expiratory muscles are actively contracting to promote expiration. The pleural pressure (*Ppl*) generated by the expiratory muscles is 25 cm H_2O. Since the static recoil pressure (*Pst*) of the lung at end inspiration was 15 cm H_2O, the pressure on the alveolus to generate expiratory airflow is 40 cm H_2O, the sum of the Ppl and Pst.

spheric pressure, and flow ceases unless a conscious effort is made to expel more air from the lungs by active contraction of expiratory muscles.

Contraction of expiratory muscles may generate an increase in intrapleural pressure to levels that exceed atmospheric pressure. This pressure is transmitted to the alveolus and promotes expiratory flow until the lung has been maximally compressed by the chest cage or airways begin to close. Thus, during an active expiratory effort, both Ppl and the Pst (l) combine to raise Palv and promote airflow (Fig. 1-11).

The characteristics of the flow generated by these pressures is obviously influenced by resistance within the airways. Flow ($\dot{V}$) in the airways is directly proportional to the driving pressure (Palv) and inversely proportional to airways resistance (Raw). This relationship can be defined by the equation $\dot{V} = \dfrac{Palv}{Raw}$. Thus, if the pressure in the alveolus [Palv = Ppl + Pst (1)] that generates expiratory flow remains constant, expiratory flow must decrease as airway resistance increases.

A number of factors influence airway resistance. First, lung volume has an important effect. As the lung increases in volume, the diameter of the airways increases proportionately. This change in airway diameter with lung inflation is caused by the tethering effect of the elastic elements of the lung parenchyma surrounding the airways. While the lung is inflated, these elements become more tense and hold the airways more widely open. Deflation relaxes the tension, and the airways narrow. At very low lung volumes airways may actually collapse if the tethering effect of the tissue supporting the airways is abnormal because of a loss of elasticity of the tissue. This relationship between airway caliber and elasticity of lung tissue is termed "interdependence."

Airway resistance is also influenced by the contractile tone of the smooth muscle in the wall of the airways. The physiology of airway smooth muscle function has been defined in recent years. It is clear that this smooth muscle is under neural influences. Beta-adrenergic activity promotes smooth muscle relaxation, whereas parasympathetic activity promotes contraction. Although not totally clear, alpha-adrenergic activity probably promotes smooth muscle contraction. In addition, the bronchial musculature is responsive to a number of chemical mediators that promote smooth muscle contraction. This subject will be discussed in greater detail later.

Dynamic airway compression is an important determinant of airway resistance during forced expiration. It has already been pointed out that, because of active expiratory muscle contraction, Ppl becomes positive during forced expiration. As a result, compression of extrapulmonary, intrathoracic airways may occur. To understand the mechanism by which this occurs, it is necessary to examine the pressure relationships that occur during a forced expiration.

Recall that the pressure which generates airflow is the alveolar pressure (Palv) and that this pressure is the sum of the static recoil pressure (Pst [l]) and pleural pressure (Ppl). During expiration, intraluminal pressure measured along the airways decreases as a result of resistance to airflow. Eventually a point is reached along the airways where the pressure within the lumen is equal to Ppl. This point has been designated the equal pressure point. The intraluminal pressure in airways downstream (i.e., mouthward) from the equal pressure point will be lower than Ppl. If the walls of the airways are exposed to Ppl, they will narrow as a result of the transmural pressure gradient. The compressed downstream segment then be-

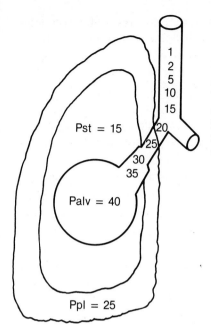

Fig. 1-12. Intrathoracic pressure relationships during an active expiratory effort illustrating schematically the concept of the equal pressure point. Since intraluminal pressure decreases downstream as a result of resistance to airflow, a point is reached at which intraluminal pressure is equal to pleural pressure (Ppl). This point is designated as the equal pressure point. Airways downstream from this point may be compressed, since the pressure outside of the airway is greater than that in the lumen.

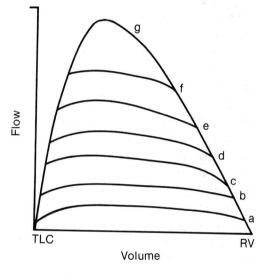

Fig. 1-13. Series of flow volume loops (*a* through *g*) recorded during vital capacity expirations of graded effort. At any given volume, a maximum flow is eventually achieved that cannot be increased by increasing the expiratory effort. For example, the flow generated by the volume represented by point *d* cannot be exceeded by simply increasing the expiratory effort used in creating curves *e* to *g*.

comes flow limiting. The driving pressure that determines maximum airflow during forced expiration is the pressure difference between Palv and the pressure at the equal pressure point. Since the pressure at the equal pressure point is Ppl, this difference (Palv − Ppl) is simply Pst (l) (Fig. 1-12).

It has already been pointed out that the Pst (l) increases with lung volume. Thus flow increases as maximum expiratory efforts are initiated from higher lung volumes. However, since Pst (l) is constant at any given volume, flow will be constant at that volume during a maximum expiratory effort regardless of the volume at which expiration is initiated. This relationship between flow and volume is best understood by examining a series of vital capacity expirations of graded effort (Fig. 1-13). For any volume, a maximum flow rate is achieved that cannot be exceeded by increasing expiratory effort. The outer envelope of this series of curves represents a maximal expiratory effort initiated at total lung capacity and defines the maximum flow that can be achieved at any lung volume.

The principles described apply to expiratory flow throughout the entire tracheobronchial tree and thus reflect the mechanical properties of the airways as a whole. In recent years characterizing differences in the mechanical properties of small and large airways has been of great interest. Two important distinguishing physiologic features of the large and small airways have practical significance. First, laminar flow regimens predominate in small airways, whereas turbulent flow regimens predominate in large airways. Laminar flow is characterized by stream lines that are always parallel to the walls of the conducting tube, whereas turbulent flow is characterized by stream lines that are totally disorganized. Laminar flow is not influenced by gas density, whereas turbulent flow is highly density dependent. Second, small airways contribute only 10% to 20% of the entire resistance to flow through the airways. Although the small airways have small individual diameters, they have a very large combined cross-sectional area simply because they are so numerous. This fact is important, since it means that a marked increase in resistance in small airways may produce only a small increase in total airways resistance and thus have little effect on expiratory flow rates.

A number of tests can be performed to evaluate the mechanical properties of the airways. Some actually measure expiratory flow rates, whereas others only indirectly assess the physiology of the airway. These tests will be described in Chapter 2.

Chapter 2

PATHOPHYSIOLOGY

Diseases of the tracheobronchial tree produce alterations in the structure and function of the airways. The functional abnormalities are of great importance primarily because they alter the distribution of ventilation within the lung and thus produce abnormalities in pulmonary gas exchange. Before considering the pathophysiology of airways disease, it is useful to consider in general terms the pathologic changes caused by airways injury so that the structure-function relationships of the airways can be kept in some perspective.

PATHOLOGIC CHANGES

The airways are particularly susceptible to injury by gases, vapor, fumes, and both particulates and pathogenic microorganisms suspended in air. Acute injury of the airway produces mucosal damage and results in increased secretory activity by submucosal glands and the secretory cells of the airways. With severe injury, the mucosal epithelium may actually be denuded down to the basal layer. Swelling of the basement membrane may occur and be accompanied by extensive edema, hemorrhage, and inflammatory cell infiltration in the lamina propria. If no further injury occurs, these mucosal changes will resolve.

With continued injury, chronic changes may be observed in the epithelial cell layer lining the airways. The earliest changes consist of metaplasia of the lining cells and an increase in the number of goblet cells. Goblet cells usually account for only 20% to 25% of the epithelial cells of large bronchi and are virtually absent in the small bronchi and bronchioles. In response to chronic injury, goblet cells may increase greatly and may be concentrated in the bronchioles. An increase in the number of basal cells and loss of the columnar organization of the epithelium may also occur. The cells themselves may eventually become large and hyperchromatic and at times may become malignant.

Hypertrophy of the submucosal glands also occurs in response to chronic injury. The deeper structures of the airway wall may also be damaged, resulting in destruction of the connective tissue, muscle, and cartilage of the submucosa. These changes may lead to scarring of the airway and partial or total obliteration of some of the small airways. In addition, destruction of the submucosal components of the airways may produce ectatic airways. To a great extent the size of the involved airway determines whether obliteration or ectasia of the airways occurs. Large airways are more likely to become ectatic, whereas small airways are more likely to be obliterated.

Under certain circumstances the mechanical properties of the airways may be altered without changes in structure. Contraction of bronchial smooth muscle, increased mucus production, and mucosal edema combine to alter airway mechanics in this form of airway injury. Two distinct mechanisms may promote these changes. First, when appropriately stimulated, mast cells located in the airway wall may release a number of chemical mediators that act directly on target tissues to produce these changes. The specific cellular events that control release of these mediators by mast cells will be discussed in detail in Chapter 3. These changes may also be produced by parasympathetic effector neuron activity. Stimulation of parasympathetic afferent fibers (irritant receptors) located in the airway epithelium initiates these neural impulses. Different sites along the tracheobronchial tree appear to respond to different stimuli. Some evidence indicates that parasympathetic reflexes may be more important in mediating these events in the large airways, whereas chemical mediators are more important in the smaller airways. These changes are completely reversible and do not lead to structural abnormalities of the airways.

PATHOPHYSIOLOGIC EFFECTS OF AIRWAY INJURY

The spectrum of pathologic changes described above may produce increased intraluminal secretions, loss of the structural integrity of the airway wall, narrowing of the airway lumen, and total obliteration of some airways. Thus the primary pathophysiologic effect of airway injury is an increase in resistance to airflow. Although the effects of increased airway resistance during expiratory flow have been greatly emphasized, increased resistance to airflow is present during both inspiration and expiration. As a result, inspiratory and expiratory flow rates must decrease if the pressure generating flow remains constant.

Increased resistance to inspiratory airflow is of great significance physiologically, since it results in an alteration of the distribution of ventilation to the gas-exchanging parenchymal tissue of the lung. The significance of the distribution of ventilation within the lung for normal gas exchange will be discussed in detail in Chapter 22. Any pathologic process that alters the distribution of ventilation within the lung will cause arterial hypoxemia. In general, the degree of hypoxemia correlates with the degree to which the ventilation of perfused alveoli is impaired.

The distribution of ventilation throughout the lung can be affected greatly by changes in the mechanical properties of individual gas-exchanging units (acini). The mechanical properties of these units are determined by the resistance to airflow into the unit and by the compliance of alveoli in the unit. Compliance can be thought of in terms of elasticity of the inflatable gas-exchanging tissue (alveoli). At any inflating pressure, the time required to inflate alveoli is determined by the resistance to airflow into the alveoli. Provided that the time for filling is adequate, the volume the alveoli expand is primarily determined by their compliance. Resistance to airflow and the elastic properties of the alveoli are relatively uniform in gas-exchanging units throughout the normal lung. Thus the time required to adequately inflate all lung units is reasonably similar. The distribution of ventilation in the normal lung is not significantly influenced by differences in the mechanical properties of the airways or alveoli.

If airways disease is present, ventilation will tend to be distributed to units with the lowest resistance to airflow, since units with higher resistance will require a longer time for filling. If the alveoli are normal, the compliance of the gas-exchanging units throughout the lung will remain nearly identical. Thus, provided that the time for inspiration is adequate to overcome delays in the filling of some alveoli because of resistance to airflow, ventilation of all alveoli will remain normal. However, if inspiratory time is inadequate to allow compensation for delayed filling of some alveoli, inhomogeneity of ventilation will occur as a result of differences in resistance to airflow in individual units. Similarly, resistance to expiratory flow may prevent complete emptying of lung units. The gas trapped in these units contributes to the total volume of gas present in the lung after a maximum expiration. Thus an increase in the residual volume of the lung is an important physiologic effect of increased resistance to expiratory airflow.

To summarize, increased resistance to airflow is the primary pathophysiologic effect of airway disease. Because of the increased resistance, inspiratory and expiratory flow rates decrease. As a result, the distribution of ventilation throughout the lung is altered, and the residual volume of the lung increases.

A number of tests have been designed to detect abnormalities in the mechanical properties of the airways. These tests are all based on the fact that injury to airways causes an increase in resistance to airflow. Since the pressure that generates flow is reasonably reproducible during a forced expiratory maneuver, the tests routinely employed in the clinical laboratory are primarily designed to directly or indirectly measure flow rates during forced expiration.

CLINICAL TESTS OF MECHANICAL PROPERTIES OF AIRWAYS
Large airways

A recording of the *forced vital capacity* (FVC) is the most common technique used to detect impairment of expiratory flow (Fig. 2-1). To perform this simple test

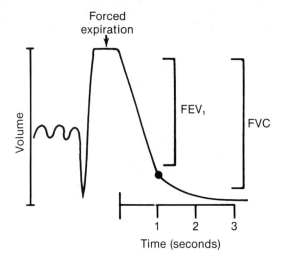

Fig. 2-1. Spirographic tracing demonstrating a forced expiratory maneuver initiated from total lung capacity. The volume expired in 1 second (FEV$_1$) and the total volume expired, the forced vital capacity (FVC), are directly measured from the tracing and used to calculate the ratio of FEV$_1$ to FVC, or FEV$_1$ %.

the patient fills the lungs maximally and then forcibly exhales. During exhalation, the expired volume is plotted against time. A number of different flow rates may be calculated from a spirometry tracing by connecting any two points on the curve and measuring the corresponding expired volume and time. In clinical practice, however, the most frequently employed index of flow obtained from this test is an indirect measurement of flow: the ratio of the forced expired volume (FEV) in 1 second to the total forced expired volume (FEV$_1$/FVC $\times$ 100, or FEV$_1$%). A value less than 75% indicates decreased flow caused by an increase in airway resistance in the large airways.

Although a number of different flow rates can be calculated from a forced spirogram, the *maximum midexpiratory flow rate* (MMEFR) is employed most often clinically (Fig. 2-2). This flow rate is calculated by measuring the volume between 25% and 75% of the FVC and the time required to exhale this volume. If the FEV$_1$% is abnormal, no special significance can be applied to a decreased MMEFR. If, however, the FEV$_1$% is normal, the MMEFR may be decreased if the rate of expiratory flow slows disproportionately as lung volume decreases during expiration. This abnormality correlates with an increase in resistance to airflow predominantly to the small airways.

Flow rates can be measured directly during a forced expiratory maneuver. A plot of instantaneous flow rates against volume over the entire range of expired volume is referred to as a *maximum expiratory flow-volume curve* (Fig. 2-3). Dur-

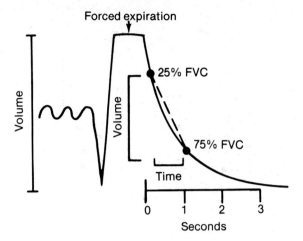

Fig. 2-2. Spirographic tracing illustrating how the maximum midexpiratory flow rate is calculated.

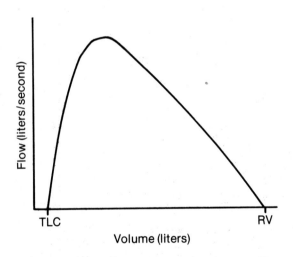

Fig. 2-3. Maximum expiratory flow volume curve. A maximum expiratory effort is initiated at total lung capacity and continued until residual volume is reached. Flow is plotted instantaneously against volume during this effort.

ing a forced expiration, flow ($\dot{V}$) initially increases rapidly as expiration begins. Peak flow is reached when 20% to 25% of the total expired volume has been exhaled. Flow then decreases throughout the remainder of the expiratory maneuver. In this test the peak flow rate may be primarily influenced by airway resistance in the large airways. The flow rate at which 50% ($\dot{V}max_{50}$) or 75% ($\dot{V}max_{75}$) of the total expired volume has been exhaled is usually measured in this test to determine the effects of decreasing lung volume on flow. If peak flow is markedly decreased, these values have little meaning. However, if peak flow is minimally decreased, disproportionate decreases in flow at these low lung volumes can reflect increased resistance to flow predominantly in the small airways.

The final method for detecting abnormalities in the mechanical properties of the large airways is to directly measure *airways resistance* (Raw) or its reciprocal, *conductance* (1/Raw). These measurements can be obtained only by using a body plethysmograph and thus are not routinely obtained in most clinical laboratories. Two points about these techniques should be remembered. First, the lung volume at which the measurement is made must be recorded, since, as discussed previously, lung volume influences airway resistance by changing the diameter of the airways. Second, these techniques cannot accurately detect increased resistance localized to the small airways, since the contribution of resistance in small airways to total airway resistance is small.

Small airways

Because of the interest in detecting increases in airway resistance predominantly in the small airways, a number of tests have been developed to assess the mechanical properties of these airways. Two of these tests, the MMEFR and the $\dot{V}max_{50}$–$\dot{V}max_{75}$, have been discussed. These tests are not entirely specific for small airways abnormalities. A mild increase in resistance in large airways would decrease peak flow and flow at low lung volumes in the same range as observed with an increase in airway resistance predominantly in small airways. Thus other methods are required to more accurately differentiate these conditions.

A comparison of the values for $\dot{V}max_{50}$ obtained while breathing an oxygen-helium mixture (20% oxygen and 80% helium) and air ($\Delta\dot{V}max_{50}$) is one method that may localize an increase in airway resistance to either large or small airways (Fig. 2-4). This test has been designed to take advantage of the difference in the flow regimens in large and small airways. As previously mentioned, laminar flow predominates in small airways, whereas turbulent flow predominates in large airways. In addition, laminar flow is uninfluenced by gas density, whereas turbulent flow is density dependent. Thus an increase in resistance in small airways should produce comparable flow rates whether air or a less dense gas mixture (oxygen and helium) is breathed. If the site of increased resistance is in the large airways, however, flow should be much higher when the less dense gas mixture is breathed. Thus a comparison of the $\dot{V}max_{50}$ obtained while breathing these two gas mixtures should localize the site of increased airways resistance. This technique is often employed in research laboratories but has little applicability in clinical laboratories because of the necessity of rigid adherence to certain technical aspects of performing these studies.

Measurement of the volume of the lungs at which airway closure occurs has

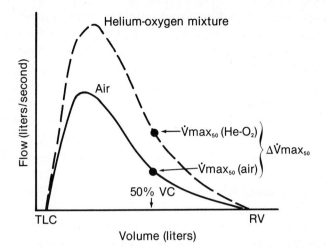

Fig. 2-4. Maximum expiratory flow volume loops obtained while breathing an air and helium-oxygen mixture. Note the difference in the curves. The method for calculating the flow rate at which 50% of the total expired volume is exhaled ($\Delta \dot{V}max_{50}$ is depicted).

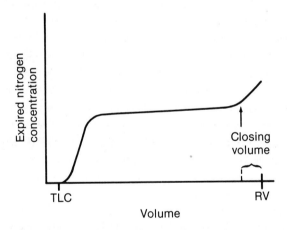

Fig. 2-5. Measurement of closing volume by the single breath oxygen technique. After a single inspiration of 100% oxygen, expired nitrogen concentration is plotted against volume during a slow expiratory maneuver initiated at total lung capacity and continued to residual volume. The point at which the expired nitrogen concentration abruptly deviates from the plateau achieved during the majority of expiration is considered the point at which airway closure begins. The closing volume can be directly measured by reference to the volume axis.

also been proposed as a test for detecting abnormalities in the function of small airways (Fig. 2-5). This test is performed by continuously plotting the concentration of nitrogen in expired gas against lung volume after the patient has inhaled a single breath of 100% oxygen. The steady state concentration of nitrogen in expired gas during exhalation is determined by the mixing of individual nitrogen concentrations in alveoli throughout the lungs, which are emptying at the same time. In the upright individual the concentration of nitrogen in alveoli in the apex of the lung is higher than that of alveoli in the base of the lung. Thus, if the alveoli in the base of the lung can no longer contribute to exhaled gas because of closure of small airways in these regions, the concentration of nitrogen in expired gas when measured at the mouth must increase. The volume at which this abrupt increase in expired nitrogen concentration occurs can be measured and is considered the *closing volume*. An increase in closing volume is considered to be indicative of small airways disease.

The final physiologic test that reflects an increase in resistance in small airways is measurement of the *frequency dependence* of the *dynamic compliance* of the lung. This technique is only used in research laboratories because of the technical considerations involved in performing the test. However, one should be aware of the theory behind this test.

The compliance of a distensible structure is defined as a change in volume for a given change in pressure ($C = \Delta V / \Delta P$). In determining the compliance of the lung, these measurements are usually made during lung deflation when flow has been interrupted. Thus the static compliance (Cst) is usually obtained. Compliance can also be measured during airflow (dynamic compliance, Cdyn). The Cdyn, however, may be influenced by resistance in small airways, since a change in volume is dependent on complete filling of all gas-exchanging units of the lung. As previously pointed out, filling of individual lung units is influenced both by the compliance of the unit and the resistance to airflow in the small airways supplying the unit. This can be mathematically represented by calculating a time constant that represents in a relative way the time required for filling of each lung unit. The time constant is defined as resistance times compliance:

$$\text{Raw} \times \text{C, or } \frac{\Delta P}{\Delta V / t} \times \frac{\Delta V}{\Delta P}$$

In the normal lung, time constants for all units are reasonably uniform. Therefore regardless of the filling time (inspiratory time), all units will fill equally. If, however, time constants of individual gas-exchanging units exhibit wide discrepancies caused by differences in resistance in small airways, lung units will fill asynchronously. Those with short time constants will fill first and those with long time constants later. Nonetheless, provided that inspiratory time is adequate, all units will fill. Thus the Cst and Cdyn will be essentially identical, since change in volume will be identical. If, however, inspiratory time is progressively decreased by increasing the respiratory rate, units with long time constants eventually may not have adequate time to completely fill. In this situation volume will decrease, and Cdyn will be lower than Cst. A fall in Cdyn as respiratory rate increases is called

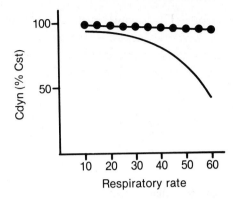

Fig. 2-6. Illustration of frequency dependence of dynamic compliance. The response in a normal individual *(line interrupted with dots)* is depicted for comparative purposes. Under normal circumstances, dynamic compliance does not decrease as the respiratory rate increases. With frequency dependence, however, dynamic compliance *(solid line)* decreases as the respiratory rate increases.

frequency dependence of Cdyn and is indicative of increased resistance in small airways (Fig. 2-6). Obviously, inhomogeneity in the compliance of individual units or increased resistance in large airways will produce similar changes. Thus Cst and Raw must be normal for accurate interpretation of the results of measurements of frequency dependence of Cdyn.

· · ·

In summary, diseases producing increased resistance in large airways result in a decrease in the $FEV_1\%$, a decrease in the peak flow rate, density dependence of flow at midvital capacity, an increase in airway resistance, and an increase in the residual volume of the lung. Disease localized predominantly to small airways results in a disproportionate decrease in flow rates at low lung volumes, a lack of density dependence of flow at midvital capacity, an increased closing volume of the lung, frequency dependence of Cdyn, and an increase in the residual volume of the lung.

Chapter 3

ASTHMA

Asthma is a disease characterized by intermittent, acute airways obstruction that is spontaneously reversible or reversible after appropriate therapy. The airflow obstruction present in other airway diseases is often partially reversible, but this should not be considered evidence that the patient also has asthma. The diagnosis of asthma should be reserved for patients with truly intermittent airways obstruction who fulfill the defined diagnostic criteria.

PATHOLOGIC FEATURES

Pathologic examination of lung tissue is of no value in the diagnosis of asthma. The pathologic changes that have been described in asthma have been observed predominantly in individuals dying of the disease, thus the pathologic features of mild asthma are not defined well. Diffuse mucous plugging of both small and large airways is usually present in patients who die of this disease. In addition, the number of mucosal goblet cells increases, hyperplasia of submucosal glands occurs, and the submucosa is infiltrated with neutrophils and eosinophils. Hypertrophy of the bronchial smooth muscle and thickening of the mucosal basement membrane may also be prominent. In some cases immunoglobulin deposits can be identified in the basement membrane.

PATHOGENESIS

A number of stimuli may precipitate acute airways obstruction. Before considering the major physiologic mechanisms in the pathogenesis of acute airways obstruction, the factors that influence patency of the airways should be considered first. Although an increase in bronchial secretions and mucosal edema contribute to airways obstruction, bronchial smooth muscle tone is the predominant determinant of the caliber of the airway lumen. With smooth muscle contraction the airway lumen is narrowed, whereas smooth muscle relaxation causes dilation of the lumen. Thus the dynamics of acute airways obstruction are primarily determined by the

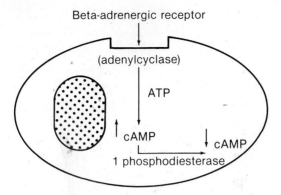

Beta-adrenergic receptor

(adenylcyclase)

ATP

cAMP

cAMP

1 phosphodiesterase

Fig. 3-1. Schematic representation of the intracellular biochemistry of the beta-adrenergic system in bronchial smooth muscle cells.

balance between physiologic mechanisms that stimulate smooth muscle contraction and those which promote smooth muscle relaxation.

Bronchial smooth muscle relaxation is mediated primarily through beta-adrenergic receptors located on the surface of these cells. In recent years the biochemical events occurring within the cell after beta-adrenergic stimulation have been described in detail. Since the rationale for certain forms of therapy used in the treatment of asthma is based on an understanding of these intracellular events, they will be described in some detail.

The interaction of beta-adrenergic agonists with molecular receptors located on the surface of the bronchial smooth muscle cell activates adenyl cyclase resulting in the generation of increased concentrations of adenosine 3': 5'-cyclic phosphate (cyclic AMP) within the cell. Cyclic AMP can be considered an intracellular messenger hormone that controls many of the biologic activities of cells in the body. Cyclic AMP promotes relaxation of the bronchial smooth muscle cell. Thus the intracellular concentration of cyclic AMP directly influences patency of the airway lumen. Although beta-adrenergic agonists are the most widely recognized agents that stimulate cyclic AMP generation, other agents, such as certain prostaglandins, also are likely to induce smooth muscle relaxation through this mechanism. Cyclic AMP is catabolized in the cell by the enzyme phosphodiesterase. The equilibrium between stimulation of cyclic AMP production and the breakdown of cyclic AMP by phosphodiesterase determines the intracellular concentration of this messenger hormone (Fig. 3-1).

The stimuli that produce acute airways obstruction are varied. Acute airways obstruction may follow inhalation of specific allergens and certain noxious fumes or gases or may be a result of certain physical factors such as exercise or exposure to cold air. In these various situations, bronchial smooth muscle contraction is mediated either by neural impulses from parasympathetic nerve fibers or by chemical mediators released by mast cells. Although these mechanisms may combine to stimulate smooth muscle contraction, for conceptual purposes mast cell mediator release may be considered to be primarily involved in allergen-induced acute airways obstruction, whereas parasympathetic nerve stimulation is involved in acute airways obstruction induced by physical factors or after exposure to noxious stimuli (Fig. 3-2).

The events involved in the release of chemical mediators by mast cells have received considerable interest in recent years. As part of an immune response to a sensitizing antigen, some individuals develop IgE-class antibody, which fixes to the surface of mast cells. On reexposure to the antigen, the interaction of antigen with the cell surface–bound IgE somehow results in degranulation of the mast cell. As part of this process, histamine, eosinophilic chemotactic factor (ECF), slow-reacting substance of anaphylaxis (SRS-A), and other mediators are released extracellularly. These mediators appear to directly stimulate mucosal edema, increased bronchial secretions, and smooth muscle contraction (Figs. 3-3 and 3-4).

Stimulation of bronchial smooth muscle by parasympathetic effector neurons appears to involve a neural arc that receives afferent impulses from fibers located in the bronchial mucosa. Although this mechanism is not specifically involved in allergen-induced acute airways obstruction, this should not be interpreted to mean that this mechanism may not at times be responsible for smooth muscle contraction in patients with a clear history of allergic asthma. These patients also may develop

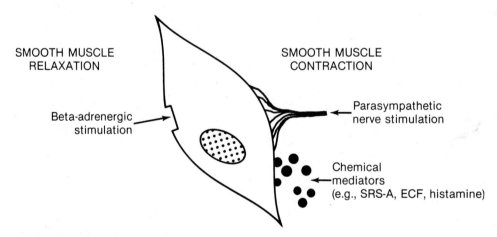

Fig. 3-2. Factors that influence bronchial smooth muscle contraction or relaxation. Beta-adrenergic stimulation is the major mechanism for promoting smooth muscle relaxation, whereas parasympathetic nerve stimulation or chemical mediators may promote smooth muscle contraction.

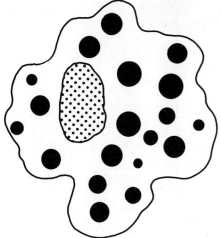

Fig. 3-3. Mast cell with numerous characteristic cytoplasmic granules.

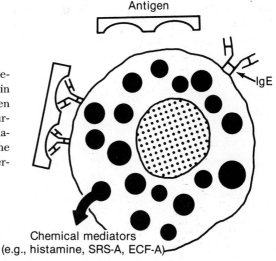

Fig. 3-4. Mechanism of mast cell degranulation mediated by immunoglobin E (IgE). The linking of specific antigen with IgE molecules bound to the surface of the mast cell triggers degranulation which results in release of the chemical mediators of immediate hypersensitivity reactions.

bronchospasm after inhalation of noxious agents, exercise, or exposure to cold air. Clearly the primary mechanism involved in promoting smooth muscle contraction is dependent on the nature of the stimulus.

As mentioned previously, the dynamics of airway patency are determined by the balance between the effect of beta adrenergic–mediated bronchial smooth muscle relaxation and factors stimulating bronchial smooth muscle contraction. Although almost everyone is exposed to the same allergens, noxious stimuli, and physical factors, for unknown reasons only a relatively small percentage of people develop asthma. Furthermore, even some individuals with IgE antibodies to specific allergens do not develop airways obstruction after antigen exposure. It has been hypothesized that patients with asthma have a relative deficiency in beta-adrenergic activity that does not allow them to maintain bronchial smooth muscle relaxation after exposure to stimuli which promote smooth muscle contraction. As a result, such individuals are more susceptible to the development of airways obstruction.

ETIOLOGIC FACTORS

In the majority of patients with asthma, an attack occurs after inhalation of an allergen; exposure to noxious gases, fumes, or cold air; or exercise. However, it is often difficult to clearly identify the precipitating factor in any individual episode. Although there has been great interest in the immunologic basis of asthma, it is unusual to identify the specific allergen that is responsible for precipitating asthma in the majority of adults. Nevertheless, it is important to attempt to identify an environmental allergen that may be responsible for precipitating an asthma attack, since it may then be possible to prevent episodes by avoiding contact with the antigen. If the antigen is somewhat ubiquitous, such as grass, tree, or plant pollens, avoiding contact may not be possible. However, if the antigen source is a pet, household plant, or other domestic object, the patient's reaction may be greatly lessened by removing the object.

In this context it is extremely important to recognize that asthma may be related to the individual's occupational environment. Occupational asthma may be caused by exposure to antigens to which the patient has been sensitized at work or to chemicals or dust that may stimulate acute airways obstruction through nonimmune mechanisms. Probably the best example of occupational asthma is seen in individuals who inhale cotton, flax, or hemp dust. A component of these dusts can directly release histamine into the lung and thus produce acute airway obstruction. This is potentially an extremely important problem since cotton is such an important fiber in our society. A number of examples of immune-mediated occupational asthma exist. Asthma has developed in workers sensitized to bacterial enzymes used in the production of detergents and in workers sensitized to wood dusts, platinum, nickel, or toluene di-isocynate. Acute airways obstruction may also occur after antigen exposure in individuals with extrinsic allergic alveolitis. Thus immune-mediated asthma may also develop in individuals who are exposed to a variety of thermophilic actinomycetes, molds, or animal proteins in their occupation.

Some patients develop asthma only after exertion. In the majority of these individuals, parasympathomimetic stimulation of bronchial smooth muscle contraction appears to be the predominant mechanism involved in the production of acute airways obstruction. However, mast cell mediator release may also occur in this situation. The explanation for this is unclear. Exposure to cold air is a common precipitating factor in many patients with asthma. This response appears to be directly related to the effect of the low humidity of cold air on afferent receptors in the bronchial mucosa. In this form of asthma smooth muscle contraction is clearly mediated by parasympathetic neural stimulation.

PHYSIOLOGIC ABNORMALITIES

A decrease in expiratory flow rates is the predominant physiologic abnormality observed in asthma. The magnitude of the decrease in the FEV_1 to FVC ratio generally reflects the severity of the episode. In addition, the vital capacity usually decreases, and the residual volume and total lung capacity (TLC) increase significantly. The TLC should increase only if the compliance of the lung increases. The increased TLC would imply that acute alterations in the mechanical properties of the lung occur in asthma and that these changes may be reversed rapidly with appropriate therapy. No rational basis exists for the occurrence of such changes during an episode of asthma.

Abnormalities in gas exchange also occur during an acute asthma attack. As a result of ventilation-perfusion mismatching, the arterial oxygen tension decreases. During most episodes total alveolar ventilation increases, thus the arterial carbon dioxide partial pressure (P_aCO_2) decreases. As the severity of airways obstruction increases, alveolar ventilation begins to fall and may eventually become inadequate. As a result, the P_aCO_2, which may range from 25 to 35 mm Hg during the initial stages of an asthma attack, may increase slowly. Ultimately the patient may develop hypercapnia.

During therapy, the lung volumes may revert to normal before the FEV_1 to FVC ratio increases. Eventually, however, this ratio also becomes normal. Between episodes, routine pulmonary function tests are usually completely normal in patients with pure asthma. However, more sophisticated physiologic tests may reveal abnormalities consistent with impairment of airflow at the level of small airways (terminal bronchioles). The changes that may be detected are an increase in the alveolar-arterial oxygen gradient, an increased closing capacity, frequency dependence of dynamic compliance, and decreased flow rates at low lung volumes. These changes may persist for many years and may be present in adults who have not had an attack of acute airways obstruction since childhood. The reason for these persistent abnormalities in the mechanical properties of the small airways is unclear.

CLINICAL MANIFESTATIONS

In the majority of patients, asthma attacks are self-limited or respond rapidly to appropriate therapy. In more severe episodes, airways obstruction tends to be slowly progressive over a period of days. In fact, it is uncommon for an individual to develop status asthmaticus, a state in which airways obstruction is not responsive to standard therapy, unless the duration of the episode has exceeded several days. In the great majority of patients, progressive shortness of breath is the predominant symptom during an acute attack. Cough is frequently present, and some patients complain of audible wheezing.

On physical examination, the patient is usually anxious, uses accessory muscles of respiration to breathe, and is tachypneic. Auscultation of the lungs reveals diffuse, inspiratory and expiratory wheezes. As the severity of airways obstruction increases, wheezes may decrease in intensity, may become high-pitched in quality, and, at times, are barely audible. With increasing airways obstruction, hyperinflation of the lungs becomes marked. At this stage intercostal muscle retraction and a prominent pulsus paradoxus may become evident. If the episode persists for a prolonged period, the patient frequently becomes fatigued and confused.

With successful therapy, the clinical manifestations of asthma resolve in an orderly manner. Intercostal retraction and pulsus paradoxus are the first signs to disappear. As further improvement occurs, the patient becomes asymptomatic, and finally wheezing disappears. As a general rule, patients become asymptomatic when pulmonary function tests have returned to 60% to 70% of baseline values. Thus subclinical airways obstruction is still present at this stage. Because airways obstruction has not completely reversed by the time the patient is asymptomatic, symptoms may recur if therapy is abruptly discontinued. Subclinical airways obstruction may persist for weeks after an acute asthma attack. As a result, patients may complain of exertional dyspnea for a long time after recovery from an acute episode.

DIAGNOSIS

The diagnosis of asthma is based on an appropriate history and clinical or laboratory evidence that the patient has reversible airways obstruction. Standard laboratory studies are of little value in the diagnosis of the disease. During an acute episode, peripheral blood and sputum eosinophilia is observed in the majority of patients. Less frequently, Curschmann spirals or Charcot-Leyden crystals are observed in the sputum. All other routine laboratory studies are usually normal.

Occasionally patients will be seen first during a remission period. Despite a suggestive history, it may be impossible to make an accurate diagnosis of asthma during this period. In this situation, however, several diagnostic studies may prove useful. First, demonstrating that the patient is atopic and thus potentially susceptible to develop airways obstruction after antigen exposure may be valuable. The atopic individual will have IgE-class antibody against potential allergens. To document atopy, the standard skin test antigens should be applied intradermally. The development of an immediate wheal and flare reaction at the antigen site is strong evidence that the individual has IgE-class antibody directed against the inciting antigen. Measurement of serum IgE levels is also a useful way of identifying atopic individuals, since few other conditions increase the serum concentration of IgE.

Occasionally, reproduction of an asthma attack may be desirable for diagnostic purposes. This can be accomplished in one of two ways. First, the individual can be exposed to an inhalation challenge if an allergen preparation is available. Patients with IgE-mediated asthma will develop clinical and physiologic evidence of airways obstruction in the laboratory within 30 minutes of an inhalation exposure to the allergen to which they are sensitized. This test is highly diagnostic when positive. It is limited both by the inability to identify specific allergens that may be important in precipitating asthma in most adult patients and by the lack of appropriate antigens for testing purposes.

Inhalation of chemical mediators known to provoke airways obstruction is the second method for inducing an asthma attack in the laboratory. In this test, histamine, methacholine chloride (Mecholyl), or prostaglandin can be employed. Individuals with asthma develop airways obstruction at concentrations of these mediators, which are much smaller than those required to provoke airways obstruction in nonasthmatic individuals. Thus this test is useful in confirming whether an individual has asthma but provides no information about the specific antigen involved in precipitating attacks.

Routine pulmonary function tests performed before and after inhalation of standard bronchodilator drugs may also have diagnostic value. This approach is of most value when the patient is seen during a period of airways obstruction. Complete reversibility of the airways obstruction after inhalation of bronchodilators is strong evidence that the patient has asthma. Partial reversibility is of little value in the diagnosis, since this type of response can be seen in individuals with airways obstruction caused by other airway diseases. This approach obviously has little value in patients in remission with normal pulmonary function studies at the time they are seen.

TREATMENT

In considering the treatment of asthma, prophylactic therapy and therapy to reverse acute airways obstruction must be discussed separately. Clearly, the prevention of an acute attack would be the ideal approach to the management of the patient with asthma. Hyposensitization therapy has long been used as a form of preventive therapy. Although not of proven value in asthma, this form of therapy has been effective in the prevention of ragweed hay fever, and a scientific basis for its efficacy has been proposed. Like allergic asthma, IgE-mediated, mast cell degranulation is thought to be the principal mechanism involved in the pathogenesis of hay fever. During the administration of ragweed antigen, IgG antibodies are produced that prevent the binding of the antigen to the IgE attached to the surface of the mast cell. As a result, degranulation of the mast cell is prevented. Despite the theoretical basis for this treatment, its value in asthma has yet to be convincingly demonstrated. It is the clinical impression of many allergists that this form of therapy is beneficial in children but has little value in adult patients.

Disodium chromoglycate prevents asthma attacks in some patients. This drug prohibits the degranulation of mast cells despite the interaction of antigen with IgE on the surface of the cell. The mechanism by which the drug inhibits mast cell degranulation is unknown. At present the value of this form of therapy is limited for several reasons. First, the drug is useful only in patients with allergic asthma, which is relatively uncommon in adults. In addition, the drug has to be administered by inhalation at frequent intervals, so that for patients who only have sporadic episodes of asthma, disodium chromoglycate is not useful. Despite these limitations, this form of therapy is effective in preventing asthma attacks in selected patients with allergic asthma.

The treatment of acute asthma often requires a combination of drugs such as the beta-adrenergic agonists, methyl xanthines, and corticosteroids. A large number of beta-adrenergic agonists are available for use. These drugs produce bronchodilation by stimulating beta receptors on the surface of the bronchial smooth muscle cell. Since beta-adrenergic receptors are also present on cardiac muscle cells, tachycardia and hypertension may be observed during their use. Because pharmacologic effects limit to some degree the usefulness of these drugs in the treatment of acute asthma, drugs that selectively stimulate the beta-2 receptors of the bronchi have been developed. Despite theoretical advantages, the cardiovascular side effects observed with the general beta-adrenergic stimulants have not been completely eliminated. Nevertheless, the use of beta-2 agents has practical advantages. Manipulation of the catecholamine structure to increase the beta-2 specificity of the compound also makes the drug less susceptible to enzymatic degradation. As a result, the duration of action of the beta-2 agonists is prolonged. The increased duration of action is a real advantage when oral agents are used as part of the therapy of asthma. Muscle tremor is the only side effect of these drugs that does not occur with general beta agonists.

The xanthine derivatives are also regularly used in the treatment of acute asthma. The xanthines also produce bronchodilation by increasing cyclic AMP in bronchial smooth muscle cells. In contrast to the beta-adrenergic agents, however, the xanthines inhibit the metabolism of cyclic AMP by phosphodiesterase. Gastrointestinal side effects, arrhythmias, and hypotension are the most frequently observed toxic effects during the parenteral administration of theophylline.

In recent years the bronchodilating effect of theophylline has demonstrated a direct relationship to the serum concentration of the drug. In general, increasing blood levels result in greater bronchodilation. This relationship is limited, however, by the predictable development of toxicity when the serum concentration exceeds 20 µg/ml. Therapeutic blood levels can be achieved most rapidly by administering an intravenous loading dose of aminophylline followed by a constant rate of infusion of the drug. The amount of the loading dose and the rate of infusion can initially be calculated on the basis of the patient's weight. However, the half-life of theophylline is well recognized as extremely variable in normal individuals and is affected by other medical conditions. For example, heart failure and chronic liver disease increase the half-life. Since the serum concentration is dependent on the half-life of the drug, marked variation in serum levels may occur if empiric dosage schedules are used. Serum levels must be measured to guarantee optimum therapy and avoid the toxic effects of the drug.

Sustained release preparations have recently been introduced for oral therapy. Because the theophylline in these preparations is continuously absorbed from the intestine over a period of hours, the kinetics observed after ingestion are similar to those observed with continuous intravenous infusion of the drug. As a result, consistent blood levels can be achieved with these preparations, and the drug can be administered less frequently than other oral preparations require. Thus this kind of preparation has practical advantages for the outpatient management of asthma.

The corticosteroids are also of great benefit in the treatment of acute asthma. Although the exact mechanism that aborts episodes of acute airways obstruction has not been clearly defined, these drugs are of great value in patients with status asthmaticus. Some patients with asthma require steroids on an outpatient basis to control their disease. Long-term systemic steroid therapy is accompanied by a number of severe side effects that limit its value. In recent years, steroid preparations that can be inhaled have been developed for clinical use. These agents have the benefit of being effective in controlling the patient's disease while not exposing the patient to the side effects of long-term daily oral therapy. Although more studies are required to demonstrate clearly the relative safety of this therapy, it seems reasonable to recommend this as the most effective way of managing steroid-dependent patients at the present time.

When severe episodes of airways obstruction lead to the development of respiratory failure, endotracheal intubation and mechanical ventilation may be required. In general, patients with asthma should be considered candidates for mechanical ventilation at a P_aCO_2 less than that which would be considered an indication for similar therapy in patients with either chronic bronchitis or emphysema. Since hypocapnia is usually present during acute bronchospasm, the development of any degree of hypercapnia represents a significant deterioration in total alveolar ventilation. The development of a P_aCO_2 in excess of 50 mm Hg should be considered a grave prognostic sign, and intubation and mechanical ventilation must be considered.

Other general measures are usually included in the management of acute asthma. Although its value as an integral part of therapy has not been clearly demonstrated, hydration may be of some value when inspissated bronchial secretions are present in patients with severe attacks. In some patients, airways infection is an important contributing factor in the pathogenesis of the disease. Therefore, broad-spectrum antibiotic therapy may be beneficial in selected patients. As a general rule, sedatives or other drugs that suppress central ventilatory drive should not be administered to patients during an acute asthma attack. Suppression of ventilatory drive may lead to progressive respiratory failure and complicate the management of the patient profoundly.

Chapter 4

BRONCHIECTASIS

Bronchiectasis is a disease characterized by permanent, abnormal dilation of the bronchi caused, at least in part, by destructive changes in the bronchial wall. The extent, severity, and appearance of the dilated bronchi varies considerably from case to case.

PATHOLOGIC CHANGES

Microscopically bronchiectasis is characterized by destructive changes involving all components of the bronchial wall. Destruction of the smooth muscle and cartilage of the bronchial wall are probably most important from a structural standpoint. However, the epithelial lining and the submucosal glands are also involved in the disease, and these changes may lead to significant functional abnormalities in airway clearance mechanisms. Mucosal ulcerations are common, and the normal bronchial columnar epithelium is often replaced by nonciliated squamous epithelium. Inflammatory cells and areas of necrosis are also frequently present in the bronchial wall, and the amount of peribronchiolar lymphoid tissue may be increased. In some cases the bronchial arteries are hypertrophied, and the bronchial artery to pulmonary vein anastomoses are grossly enlarged. In addition to the pathologic changes in the airways, focal abnormalities may also be present in the lung parenchyma. Atelectasis and areas of acute or chronic organizing pneumonia may occur distal to the involved airways.

Bronchiectasis can be classified grossly into four major categories based on the extent of anatomic involvement. This type of classification is useful for roentgenographic classification of the disease. *Cylindrical bronchiectasis* is characterized by uniform dilation of bronchi and abrupt termination of the lumen of some airways by mucous plugs. The number of subdivisions of bronchi is anatomically normal, and little obliteration of bronchioles occurs. *Varicose bronchiectasis* is the most common form of the disease. In this type, irregular areas of dilation are separated by areas of relative narrowing, producing a resemblance to venous varicosities.

Fewer than ten generations of bronchi are usually grossly visible, and extensive obliteration of bronchi and bronchioles occur distal to these patent airways. *Saccular (cystic) bronchiectasis* is characterized by termination of bronchi only after several generations evolve into large cystic areas. The bronchi and bronchioles distal to these areas are almost totally obliterated. The extensive loss of parenchyma occurring in this form of the disease is indicated by the fact that, although the cysts occur at the level of the third to fifth generation of bronchi, they are generally located subpleurally. *Proximal bronchiectasis* is seen only in association with mucoid impaction of the bronchus. It involves only the first few generations of bronchi, and unlike other forms of bronchiectasis, the bronchi and bronchioles distal to these areas are entirely normal; no significant loss of lung parenchyma occurs.

PATHOGENESIS

Although the pathogenesis of bronchiectasis is not clear, both genetic factors and infections of the lung appear to predispose to the development of the disease. Bronchiectasis often is present in cystic fibrosis and Kartagener syndrome, both of which are systemic, genetic disorders. In some patients, infection is an important contributing factor in the pathogenesis. This relationship is clear in cases in which localized bronchiectasis develops in areas of prior pulmonary infection. Bronchiectasis is also associated with congenital hypogammaglobulinemia. However, recurrent infections, rather than a genetically determined abnormality of the bronchi, probably are primarily responsible for the development of bronchiectasis in these cases. In the majority of cases of generalized bronchiectasis, an obvious predisposing factor cannot be identified. Since these cases usually date from childhood, infection in infancy or early childhood often is assumed to be the cause.

The sequence of events that leads to the destruction of the bronchial wall in bronchiectasis has not been described. Abnormalities in the structure of the bronchial wall may be present in individuals who develop this disease. Similarly, abnormalities in either the ciliary function of the ciliated mucosal cells or the biochemical constituents of mucus might conceivably play a role in the development of the disease.

CLINICAL MANIFESTATIONS

Cough, sputum production, and hemoptysis are the most common symptoms of bronchiectasis. Although these symptoms and the extent and severity of the disease generally are related, some patients with extensive disease may have few symptoms. Sputum production, when present, may vary considerably from day to day. In many patients, sputum production is most marked in the morning. Patients who do not have cough and sputum production are often referred to as having "dry bronchiectasis." Hemoptysis may be the initial symptom in these patients. Patients with extensive bronchiectasis may complain of dyspnea on exertion. If the disease is untreated, progressive destruction of lung tissue and impairment of gas exchange may lead to the development of cor pulmonale.

Physical examination of the chest may be entirely normal. However, most patients with bronchiectasis have coarse rales or rhonchi over the involved areas of lung. Digital clubbing and peripheral cyanosis are often present in patients with extensive, chronic disease. Findings of cor pulmonale may be present in advanced cases.

Two unusual but extremely important extrathoracic complications of bronchiectasis exist. A brain abscess may develop in patients with bronchietasis and chronic suppurative parenchymal infection as a result of hematogenous seeding of a pathologic organism to the brain. This complication may have catastrophic effects if it is not recognized early and appropriate therapy instituted rapidly. Amyloidosis

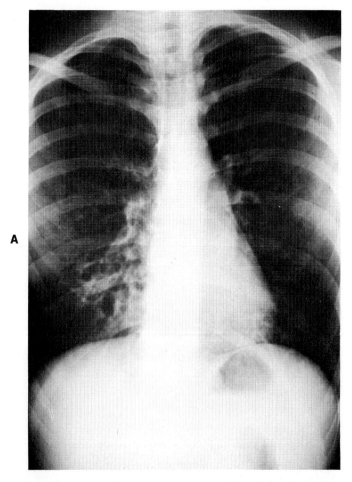

Fig. 4-1. A, Cystic bronchiectasis with cystic changes in the right lower lung field.

may develop in patients with extensive, chronic disease. This complication should be considered whenever patients with bronchiectasis develop clinical manifestations of visceral organ dysfunction during the course of their disease.

ROENTGENOGRAPHIC MANIFESTATIONS

The plain chest roentgenogram is abnormal in the majority of cases of bronchiectasis. A variety of abnormalites may be present. In many cases, linear markings are increased in the area of involvement presumably as a result of peribronchiolar fibrosis. Crowding of vascular markings because of loss of volume may also be present in involved areas. Ill-defined, patchy areas of infiltration caused by chronic infection of the lung parenchyma may be observed in some cases. In cases of saccular bronchiectasis, cystic structures may be visible on the plain roentgenogram (Fig. 4-1). These cysts may be several centimeters in diameter and occasion-

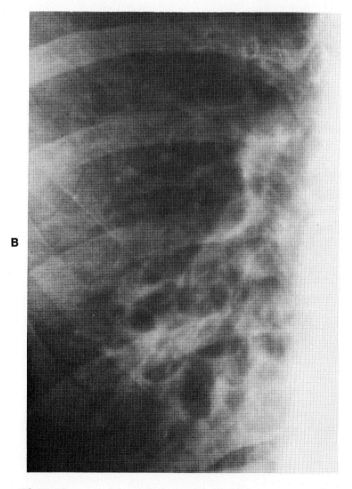

B

Fig. 4-1, cont'd. B, Close-up of the right lower lung field demonstrating the cystic changes.

ally may contain air fluid levels. These cysts are often appreciated better on the lateral roentgenogram. Some patients may exhibit evidence of marked hyperinflation of the lungs with depression of the diaphragm and an increase in the retrosternal air space.

Although the diagnosis of bronchiectasis may be strongly suspected on the basis of the plain roentgenogram, a bronchogram is essential to document the diagnosis. The bronchogram not only has diagnostic value but also defines the extent of the disease. For this reason a bronchogram is absolutely essential for any patient being considered for surgical resection of an involved area of lung.

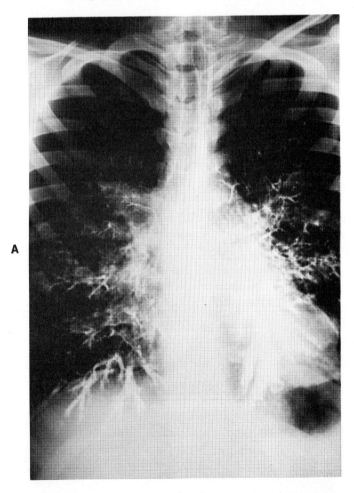

A

Fig. 4-2. A, Bronchogram demonstrating cylindrical bronchiectasis in the right lower lobe and varicose bronchiectasis in the left lower lobe. Note not only the characteristics of the bronchi in these two forms of bronchiectasis but also the greater degree of volume loss associated with varicose bronchiectasis.

The bronchographic findings correlate well with the gross pathologic changes previously described. The presence of cylindrical, varicose, saccular, or proximal bronchiectasis may be accurately identified by bronchography (Figs. 4-2 and 4-3). The only significant disparity between the anatomic and bronchographic findings is the level at which bronchi appear to be obliterated. In most cases several generations of intact bronchi exist beyond the point at which obstruction is apparent on the bronchogram. This is caused by the inability of the bronchographic contrast material to fill bronchi obstructed by mucous plugs. Deep inspiration and vigorous coughing before the procedure may result in more complete filling of the bronchial tree. However, this is usually most effective in cases in which minimal disease is present.

Reversible bronchial dilation resembling cylindrical bronchiectasis may occur during the course of pneumonia. The changes are usually mild and disappear with complete resolution of the pneumonia. The only significance of this observation is that an inaccurate diagnosis of cylindrical bronchiectasis may be made if a bronchogram is performed during or soon after an acute pneumonia. Cystic or varicose changes do not occur during the course of acute pneumonias.

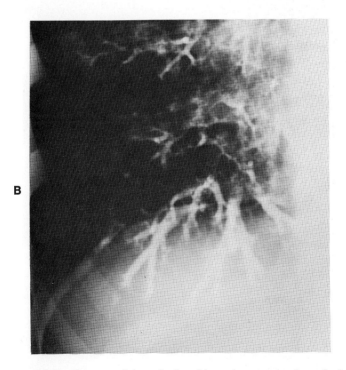

Fig. 4-2, cont'd. B, Close-up of the cylindrical bronchiectasis in the right lower lobe.

Continued.

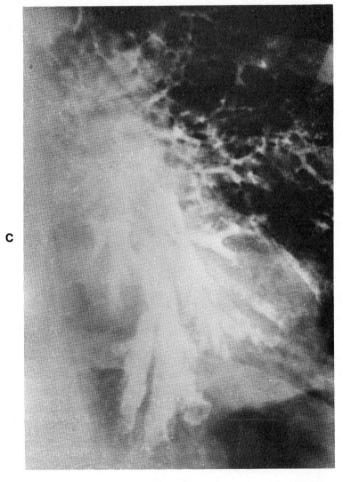

Fig. 4-2, cont'd. C, Close-up of the varicose bronchiectasis in the left lower lobe.

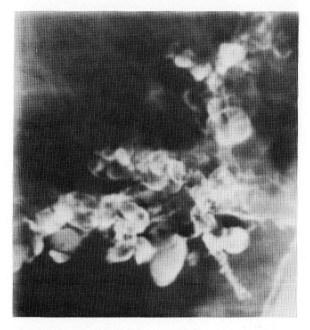

Fig. 4-3. Close-up of a bronchogram showing changes of cystic bronchiectasis in the right upper lobe.

PHYSIOLOGIC MANIFESTATIONS

The physiologic abnormalities that occur in patients with bronchiectasis vary greatly. This is not surprising, since the extent of the disease may vary from localized, cylindrical changes to diffuse, saccular changes. Thus the physiologic abnormalities occurring in this disease can only be discussed generally.

A decrease in expiratory flow rates is a common abnormality in patients with bronchiectasis. This is partly caused by loss of the functional integrity of the airways when the cartilage and muscle of the bronchial wall are destroyed. In addition, diffuse mucous plugging of the lumen of the airways probably also contributes to the decrease in expiratory flow rates. A decrease in the vital capacity is also frequently present in this disease. In mild cases it may reflect a recompartmentalization of the lung volumes as a result of the increase in the residual volume that accompanies airways obstruction. However, in severe cases lung parenchyma distal to chronically obstructed airways is lost. As a result, the vital capacity and residual volume may be decreased.

Gas exchange may be severely deranged as a result of the shunting of blood through areas of nonventilated lung that are distal to obstructed or destroyed airways. Thus severe hypoxemia may be present in patients with extensive saccular disease. Hypercapnia may develop as the disease progresses.

Excessive shunting of bronchial artery blood into the pulmonary circulation may occur and produce markedly enlarged bronchial artery–pulmonary artery anastomoses. As the anastomoses increase in size, systemic blood may actually flow retrogradely into pulmonary arteries. Pulmonary artery blood flow may be markedly decreased in these areas because of the pressure differential between the pulmonary and systemic circulations. Hypoperfusion of such areas can be detected by standard lung scans. Similarly, arteriograms may demonstrate decreased flow to such severely involved areas.

DIAGNOSIS

In virtually all cases, the diagnosis of bronchiectasis must be based on bronchographic findings. The only exceptions might be patients with a congenital disease associated with bronchiectasis who have characteristic clinical and roentgenographic manifestations of the disease. Even in such cases, however, a bronchogram may be important to define the extent and severity of the disease.

TREATMENT

Two major principles are involved in the treatment of patients with bronchiectasis. First, treatment of pulmonary infection is extremely important. This probably not only preserves parenchymal tissue, but also minimizes the likelihood of the development of a brain abscess or amyloidosis. Although appropriate antibiotics should be selected on the basis of the results of sputum cultures, this may not be possible at all times, and broad-spectrum antibiotics will have to be employed empirically or on a regular basis if purlent bronchitis or pneumonia recur frequently.

The use of physical measures to promote clearance of secretions is the other important aspect of the treatment of bronchiectasis. Postural drainage and chest physical therapy may be beneficial in patients with either localized or diffuse disease who produce significant quantities of sputum. A treatment program must be individualized for each patient. Obviously patients with dry bronchiectasis are unlikely to benefit from such therapy.

In addition, some patients benefit from the use of oral or inhaled bronchodilators. These agents are generally of most value in patients with mild bronchiectasis who have associated bronchitis. Once the disease has progressed to destruction and obliteration of the bronchial wall, pharmacologic agents are unlikely to be of value.

Serial pulmonary function studies may be useful in assessing the response of the patient to therapy. In some patients, improvement in lung function may be dramatic after a good therapeutic regimen has been in use for several weeks. Thus the patient's subjective response to therapy should be complemented by evaluation of lung function.

The role of surgery in the management of bronchiectasis is now limited. Surgical resection of involved areas of lung was a common practice in the past. However, experience has shown that surgery frequently failed to reverse the course of the disease. In fact, bronchiectasis often developed or became more severe in uninvolved areas of the lung after resection of involved lung. With the advent of effective antibiotic therapy and good physical measures to promote clearance of secretions, the great majority of patients with localized bronchiectasis can be managed medically. However, occasionally a patient with localized disease may continue to have recurrent parenchymal infection or recurrent episodes of significant hemoptysis. Such patients probably represent the only group who should be considered for surgical resection. Resection of areas of lung that are the site of life-threatening hemoptysis is the only reason for surgery in patients with diffuse disease. Great care must be taken to clearly identify the site of bleeding by bronchoscopy before resection. Frequently lung function is so impaired in such patients that the morbidity associated with the procedure is significant.

SPECIFIC ENTITIES
Kartagener syndrome

Kartagener syndrome consists of the triad of situs inversus, chronic sinusitis, and bronchiectasis. Although the entire syndrome may occur in more than one family member of the same generation, other family members may have only isolated bronchiectasis, situs inversus, sinusitis, or any combination of these abnormalities. Although other developmental abnormalities have been associated with this syndrome, they occur only sporadically. This syndrome has not been observed in two consecutive generations. Thus the defect probably is transmitted as a mendelian recessive trait with variable expressivity.

Because of the familial nature of this syndrome, a number of theories have been proposed to explain the defect that leads to the development of bronchiectasis. Nevertheless, abnormalities in either the components of the bronchial wall or bronchial secretions that might predispose to the development of bronchiectasis have not been described. Recently, however, a defect in the ultrastructure of the cilia of the bronchial mucosal cell resulting in a loss of normal ciliary function has been described in patients with this syndrome.

The clinical and roentgenographic manifestations of the bronchiectasis that occurs in this syndrome are identical to those observed in other forms of bronchiectasis. Other than the presence of situs inversus, no diagnostic features of this syndrome exist.

Cystic fibrosis

Cystic fibrosis is a hereditary disease characterized by a general dysfunction of exocrine glands. Although all exocrine glands are probably affected in this disease, the most important sites of involvement are the pancreas and the bronchial wall. The disease is transmitted as an autosomal recessive trait. The incidence of

the disease has been estimated to be 1 in 2000 live births for a caucasian population. The incidence is much lower in blacks. The disease is a major cause of chronic
respiratory disease in children. Pulmonary infection and chronic respiratory failure
are the most common causes or morbidity and mortality in this disease. Although
cystic fibrosis was initially considered to be invariably and rapidly fatal, many patients are surviving well into their teens and early adulthood. Furthermore, milder
forms of the disease compatible with long survival are being recognized with increasing frequency. This discussion will be concerned only with the pulmonary
manifestations of cystic fibrosis.

Bronchiectasis is present in the majority of individuals by the time they reach
the second decade of life. Newborn infants with cystic fibrosis who die shortly after
birth have normal lungs. Thus the pulmonary pathologic changes so characteristic
of the disease are not congenital. Current theory focuses on abnormalities in bronchial secretions or defects in bronchial clearance mechanisms as causes for the development of the pathologic changes in the airways. Because of abnormal clearance
of secretions, mucous plugging of small airways leads to infection and tissue damage. This sequence of events is progressive and ultimately leads to obliteraton of
bronchioles and small bronchi and the development of peribronchiolar fibrosis and
chronic organizing pneumonia. In some patients, air trapping or emphysema may
develop distal to obstructed airways and lead to marked hyperinflation of the lungs.
The progressive nature of the airways obstruction and the progressive loss of lung
parenchyma may eventually lead to death. Approximately 95% of the deaths in
patients with cystic fibrosis who survive infancy are caused by chronic pulmonary
disease.

The clinical, roentgenographic and physiologic manifestations of the lung involvement when bronchiectasis has developed are similar to those of patients with
other forms of severe, extensive bronchiectasis. Early in the course of the disease,
atelectasis caused by airways obstruction may be the only abnormality present on
the chest roentogenogram. At times this is associated with roentgenographically
visible mucoid impaction. Spontaneous pneumothorax and pneumomediastinum
may develop in some patients. At times these may be asymptomatic and detected
only on a routine chest roentgenogram.

The early and advanced stages of the disease are characterized by recurrent
pneumonias. In recent years, *Pseudomonas aeruginosa* has become the organism
isolated most frequently from the respiratory tract of patients with this disease.
Once this organism appears in the secretions, it is extremely difficult to eradicate
even with the most effective antibiotics. *Staphylococcus aureus*, once the most
common isolate, is now observed with decreasing frequency. *Hemophilus influenzae* and other potential pathogens may be isolated occasionally.

The manifestations of the clinical course of pulmonary involvement in cystic
fibrosis are quite variable. As previously mentioned, some patients may have min-

TABLE 3
Manifestations of cystic fibrosis in adults

Abnormality	Appropriate incidence (%)
Obstructive ventilatory defect	95
Pancreatic insufficiency	95
Aspermia (males)	95
Sputum culture positive for *Pseudomonas aeruginosa* or *Staphylococcus aureus*	90
Sinusitis	90
Hemoptysis	60
Intestinal obstruction	20
Pneumothorax	15
Cholelithiasis	12
Glycosuria	8
Biliary cirrhosis	5
Intussusception	5

imal symptoms and may be diagnosed in adulthood. Recent studies suggest that 3% to 4% of patients will be diagnosed in their teenage years or later (Table 3).

Diagnosis. A positive sweat test is the hallmark of the diagnosis of cystic fibrosis. A number of technical problems are involved in performing this test correctly. Pilocarpine iontophoresis with quantitive measurement of the chloride content of the sweat is the most reliable technique. A positive result should always be verified before the diagnosis is considered established. An increase in the sweat chloride content to greater than 60mEq/L is considered positive in most laboratories. Because of the variable manifestations of the pulmonary involvement of cystic fibrosis, sweat tests should be performed in teenagers or young adults in a variety of clinical settings. The presence of chronic cough, recurrent pneumonias, pseudomonas or staphylococcal pneumonia, and atelectasis should be valid indication for performing a sweat test.

Treatment. A comprehensive plan of therapy, including patient and family education, is necessary for managing patients with cystic fibrosis. As a result of pancreatic exocrine gland dysfunction, oral enzyme replacement is frequently necessary, and careful attention must be paid to the nutritional status of the patient. Treatment of the pulmonary disease requires intensive use of antibiotics and measures to improve mechanical clearance of bronchial secretions.

Chapter 5

CHRONIC BRONCHITIS

Chronic bronchitis is a disease characterized clinically by cough and sputum production. The diagnosis of this disease is based solely on a history of cough with sputum production occurring on most days of 3 consecutive months during 2 consecutive years, provided that other specific diseases associated with excess production of bronchial secretions are excluded. Since the diagnosis of chronic bronchitis is based on history alone, it is important to recognize that many patients provide an unreliable history of sputum production. This is particularly true of patients who tend to swallow secretions rather than expectorate them. Thus a casual history may greatly underestimate the true incidence of this disease.

PATHOLOGIC CHANGES
Hypertrophy of the submucosal glands of the bronchial wall is the characteristic pathologic abnormality observed in chronic bronchitis. In the normal bronchus the submucosal glands comprise approximately a third of the bronchial wall distance measured from the epithelial surface to the inner surface of the cartilage. The ratio of mucosal gland thickness to bronchial wall thickness is termed the Reid index after the pathologist who demonstrated the usefulness of this measurement for the pathologic diagnosis of chronic bronchitis. In chronic bronchitis the mean value for the Reid index is approximately twice that observed in a normal population (Fig. 5-1). However, since the range of the index in normal individuals and patients with chronic bronchitis overlaps, the pathologic diagnosis of chronic bronchitis cannot be based solely on an increase in the Reid index.

The normal bronchus contains both serum and mucus-secreting submucosal glands. In chronic bronchitis, mucus-secreting glands not only hypertrophy but also are more numerous than in the normal population. In addition to changes in the glands themselves, the necks of the gland ducts dilate as they open into the bronchial lumen. As will be discussed later, this pathologic alteration leads to a roentgenographic abnormality, which is useful in the diagnosis of the disease. Edema

52

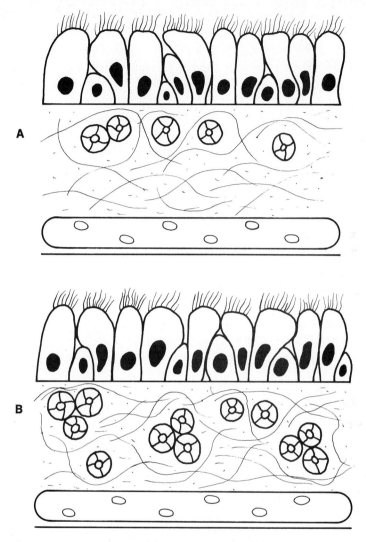

Fig. 5-1. A, Schematic representation of the normal relationship between the thickness of the bronchial submucosal gland layer and the thickness of the bronchial wall. **B,** Schematic representation of the changes in the bronchial submucosal gland layer that occur in chronic bronchitis.

and infiltration of the submucosa by mononuclear inflammatory cells are also present to variable degrees.

Two major changes occur in the mucosa in chronic bronchitis. First, squamous metaplasis of the mucosal epithelium occurs frequently. Areas of metaplasia may occur in the mucosal epithelium lining both bronchi and bronchioles. In addition, the number of goblet cells is increased in the epithelial layer. The increase in these cells is most strikingly observed in the epithelium lining bronchioles, since they normally are not present in the bronchiolar epithelium.

The pathologic changes that occur in the small bronchioles should be emphasized, since the small airways may be the initial site of involvement in this disease. Since submucosal glands are not present in bronchioles, the characteristic hypertrophy of these glands is not observed at this level of the tracheobronchial tree. Squamous metaplasia of the epithelium, infiltration of the wall by chronic inflammatory cells, and an increase in connective tissue in the bronchiolar wall appear to be the earliest changes in the bronchioles. As the disease progresses, a further increase occurs in connective tissue and smooth muscle in the wall of the bronchiole. Goblet cell metaplasia of the lining epithelium occurs as the disease progresses even further. Peribronchiolar inflammation and fibrosis may be prominent in some cases. In the most severe cases the number of small bronchioles in the lung is markedly decreased. The process involved in obliteration of these bronchioles is unclear.

EPIDEMIOLOGIC FACTORS

Approximately 20% of adult men and less than 10% of adult women in the United States have chronic bronchitis. Clearly cigarette smoking is the major factor related to the development of this disease. This relationship has been confirmed by studies conducted in countries around the world. The exact mechanism by which cigarette smoking leads to the development of chronic bronchitis is unclear. However, cigarette smoke produces an abrupt increase in airway resistance in normal subjects and interferes with the ciliary action of bronchial mucosal cells.

Specific occupations also seem to be associated with an increased risk of developing chronic bronchitis. Cigarette smoking is common in most workers; thus it is difficult to clearly identify a potentially important occupational exposure that may cause chronic bronchitis, since the number of cases produced is often trivial in comparison to those caused by cigarette smoking. For the same reason, determining whether smoking and an occupational exposure may act synergistically in producing chronic bronchitis is extremely difficult. Despite these limitations, coal workers, grain workers (millers and bakers), and individuals exposed to cotton, hemp, or flax dust may develop a form of occupational bronchitis. The mechanism by which these various dust exposures cause chronic bronchitis is unclear. Individuals exposed to grain, cotton, hemp, or flax dust may also develop asthma or, occasionally, a form of hypersensitivity pneumonitis, suggesting that immune mechanisms may also be important in the pathogenesis of some cases of occupational bronchitis.

Air pollution also appears to contribute to the development of chronic bronchitis. Chronic bronchitis is more common in nonsmoking individuals who reside in polluted urban centers than in similar individuals residing in nearby rural areas. This seems to be true in all industrialized countries. Sulfur dioxide appears to be the major chemical component of polluted air that is responsible for the development of chronic bronchitis.

CLINICAL MANIFESTATIONS

Cough and sputum production are the major clinical manifestations of chronic bronchitis. The volume of sputum may vary considerably among patients. In most patients, the greatest volume is raised in the first hour after rising in the morning. Hemoptysis occurs in a large percentage of patients at some time during the course of their disease. Although the volume of blood raised is usually not great, it may occasionally exceed 100 ml in a 24-hour period.

The majority of patients with chronic bronchitis do not complain of dyspnea during exertion. However, progressive impairment of lung function occurs in approximately 10% of the patients, and dyspnea during exertion is uniformly present in these patients. Since the great majority of these patients develop emphysema, it is difficult to determine whether the dyspnea experienced by these patients is due to progressive airways disease or emphysema. With progressive impairment of lung function, manifestations of cor pulmonale and repeated episodes of respiratory failure may develop. If a patient is first seen at this stage of the disease, the diagnosis of chronic bronchitis may be overlooked because patients tend to raise smaller volumes of sputum or stop raising sputum altogether as the disease progresses. This appears to be caused by the fact that patients stop smoking cigarettes as they become more symptomatic. Thus the patient's history of sputum production should be recorded carefully before chronic bronchitis is excluded as an important component of the patient's disease.

Physical findings vary depending on the severity of the disease when the patient is examined. Patients with very mild disease may have no abnormal findings. However, coarse rhonchi and wheezes are audible over the lungs in most patients. In some patients these abnormal breath sounds are audible only during a forced expiration. Rales are usually not present. If emphysema is present, the breath sounds may be decreased in intensity and hyperresonance to percussion over the thorax may occur. In patients with severe disease, findings of cor pulmonale may be present. Alterations in the heart sounds or palpatation of a right ventricular lift in such patients caused by hyperinflation of the lungs is difficult to judge. However, an accentuated pulmonic valve closure sound, a right-sided S_3, or a murmur of tricuspid insufficiency may be audible in some patients. Distended neck veins, hepatomegaly, and peripheral edema are common findings in patients with right ventricular failure. Cyanosis of the fingers and toes is usually present. Digital clubbing is rare in chronic bronchitis.

ROENTGENOGRAPHIC MANIFESTATIONS

The chest roentgenogram is normal in the majority of patients with chronic bronchitis. However, several roentgenographic abnormalities may be present in this disease. In some cases, parallel linear markings, so-called tram lines, may be observed radiating from the hilar region into the lower lung fields. Although the basis for these lines is unclear, some radiologists have proposed that they represent visualization of bronchial walls that have become thickened as a result of peribronchiolar fibrosis. This finding is often subtle and also may be seen on the chest roentgenogram of some normal individuals. Thus it is not a particularly useful roentgenographic sign for the diagnosis of chronic bronchitis.

A general increase in lung markings on the chest roentgenogram, often termed "dirty lungs," has also been described in chronic bronchitis. Although the reason for the increased number of markings is unclear, they have been attributed to areas of chronic inflammation and fibrosis in peribronchiolar regions of the lung. These abnormal markings are not specific for chronic bronchitis. Increased markings of this type may also be observed in patients who have both chronic bronchitis and emphysema. Although a pattern of arterial deficiency (hyperlucency of lung fields) is usually associated with emphysema, increased number of markings on the chest roentgenogram do not exclude the presence of rather far advanced emphysema.

The demonstration of "bronchial diverticulosis" by bronchography is possibly the most diagnostic roentgenographic sign of chronic bronchitis. The characteristic hypertrophy of the submucosal glands that occurs in this disease is accompanied by enlargement and dilation of the gland ducts. These enlarged ducts appear as diverticuli of the bronchial wall when the lumen is filled with contrast material.

In addition to the enlarged gland ducts, a bronchogram may also demonstrate incomplete filling of the airways as a result of the accumulation of secretions in the distal airways. Since the diameter of the airways is normal, the exclusion of the presence of bronchiectasis is important. Bronchograms are usually not performed as part of the routine diagnostic evaluation of a patient with chronic cough and sputum production. However, since the symptoms of both diseases may be identical, a bronchogram occasionally may be necessary to differentiate bronchitis and diffuse bronchiectasis or to detect localized areas of bronchiectasis in a patient with chronic bronchitis.

PHYSIOLOGIC MANIFESTATIONS

The physiologic abnormalities observed in patients with chronic bronchitis are dependent on the severity of the disease at the time the studies are performed. In many patients with chronic bronchitis, routine clinical pulmonary function tests are normal. However, more sophisicated physiologic studies would reveal abnormalities in the majority of patients that reflect pathologic changes in the small airways.

These abnormalities include a decrease in the maximum midexpiratory flow rate, a decrease in flow rates at low lung volumes, and an increase in the closing volume or closing capacity of the lung. In addition, the residual volume may be increased at this stage. As the residual volume increases, the vital capacity falls proportionately. As a result the total lung capacity (TLC) remains normal. Gas exchange is also abnormal in the majority of patients because of mismatching of ventilation and perfusion. Since these abnormalities may be relatively minor, measurement of the alveolar-arterial oxygen gradient is usually the best method for detecting abnormal gas exchange.

As the disease progresses, routine pulmonary function tests become abnormal. The forced expired volume to forced vital capacity (FEV_1 to FVC) ratio decreases, and the residual volume increases further. The TLC usually remains normal. The single breath diffusing capacity is usually normal or only mildly decreased. Resting hypoxemia develops at this stage. As the disease progresses further, hypoxemia may become more marked and hypercapnia may develop. As previously mentioned, emphysema is also present in the majority of patients with severe disease. Thus physiologic studies may reflect the combination of both diseases. A great decrease in the single breath diffusing capacity and an increase in the TLC generally indicate the presence of emphysema (see Chapter 9).

CLINICAL COURSE

The clinical course of chronic bronchitis is quite variable. Accurately reconstructing the natural history of the disease is difficult, since most clinical studies have been of relatively short duration and have focused predominantly on symptomatic patients with obvious physiologic abnormalities. The results of these studies have shown that the majority of patients with pulmonary function abnormalities have progressive deterioration of lung function over many years. If this rate of deterioration in lung function is extrapolated backward, the great majority of patients appear to have normal routine pulmonary function tests at age 30. Obviously, patients who do not have progressive deterioration in lung function in later years also have normal function at this age. For purposes of discussion, therefore, it is reasonable to conclude that the majority of patients with chronic bronchitis do not have significant abnormalities in standard clinical tests of lung function at age 30. As pointed out previously, however, most of these patients probably have physiologic abnormalities consistent with pathologic changes in the small bronchioles.

In the majority of patients, the deterioration in lung function studies that occurs throughout their lives clearly is no greater than that observed in the population as a whole. Thus chronic bronchitis does not produce abnormalities in routine clinical pulmonary tests in the majority of patients. About 10% to 20% of patients, however, demonstrate more rapid deterioration in lung function than the rest of the population. These patients exhibit a fairly constant deterioration in lung function on a yearly basis. Some of them ultimately develop cor pulmonale and respiratory failure (Fig. 5-2).

There are several important facts about the clinical course of this group of patients. First, these patients often have recurrent clinical episodes of increased cough and changes in the characteristics of their sputum production that appear to reflect acute exacerbations of bronchitis. Second, most patients probably develop emphysema during the course of their disease.

The pathogenesis of the acute exacerbations of bronchitis observed in these patients is unclear. These episodes presumably are caused by infection of the respiratory tract. However, despite the fact that careful bacteriologic studies have been done both in the United States and abroad, it has not been possible to substantiate this theory. Although *Hemophilus influenzae, Streptococcus pneumoniae,* and other organisms can be grown from the sputum of patients with chronic bronchitis, their presence does not correlate with these acute episodes. These organisms are often present when the clinical course of the disease is stable and are often absent during acute exacerbations. Studies to detect infection with viruses or *Mycoplasma pneumoniae* during acute exacerbations have also not been successful. Thus no clear evidence shows that infection definitely plays a role in these exacerbations.

Although lung function deteriorates during these episodes, this appears to contribute little to the progressive deterioration of lung function that occurs during the course of the disease. Pulmonary function tests have been shown to return to baseline values after recovery from the acute exacerbations. This sequence of events seems to follow each episode regardless of its frequency and severity.

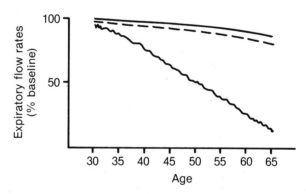

Fig. 5-2. Natural course of the changes in expiratory flow rates in patients with chronic bronchitis. Changes in the normal population with aging depicted by the solid line. Changes in the majority of patients with chronic bronchitis (80% to 90%) are depicted by the interrupted line. A minority of patients (10% to 20%) with chronic bronchitis have a progressive decrease in expiratory flow rates throughout life.

The episodes are important for two reasons. First, in patients with severe disease, an acute exacerbation of bronchitis may precipitate an episode of respiratory failure. As a result, these episodes contribute significantly to the morbidity and mortality. Second, these episodes may lead to an inaccurate prognosis in individual patients. The projected duration of survival for patients with chronic bronchitis is directly related to the degree of baseline functional impairment at the time of evaluation. Since an acute exacerbation may temporarily result in a dramatic deterioration of lung function, a patient who is evaluated during such an episode may be thought to have a much greater impairment of baseline physiologic status than truly present. Thus patients should be evaluated only for prognostic purposes after they have received optimal treatment for acute exacerbations of the disease.

As previously mentioned, the majority of patients with chronic bronchitis who have progressive deterioration of lung function probably develop emphysema during the course of the disease. Although chronic bronchitis alone may lead to the development of cor pulmonale and respiratory failure, this occurs only occasionally. Severe pathologic changes in bronchioles are the most consistent findings in this group of patients. Similar pathologic changes are also prominent in the patients with chronic bronchitis and emphysema who develop cor pulmonale and respiratory failure. Clearly, progressive pathologic changes in bronchioles and the development of emphysema are the two determinants of the severe physiologic impairment that is associated with the development of cor pulmonale and respiratory failure. Thus the pathologic changes in large airways have little correlation with the development of respiratory failure and cor pulmonale.

Serial chest roentgenograms provide an insensitive method of following the course of chronic bronchitis. In some patients, changes caused by the development of emphysema may be observed on serial roentgenograms obtained over many years. However, in general the chest roentgenogram does not reflect the changes that occur in lung function during the course of the disease. Thus clinical pulmonary function tests must be obtained to document progression of the disease.

As previously mentioned, the long-term prognosis of the disease is directly related to the degree of physiologic impairment present at evaluation. The FEV_1 has proved to be extremely useful for prognostic purposes. Symptomatic patients with an initial FEV_1 greater than 1.25 L have a 50% survival rate of almost 10 years. In contrast, patients with FEV_1 of less than 0.75 L have a 50% survival rate of less than 4 years. Within any group of patients with similar initial values, the rate of lung function decline also has prognostic significance. Obviously the more rapid the decline in lung function, the worse the prognosis.

Episodes of respiratory failure are not incompatible with long survival. Approximately a third of patients survive for 2 years or longer after an episode of respiratory failure. This is probably explained by the fact that in some patients an acute exacerbation of bronchitis, which is completely reversible with appropriate therapy, is responsible for the episode of respiratory failure.

TREATMENT

No specific treatment is effective in reversing the pathologic changes of chronic bronchitis once the disease is clincially apparent. However, a preclinical stage of the disease may exist in which only small airway involvement is present. This concept is of interest, since evidence shows that disease localized to small airways is reversible. For instance, physiologic abnormalities consistent with disease in small airways in smokers may reverse with smoking cessation. Smoking cessation does not result in improvement in abnormal routine function tests in the majority of patients. Nevertheless, cessation of smoking is the most important aspect of the management of patients with clinically apparent chronic bronchitis. The frequency of cough and the volume of sputum decrease in most patients who stop smoking.

Bronchodilators may be of value in many patients with chronic bronchitis. Some degree of airway obstruction reversibility can be demonstrated in the pulmonary function laboratory after inhalation of a bronchodilator. Although no direct correlation exists between the ability to demonstrate response in the laboratory and clinical improvement from oral or inhaled bronchodilators, the results of these studies suggest that the majority of symptomatic patients with chronic bronchitis who have significant functional abnormalities may benefit from bronchodilator therapy.

Inhaled bronchodilators should be administered cautiously in patients with chronic bronchitis for the following reasons. First, some patients may develop paradoxical bronchospasm after inhalation of any drug, even a bronchodilator. This is possibly caused by the direct irritant effect of the propellant used in the inhaled preparation. Second, many patients with chronic bronchitis are in the age group in which coronary artery disease and other cardiac disorders are common. In these patients the cardiovascular effects of inhaled bronchodilators may lead to serious complications. Thus inhaled bronchodilators should be used conservatively and only after oral bronchodilator therapy has been shown to be ineffective.

Some patients with chronic bronchitis may have dramatic reversibility of their disease during corticosteroid therapy. Predicting which patients will respond to corticosteroids in this manner is extrememly difficult. However, the presence of eosinophilia, recurrent episodes of acute bronchospasm, or a family history of asthma are factors that tend to be correlated with corticosteroid responsiveness. Clearly, corticosteroids should not be administered on a chronic basis in such patients. If possible, however, appropriate patients should receive a trial of corticosteroid therapy with careful monitoring of the response by serial physiologic testing.

The relationship between bacterial infection and acute exacerbations of bronchitis has already been discussed. Despite the fact that a clear relationship cannot be demonstrated, antibiotics often are administered during an acute exacerbation. In recent years a number of clinical studies have been performed to determine whether antibiotic therapy is effective in decreasing the morbidity associated with these acute clinical exacerbations. Although the results are far from conclusive, they at least suggest that some patients may be helped by this therapy. Since the results of sputum cultures are of little value in identifying specific pathogens in this situation, the choice of antibiotics must be made empirically. Erythromycin, tetracycline, penicillin, or a semisynthetic analog of penicillin are usually administered in this clinical setting. Although antibiotics often are prescribed on a regular basis for a short period each month, such therapy has very little rational. It is far better to treat patients when acute exacerbations are clinically evident rather than prescribe antibiotics as part of a prophylactic regimen.

Patients with cor pulmonale should obviously be treated aggressively in an attempt to maintain optimum cardiac function. Diuretics are frequently beneficial in these patients. Although some patients appear to respond favorably to administration of digitalis, caution must be exercised in using this drug because of the increased risk of developing cardiac arrhythmias in patients who are hypoxemic. In addition to these standard approaches for cor pulmonale, continuous oxygen has recently received some attention as a useful adjunct to other therapies in these patients. This therapy appears to decrease the number of episodes of cardiac decompensation in some patients and may also provide relief of symptoms caused by severe hypoxemia. However, oxygen administration has not had any clear effect on long-term survival. Recently, studies to determine the beneficial effect of oxygen administered nocturnally have been initiated. The results of these studies are not yet available.

Chapter 6

BRONCHIAL NEOPLASMS

A large variety of benign and malignant neoplasms arise in the lung. Detailed description of all these entities is beyond the scope of this dicussion. This chapter will be concerned only with neoplasms of some clinical importance that appear to arise from the bronchial wall.

BRONCHOGENIC CARCINOMA

Bronchogenic carcinoma is a major medical problem in the United States. At a time when mortality for most malignant tumors is decreasing, the mortality for lung cancer continues to increase. More than 80,000 persons will die from this disease in the coming year. About 30% of all male cancer deaths and 7% of all female cancer deaths are caused by this tumor. In men the number of deaths from bronchogenic carcinoma alone is greater than the combined deaths attributed to the five next most common forms of cancer. In women the number of deaths is increasing each year and is currently exceeded only by those caused by breast, colon, and rectum carcinomas (Fig. 6-1).

Pathologic features

Bronchogenic carcinoma has been classified into four major pathologic categories: (1) epidermoid or squamous cell carcinoma, (2) small cell carcinoma, (3) adenocarcinoma, and (4) large cell carcinoma. The histopathologic features that characterize each histologic tumor type are beyond the scope of this discussion. However, even among experienced pathologists, significant interobserver and intraobserver variability exists in classifying lung tumors. Although reasonable agreement occurs when dealing with well-differentiated adenocarcinoma and epidermoid carcinomas, significant disagreement occurs when the tumor is a large or small cell carcinoma. The disagreement is even more pronounced when dealing with an undifferentiated epidermoid carcinoma or undifferentiated adnocarcinoma. In addition, the histologic pattern may vary significantly within a single tumor. Despite

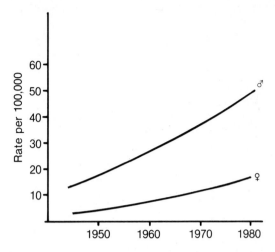

Fig. 6-1. Death rates caused by bronchogenic carcinoma in men and women during the last 30 years. Although the number of deaths in men far exceeds the number in women, the rates are progressively increasing in both sexes.

these limitations in making an exact pathologic diagnosis, the histologic tumor type has definite prognostic significance and influences the therapeutic approach to the patient. Each of these forms of lung cancer has certain characteristic clinical and roentgenographic features.

Squamous cell carcinoma accounts for 40% to 50% of all primary bronchogenic carcinomas. These tumors appear most often as hilar or perihilar masses (Fig. 6-2). They are the most common form of lung cancer to undergo cavitation. Because of their central location, a high percentage of cases can be diagnosed by sputum cytologic examination at the time of bronchoscopy. Although these tumors grow rapidly, they tend to stay localized to the thorax and thus have higher resectability and survival rates than other cell types.

About 20% to 30% of all lung cancers are small cell carcinomas, the most malignant form of bronchogenic carcinoma. These tumors generally are hilar lesions and are frequently associated with massive mediastinal adenopathy (Fig. 6-3). Systemic metastases are almost invariably present at the time of inital diagnosis. Therefore these tumors are not amenable to surgical resection. In most centers the diagnosis of small cell carcinoma is considered evidence of inoperability, even if distant metastases cannot be documented. Ectopic hormone production is most frequently associated with these tumors. Of all the forms of lung cancer, small cell carcinoma is the most responsive to radiotherapy and chemotherapy. However, despite favorable response rates, long-term survival rates are affected little by these forms of therapy.

Adenocarcinomas also account for 20% to 30% of primary bronchogenic car-

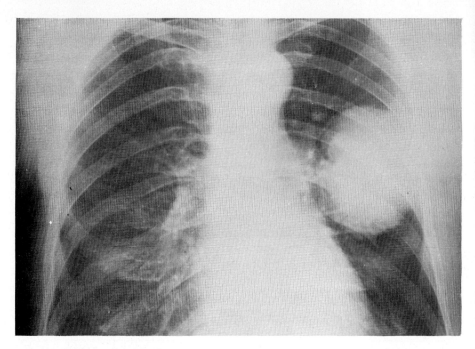

Fig. 6-2. Squamous cell carcinoma evident as a large parenchymal mass.

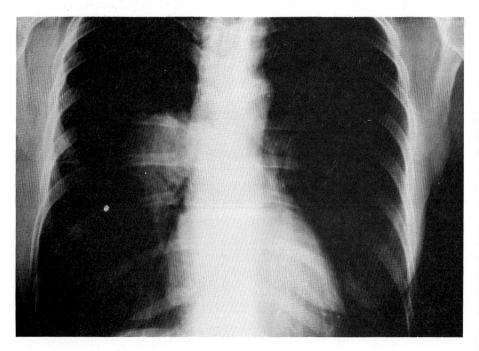

Fig. 6-3. Undifferentiated small cell carcinoma growing as a right hilar mass.

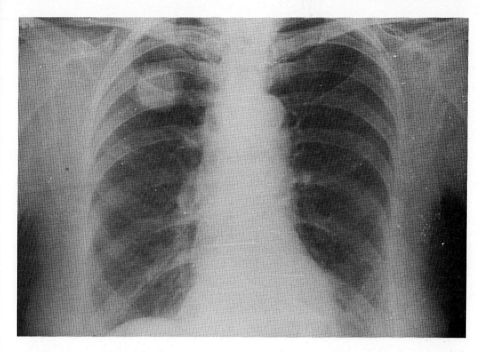

Fig. 6-4. Adenocarcinoma evident as a large solitary lesion in the periphery of the right upper lobe.

cinomas. These tumors most often are masses in the periphery of the lung (Fig. 6-4). Because of their location, they are not often diagnosed by bronchoscopy or sputum cytologic examination. The degree of histologic differentiation of these tumors is of prognostic significance. Well-differentiated, peripheral adenocarcinomas less than 4 cm in diameter have the highest 5-year survival rates of all forms of lung cancer. Since systemic metastases tend to occur early with poorly differentiated adenocarcinomas, these tumors have a poor prognosis. Pleural effusions occur most often with this form of lung cancer.

Large cell carcinoma, in its clinical and roentgenographic presentation and biologic activity, tends to mimic undifferentiated adenocarcinoma. This particular tumor has no distinctive features.

Epidemiologic factors

The incidence of bronchogenic carcinoma is determined largely by exposure to carcinogenic agents. The most important carcinogen in our society is cigarette smoke. The relationship between cigarette smoking and the development of lung cancer is strongly suggested by epidemiologic data. Nonsmokers comprise a very small percentage of patients with lung cancer. In addition, squamous cell carcinoma and small cell carcinoma, the most common types of cancer in smokers, occur only

TABLE 4
Histologic classification of bronchial tumors in smokers and nonsmokers

	Approximate incidence (%)	
Cell type	Smoker	Nonsmoker
Squamous cell	40	15
Small cell, undifferentiated	25	5
Adenocarcinoma	25	55
Large cell, undifferentiated	10	10
Carcinoid	1	15

rarely in nonsmokers. Adenocarcinoma accounts for greater than 50% of all primary lung tumors in nonsmokers. Thus smoking apparently influences both the incidence of lung cancer and the histopathologic types of tumors that are encountered (Table 4).

Since cigarette smoking is such a dominant factor in society, identifying other environmental carcinogens that may play a role in the development of lung cancer is difficult. Nevertheless, exposure to arsenic, nickel, chromium, hematite, asbestos, mustard gas, and radioactive minerals has been shown to be associated with an increased risk of developing lung cancer. Squamous cell carcinoma has been the most common form of lung cancer identified in patients exposed to nonradioactive carcinogens. Small cell carcinoma is the most prevalent form of lung cancer in individuals who mine uranium or other radioactive minerals. A marked synergistic effect exists between cigarette smoking and either uranium or asbestos exposure. Although the incidence of lung cancer is only slightly increased in persons exposed to uranium or asbestos who are nonsmokers, it is markedly increased in those who are exposed to these substances and also smoke.

Recent evidence suggests that the risk of developing lung cancer associated with cigarette smoking is related to the concentration of the enzyme aryl-hydrocarbon decarboxylase, which metabolizes hydrocarbons to highly carcinogenic metabolites. Persons who develop bronchogenic carcinoma generally have higher levels of this enzyme than individuals with similar smoking histories who do not have lung cancer.

Certain types of lung disease may also be a factor in the development of lung cancer. Several studies have suggested that an increase in the incidence of bronchogenic carcinoma occurs in patients with chronic fibrosing alveolitis. Adenocarcinomas are the most common tumors found in these patients. An increased incidence of lung cancer also may occur in patients with bullous lung disease. The apparent association of bronchogenic carcinoma with chronic bronchitis or emphysema is probably related to the fact that cigarette smoking is associated with each of these diseases.

Clinical manifestations

The clinical manifestations of lung cancer are determined by the local effects of the tumor within the thorax, the presence of disseminated metastases, or the systemic biologic effects of the tumor:

Intrathoracic
Bronchial
    Cough and hemoptysis
    Bronchial obstruction
        Atelectasis
        Obstructive pneumonitis
Mediastinal extension
    Superior vena cava syndrome
    Recurrent laryngeal nerve paralysis
    Phrenic nerve paralysis
    Pericardial involvement
        Pericardial effusion
        Cardiac arrhythmia
Chest wall extension
    Horner syndrome
    Pleural effusion
    Rib erosion
    Brachial plexus involvement

Extrathoracic
Bones
    Localized pain
    Pathologic fracture
Liver
    Hepatomegaly
    Pain
    Ascites
    Jaundice
Brain
    Headache
    Seizures
    Focal signs
    Personality changes
Skin
    Palpable lesions

Symptoms caused by the local effects of the tumor within the thorax may be predominantly pulmonary or extrapulmonary. The most common pulmonary symptoms are those caused by irritation of the bronchial mucosa—cough, sputum production, or hemoptysis. In addition, obstruction of a major bronchus may result in atelectasis or a distal obstructive pneumonitis, thus causing symptoms indistinguishable from those of a primary pneumonia.

The local extrapulmonary manifestations of lung cancer result from direct extension or metastasis of a tumor to vital intrathoracic stuctures. Involvement of the pleural space may produce a large pleural effusion resulting in progressive dyspnea. Superior vena caval syndrome, left recurrent laryngeal nerve paralysis, or phrenic nerve paralysis may be caused by direct extension of the tumor or by encroachment on these structures by mediastinal node metastases. Involvement of the pericardium and heart may produce a pericardial effusion or arrythmias. Chest wall involvement may cause pain by involvement of the parietal pleura, extension to peripheral nerves, or erosion of bones. Horner syndrome may occur when a superior sulcus tumor extends into the sympathetic ganglion. Brachial plexus involvement by a superior sulcus tumor may also cause pain and muscle atrophy of the shoulder and arm.

Systemic metastases may produce a variety of symptoms. The most common systemic symptoms are those caused by metastases to the brain, bones, and liver. Central nervous system involvement may be manifested by headaches, personality change, seizures, or focal neurologic deficits. Bone involvement is almost always manifest by pain. Liver involvement may occasionally cause jaundice. Although adrenal metastases are present in a high percentage of cases at postmortem examination, clinical manifestations of adrenal involvement are rarely ever recognized.

A number of systemic manifestations of lung cancer cannot be attributed to the local effects of systemic metastases. Although the pathogenesis of some of these manifestations is known, the cause in many cases remains obscure. These varied manifestations include weight loss, anorexia, fatigability, hypertrophic pulmonary osteorathropathy (Fig. 6-5), and the paraneoplastic endocrine and neurologic syndromes.

The paraneoplastic endocrine syndromes are caused by the synthesis and secretion by bronchogenic carcinomas of a variety of polypeptides that are identical to, or similar to, normally produced hormones (Table 5). Although these syndromes may be associated with all forms of bronchogenic carcinoma, the majority are associated with small cell carcinoma. The major exception is the association of parathormone secretion with squamous cell carcinoma. This syndrome may obviously lead to hypercalcemia. Adrenocorticotropic hormone (ACTH) secretion is probably the most common form of ectopic hormone production associated with bronchogenic carcinoma. In contrast to the effects of hypercortisonism in normal individuals, excess ACTH secretion in patients with lung cancer is exhibited by predominantly severe hypochloremic alkalosis.

At the time of diagnosis, patients with bronchogenic carcinoma may be asymptomatic or have any combination of local, systemic, or metastatic symptoms. Approximately 10% of the patients will be asymptomatic, and 30% will have either pulmonary symptoms, systemic symptoms, or symptoms attributed to metastatic disease. Prognostic significance can be attached to these various clinical presenta-

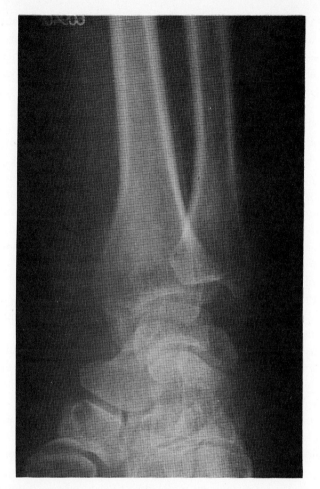

Fig. 6-5. Hypertrophic pulmonary osteoarthropathy with the prominent periosteal elevation over the distal radius and ulna.

TABLE 5

Ectopic hormone secretion associated with bronchogenic carcinoma

Hormone	Predominant cell type
Adrenocorticotropic hormone	Small cell
Parathormone	Squamous cell
Antidiuretic hormone	Small cell
Melanocyte-stimulating hormone	Small cell
Calcitonin	Small cell
Serotonin	Small cell
Human chorionic gonadotropin	Large cell
Growth hormone	Adenocarcinoma

tions. In any group of patients with nearly identical lesions and similar cell types, patients who are asymptomatic will have a more favorable prognosis than patients with symptoms. Patients with pulmonary symptoms alone have a better prognosis than individuals with systemic symptoms. Patient with metastatic symptoms at the time of diagnosis have the worst prognosis.

Diagnosis

Although a presumptive diagnosis of lung cancer can usually be made on the basis of the roentgenographic manifestations of the tumor, a variety of tests are employed to make a specific histologic diagnosis. In recent years, new techniques have been developed that have made accurate diagnosis of lung cancer possible in the great majority of patients without performance of a thoracotomy. Currently, only 10% to 15% of patients require an exploratory thoracotomy for diagnosis alone.

Cytologic examination of expectorated sputum is the only noninvasive technique available for the diagnosis of lung cancer. The percentage of cases in which a specific histologic diagnosis can be made by this technique depends on a number of variables. Proper collection and processing of the sputum sample and the diagnostic skill of the cytologic technician screening the samples are important. In addition, the location and histologic type of the tumor influence the percentage of cases that can be diagnosed by cytologic analysis. Nevertheless, the presence of malignant disease can be documented in a majority of patients by this technique, and an experienced cytologist can make a specific histopathologic diagnosis in a high percentage of cases.

The introduction of flexible fiberoptic bronchoscopy has had a major impact on the diagnosis of bronchogenic carcinoma. Bronchial brush or forceps biopsy through the flexible instrument has greatly increased the number of cases of lung cancer that can be diagnosed by endoscopic examination. Since the flexible fiberoptic instrument can be introduced under direct vision into segmental and subsegmental airways, this procedure has a great advantage over endoscopic examination, in which the rigid bronchoscope is used. When a lesion is visible through the flexible bronchoscope, a histologic diagnosis of the specific cell type can be made in 80% to 85% of cases. When the lesion is not directly visible, brush biopsy under fluoroscopic control will yield a positive diagnosis in 50% to 60% of cases.

Other invasive biopsy procedures will be required to make a specific diagnosis in selected patients. Any obvious site of a metastasis that is readily accessible should be biopsied. However, only a third of patients have clearly demonstrable metastatic disease at the time of initial examination, and in many of these patients the site of metastatic disease is not accessible to direct biopsy. In selected cases, mediastinoscopy, bilateral scalene node biopsy, or bone marrow biopsy may be useful. Mediastinoscopy is postive in approximately 40% of patients considered resectable who undergo this procedure before thoracotomy. Bilateral scalene node biopsy may also be useful in an occasional highly selected patient. This procedure may be positive in as many as 20% of cases, even in the absence of palpable nodes. Bone marrow biopsy is also a valuable diagnostic technique in selected patients. In approximately 50% of patients with small cell carcinoma, a single bone marrow biopsy will be diagnostic. About 10% of patients with adenocarcinoma will have a positive bone marrow biopsy, whereas the yield is negligible in patients with squamous cell carcinoma. Percutaneous needle biopsy of the lung or percutaneous needle aspiration may be performed for diagnostic purposes but should only be employed if the patient is considered inoperable.

Staging evaluation

An intelligent approach to the management of patients with lung cancer must be based on an adequate evaluation of the extent of the disease. As has been emphasized previously, the majority of patients have mediastinal or systemic metastases at the time of diagnosis. A thorough staging evaluation should be performed before patients are subjected to surgery so that patients who are unresectable will not experience the unnecessary morbidity, and even mortality, associated with thoracotomy. From a practical standpoint, it is important to determine whether a patient with lung cancer has disease that is apparently localized to the lung parenchyma or whether mediastinal node or extrathoracic metastases are present.

The value of mediastinoscopy in detecting mediastinal node metastases has been mentioned previously. About 30% to 40% of patients considered potential candidates for resectional surgery will have mediastinal node metastases demonstrated by this technique. In general, mediastinoscopy has a high yield in patients with lesions in the hilum or parahilar region or in patients with undifferentiated tumors. False negative mediastinoscopies occur in 10% to 15% of patients who have mediastinal node involvement. In the majority of these cases the tumor is located in the left upper lobe or left hilum. These lesions metastasize to mediastinal nodes located near the aorta and are inaccessible to the mediastinoscope.

The importance of detecting mediastinal node metastases has been well documented. The presence of mediastinal node involvement should be considered a contraindication for surgery except in unusual circumstances. Several studies have demonstrated that the presence of mediastinal node metastases carries as poor a prognosis for long-term survival as does the presence of clinically demonstrable systemic metastases. Thus resection of tumors in patients with evidence of mediastinal involvement would not be expected to increase long-term survival rates.

In the absence of symptoms attributable to a specific metastatic site, diagnostic techniques to detect extrathoracic metastases are, for the most part, grossly inadequate. The most common sites of metastases are the brain, bone, liver, and adrenal glands. Brain scans are positive in approximately 5% of patients with no symptoms of central nervous system metastatic disease and in only 50% to 60% of patients who have central nervous system symptoms. Electroencephalograms and lumbar puncture do not increase the sensitivity of detecting central nervous system metastases. The availability of computerized tomography may increase the yield of detecting brain metastases. Liver scans have also been shown to be of little value in assessing patients with bronchogenic carcinoma. Both false positive and false negative scans occur. Peritoneoscopy with direct needle biopsy of the liver has been demonstrated to be the most specific and sensitive technique for detecting liver metastases. Bone marrow biopsy is the most sensitive technique for detecting bone metastases. Bone scans are somewhat complementary and will be positive in 15% of patients with a negative biopsy. Roentgenographic surveys for bone metastases are positive in only 5% of patients with a positive biopsy. At present, no satisfactory diagnostic techniques are able to detect adrenal metastases.

Treatment

The overall 5-year survival rate for patients with bronchogenic carcinoma is between 5% and 10% (Fig. 6-6). Clearly, no single form of therapy has been highly successful in the management of this disease. Treatment must be individualized to the specific patient. The approach to therapy must be based on knowledge of the extent of the disease and, if possible, the histologic tumor type.

In general, surgical resection of a tumor localized to the lung is the only form of curative therapy. The inadequacy of staging procedures in correctly identifying patients with truly localized disease is illustrated by the fact that less than 50% of the patients with apparently localized peripheral nodules survive 5 years. Nevertheless, patients with bronchogenic carcinoma who do not have demonstrable intrathoracic or systemic metastases should be considered candidates for surgical resection.

The presence of mediastinal node metastases is associated with as poor a prog-

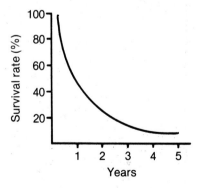

Fig. 6-6. Approximation of the survival curve from the time of diagnosis for all patients with bronchogenic carcinoma.

nosis as is the presence of obvious systemic metastases. Patients with mediastinal node metastases who have undergone resectional surgery have 5-year survival rates of less than 10%. The use of adjuvant chemotherapy or radiotherapy in patients demonstrating mediastinal node metastases has not had a significant effect on mean survival rates, except possibly in patients with squamous cell carcinoma. Recent studies have suggested that the combination of resectional surgery and radiation will result in a 5-year survival rate of between 20% to 30% in patients with squamous cell carcinoma who are known to have mediastinal node involvement.

With the exception of patients with squamous cell carcinoma, radiotherapy should be considered a form of palliative therapy and thus reserved for use in patients with symptoms directly relted to local tumor growth. Symptoms caused by bronchial obstruction, hemoptysis, bone pain, and central nervous system involvement are generally responsive to local radiotherapy.

The experience with systemic therapy has, for the most part, been disappointing. Multiple chemotherapeutic regimens are currently undergoing intensive investigation. To date, the greatest success has been achieved in the treatment of small cell carcinoma. Mean survival in patients with small cell carcinoma generally ranges between 3 and 6 months from the time of diagnosis. Combined chemotherapeutic protocols, however, have extended mean survival time to longer than a year. In patients with other cell types, equally successful regimens have yet to be demonstrated.

Another form of palliative therapy that should be considered is the use of corticosteroids for the management of patients with symptomatic brain metastases. The value of this therapy has been recognized clinically for some time. Recent studies demonstrating that steroids have an effect on the regulation of blood flow and control of edema in the region of brain metastases have provided a scientific basis for this clinical observation. Steroids may be used alone or in conjunction with local radiotherapy for controlling central nervous system symptoms resulting from brain metastases.

In patients with hypercalcemia, appropriate therapy to lower the serum calcium may also relieve disturbing symptoms and improve the patient's well-being. Acute therapy usually consists of maintaining a forced diuresis, either alone or in conjunction with oral phosphate therapy. The type of chronic therapy employed depends on the pathogenesis of the hypercalcemia. Chronic adminstration of steroids, mithramycin, or indomethacin may be beneficial in specific patients.

Immunotherapy is the newest form of treatment to be investigated in bronchogenic carcinoma. Most current studies are evaluating the effect of the systemic administration of BCG (bacille Calmette Guérin) or other nonspecific adjuvants on tumor rejection. This form of therapy is strictly experimental, and no definite conclusions can be drawn about its value at this time.

BRONCHIAL ADENOMAS

The bronchial adenomas are a group of four different histologic types of tumors that arise from the bronchial wall. These tumors comprise 6% to 10% of all primary bronchial tumors. The term "adenoma" implies that the tumors are benign and arise from mucus-secreting cells of the mucosal glands of the bronchial wall. Neither of these implications is completely true. Some of the tumors in this group clearly have low-grade malignant potential. Furthermore, the most common of these tumors, the carcinoid tumor, clearly does not arise from a mucus-secreting cell. Cylindromas, mucoepidermoid adenomas, and mucous gland adenomas, the other tumors that comprise this general group, do arise from mucus-secreting cells. Carcinoid tumors comprise 85% to 90% of all bronchial adenomas and will be discussed in greatest detail.

Carcinoid adenomas

Microscopically, pulmonary carcinoids resemble the carcinoid tumors of the intestine. They are composed of small, uniformly staining cells that arrange themselves in clumps, trabeculae, or tubules. Argentaffin granules are occasionally observed in these tumors. Mitotic figures are virtually absent, thus assessment of the degree of malignancy of the tumor from its histologic appearance may be impossible. The stroma of the tumor occasionally undergoes hyaline change, calcifies, or even ossifies.

Grossly, carcinoid tumors arise most often from major bronchi and are distributed evenly between both lungs. The tumors appear as polypoid endobronchial masses or may extend from the bronchial wall deeply into the extrabronchial lung parenchyma, thus exhibiting an iceberg effect. The surface of the tumor is vascular and rarely ulcerates. The tumor may directly extend into adjacent tissues, including lymph nodes. Distant metastases occur in less than 5% of all cases. Occasionally, the tumor is a solitary parenchymal mass in the periphery of the lung or tumorlets that appear roentgenographically as multiple small nodules scattered diffusely through both lungs.

In recent years research has shown conclusively that bronchial carcinoids arise from neuroendocrine cells that are present in the bronchial epithelium and bronchial mucous glands. These cells, referred to as "Kulchitsky cells," are part of a system of cells referred to as the amine precursor uptake and decarboxylase (APUD) system, which is distributed in many tissues. The secretion of a variety of hormones by bronchial carcinoids can undoubtedly be attributed to the cellular origin of these tumors.

The clinical manifestations of carcinoid adenomas are extremely varied. Peripheral lesions usually elicit no symptoms. However, centrally located lesions produce signs and symptoms resulting from the endobronchial location of the tumor. Hemoptysis occurs in a large percentage of patients, presumably reflecting the highly vascular nature of the tumor. Cough, sputum production, wheezing, chest pain, and fever may occur as a result of obstruction of a major bronchus leading to atelectasis or obstructive pneumonitis. Physical examination may reveal a localized wheeze directly attributable to the site of the tumor. Other findings result from the parenchymal changes that occur distal to the lesion. In the majority of patients, symptoms are present for many years before the diagnosis is made.

Occasionally, a patient may exhibit signs and symptoms directly caused by ectopic hormone production by the tumor. The carcinoid syndrome, produced by secretion of 5-hydroxytryptamine (serotonin), is probably the most common endocrine syndrome associated with these tumors. This syndrome consists of prolonged attacks of any combination of flushing, nausea, vomiting, diarrhea, fever, hypotension, edema, and wheezing. Patients who develop this syndrome usually have extensive metastatic disease. Adrenocorticotropic hormone, insulin, gastrin, antidiuretic hormone, and melanocyte-stimulating hormone have also been reported to be secreted by bronchial carcinoids. Thus clinical syndromes associated with each of these particular hormones may be observed in association with these tumors.

The roentgenographic manifestations of bronchial carcinoids depend on the location and growth pattern of the tumor. As already mentioned, approximately 20% of adenomas are peripheral lung masses. These lesions are usually sharply demarcated and occasionally may calcify or ossify. No other features distinguish these tumors from other lesions that grow as solitary nodules in the periphery of the lung. If central tumors have developed as "iceberg lesions," the primary manifestation may be a hilar or perihilar mass. If, on the other hand, the lesion has grown predominantly endobronchially, the tumor itself may not be visible, but the effects of bronchial obstruction, atelectasis, or obstructive pneumonitis may be present. In the past, bronchography was a useful procedure for localizing endobronchial adenomas. Since the advent of fiberoptic bronchoscopy, bronchography is employed only occasionally.

The diagnosis of a bronchial carcinoid requires, in almost all cases, pathologic examination of tissue obtained from the tumor. Cytologic examination of expectorates sputum or washings obtained at the time of bronchoscopy are almost invariably nondiagnostic. Since the majority of adenomas are located centrally, fiberoptic bronchoscopy is an extremely valuable technique for identifying and biopsying the lesion. Because of the highly vascular nature of some adenomas, a biopsy may not be performed for diagnostic purposes. Obviously, the diagnosis of peripheral lesions or central lesions that are not biopsied will be made only after examination of resected tumor.

In patients with an endocrine syndrome, the diagnosis may be suspected, particularly if the carcinoid syndrome is present. However, since bronchogenic carcinomas are also associated with ectopic hormone production, the presence of an endocrine syndrome cannot be considered diagnostic for a carcinoid tumor. For similar reasons, routine measurement of hormone levels are of little diagnostic value. Bronchial carcinoids may secrete serotonin even in the absence of signs and symptoms of the carcinoid syndrome. Measurement of the metabolic product of sertonin, 5-hyroxyindoleacetic acid (5-HIAA), in blood or urine may occasionally be useful.

Surgical resection is the only accepted form of therapy. Since the malignant potential of the tumor is small, appropriately located central lesions may be resected and the bronchi reanastomosed, thus salvaging lung tissue. This procedure is of most value with localized endobronchial lesions.

Cylindroma

Adenoid cystic carcinomas (cylindromas) are approximately 10% as common as bronchial carcinoids. These tumors grow by direct extension along the bronchial and tracheal wall and rarely occur as polyploid endobronchial lesions. They are located more often in the trachea and are more malignant and locally invasive than carcinoids. Distant metastases may occur in extrathoracic sites.

Mucoepidermoid and mucous gland adenomas

Mucoepidermoid and mucous gland adenomas are extremely unusual tumors. They do not have distinguishing clinical or roentgenographic features. The diagnosis is based on pathologic examination of appropriate tissue specimens. The mucous gland adenoma is, both morphologically and in its clinical activity, the only truly benign bronchial adenoma.

Section two

THE GAS-EXCHANGING
PARENCHYMA

Chapter 7

NORMAL STRUCTURE
AND FUNCTION

STRUCTURE

The lung is divided into a labyrinth of 300 million individual alveolar sacs (alveoli) by an interconnecting network of thin septate, the alveolar walls (Figs. 7-1 and 7-2). Each alveolar air space formed by this arrangement is in direct contact with the environment through the branching airway system described in Chapter 1. In turn the alveolar walls are perfused by an extensive capillary network (Fig. 7-3). The capillary network in the alveolar walls is so extensive that blood moves through the alveolar walls almost as a continuous sheet. Blood in the alveolar capillaries is separated from the air space by only a thin tissue barrier, the alveolar-capillary membrane (Fig. 7-4). These structural relationships are extremely important, since they result in an alveolar-capillary membrane surface area of approximately 70 m^2 for potential gas exchange between the environmental air and blood.

The parenchyma of the lung directly involved in gas exchange makes up approximately 80% of the total mass of the lung. The major airways and blood vessels comprise the remaining 20%. The gas-exchanging parenchyma consists of all the various cellular and noncellular components of the alveolar wall. To understand the structure-function relationship of both the normal and diseased lung, the function of the various components of the alveolar wall should be recognized and understood.

Following are the major cellular and noncellular components of the alveolar wall:

Cellular components	Noncellular components
Type I epithelial cell	Surfactant
Type II epithelial cell	Collagen
Fibroblast	Elastin
Endothelial cell	
Alveolar macrophage	

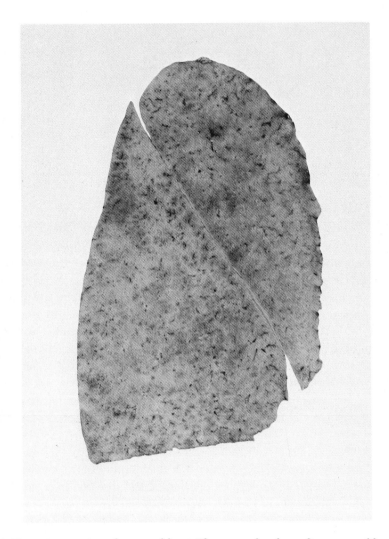

Fig. 7-1. Transverse section of a normal lung. The cut surface has a fine sponge-like appearance.

From Auerbach, O., et al.: Relation of smoking and age to emphysema: whole lung section study, N. Engl. J. Med. **286:**854, 1972.

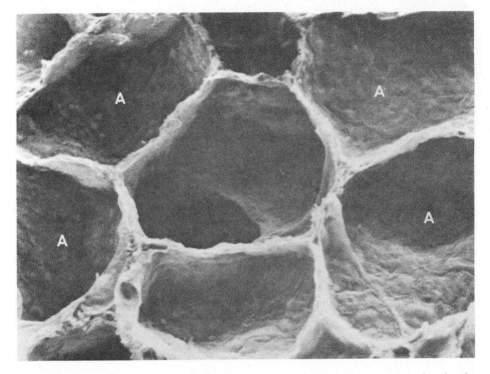

Fig. 7-2. Scanning electron micrograph of the cut surface of lung demonstrating the alveolar architecture.

From Takaro, T., Price, H.P., and Parra, S.C.: Ultrastructural studies of apertures in the interalveolar septum of the adult human lung, Am. Rev. Respir. Dis. **119:**425, 1979.

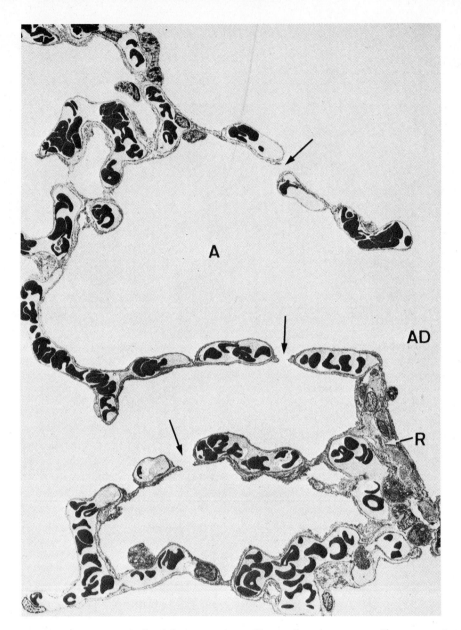

Fig. 7-3. Electron micrograph of the cut surface of lung. The extensive capillary network is contained within the alveolar walls. The wall of the alveolar duct *(AD)* is reinforced by fiber strands *(R)*. *A,* Alveolus.

From West, J.B.: Bioengineering aspects of the lung, New York, 1977, Marcel Dekker, Inc.

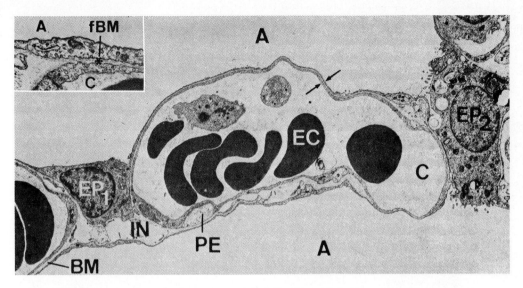

Fig. 7-4. Higher magnification of a portion of the alveolar wall demonstrating the alveolar-capillary membrane. Type I *(EP₁)* and type II *(EP₂)* epithelial cells can be identified in this section. An extremely thin membrane separates the capillary lumen *(C)* from the alveolar space. The insert demonstrates this membrane at higher magnification. *A*, Alveoli; *EC*, erythrocytes; *BM*, basement membrane; *PC*, pericytes; *IN*, interstitium.

From Bachofen, M., and Weibel, E.R.: Alterations of the gas exchange apparatus in adult respiratory insufficiency associated with septicemia, Am. Rev. Respir. Dis. **116:**589, 1977.

This is by no means a complete list. However, it includes alveolar wall components known to have an important function in the normal lung and thus must be considered when assessing the response of the alveolar wall to injury.

Cellular components of the alveolar wall

There are five major cellular components of the alveolar wall. The alveolar surface in contact with air is lined by two types of epithelial cells, designated types I and II pneumocytes, that have specific functions. The *type I pneumocyte* is characterized by very thin cytoplasmic extensions that spread over the majority of the alveolar surface. Although almost twice as many type II as type I pneumocytes exist, the cytoplasmic extensions of the type I pneumocytes line approximately 90% of the alveolar surface area. These cytoplasmic extensions are so thin that they cannot be identified by light microscopy. The type I pneumocyte contains a limited number of intracellular organelles suggesting that metabolically, the cell is relatively inactive. These characteristics suggest that the cell is anatomically specialized to provide a minimum barrier to gas diffusion and biochemically specialized to consume little oxygen. The type I pneumocyte also has limited, if any, ability to proliferate and replicate itself after injury.

The *type II pneumocyte*, or granular pneumocyte, is readily identified by the presence of lamellar cytoplasmic inclusion bodies (Fig. 7-5). In contrast to the type I pneumocyte, the type II pneumocyte has limited cytoplasm but contains abundant intracellular organelles. The type II pneumocyte has two major functions that are critical in maintaining the integrity of the alveolus. First, evidence shows conclusively that the type II pneumocyte is important in the production of surfactant, a surface active material that lines the alveolar surface. The metabolism and function of this material will be discussed in this chapter. In addition, the type II pneumocyte plays a major role in repair of the alveolar epithelium after injury. Type II

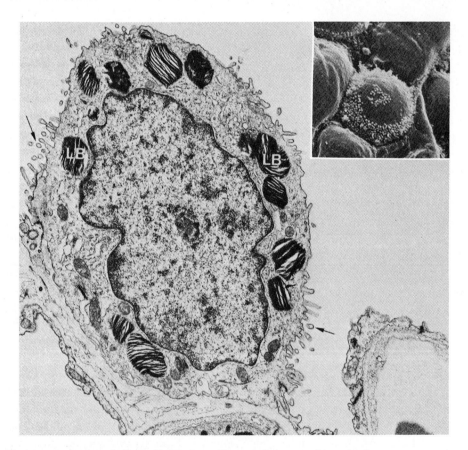

Fig. 7-5. Type II epithelial cell. *LB,* Lamellar cytoplasmic inclusion bodies.

From West, J.B.: Bioengineering aspects of the lung, New York, 1977, Marcel Dekker, Inc.

pneumocytes can readily proliferate to line the alveolar wall after type I pneumo-cytes are damaged. New type I pneumocytes apparently are derived from prolifer-ation of the type II cell.

A number of connective tissue cells are within the interstitial tissue of the alveolar wall. However, the fibroblast is the only one of these cells that will be mentioned in this discussion. The function of the fibroblast is somewhat specula-tive; however, it probably is important in the synthesis of the major connective tissue proteins found in the alveolar wall. These connective tissue proteins appear to determine the mechanical properties of the normal lung. Furthermore, the char-acteristics of protein synthesis after alveolar wall injury are extremely important in determining the pathologic and physiologic abnormalities associated with many dif-fuse diseases of the lung. Thus the fibroblast assumes great importance in the pro-cess of alveolar wall repair after injury.

The extensive intra-alveolar capillary network is lined by *endothelial cells*. The margins of adjacent cells either abut bluntly or interdigitate to form tight in-tracellular junctions. These cells are permeable to water and electrolytes but to some extent form a barrier to high molecular weight solutes. In addition, the alveo-lar-capillary endothelial cells appear to have a unique metabolic function. For many years a number of bioactive substances such as bradykinin, noradrenaline, 5-hy-droxytryptamine (serotonin), have been known to be inactivated during passage through the lung. It is now clear that the enzymes responsible for this activity are located on the surface of the alveolar-capillary endothelial cells. Electron micros-copy demonstrates that the surface of these cells is covered by irregular projections extending into the lumen of the capillary and that the cells contain enormous num-bers of pinocytotic vesicles (caveolae intracellulares) (Figs. 7-6 and 7-7). These structural arrangements greatly increase the surface area of the cells and thus in-crease their efficiency in fulfilling their metabolic function.

The *pulmonary macrophage* is distributed both within the interstitial tissue of the alveolar wall (interstitial macrophages) and in the alveolar space (alveolar macrophages). The macrophages of the lung are derived from the pool of circulating blood monocytes. Monocytes apparently migrate from the vascular space into the interstitial tissue of the alveolar wall where they either undergo structural and met-abolic changes characteristic of mature pulmonary macrophages or remain dormant with the potential for maturation at a later time. The mature macrophage eventually migrates into the alveolar space to perform its major function (Fig. 7-8). These cells are an integral part of the systemic reticuloendothelial system. They are active phagocytes and thus are important in protecting the alveolar environment against both pathogenic microorganisms and particulate matter inhaled into the lung (Fig. 7-9). These cells are also probably extremely important in modulating certain im-mune responses within the lung.

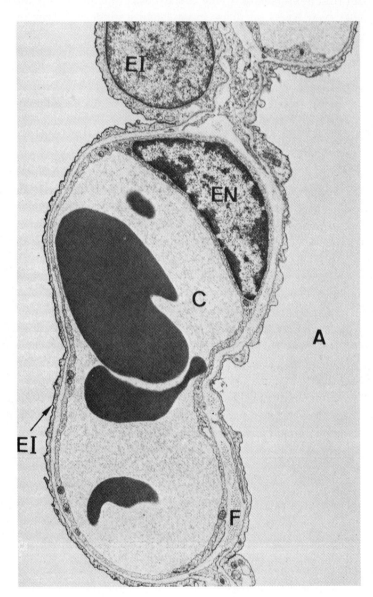

Fig. 7-6. Pulmonary capillary *(C)* showing the nucleus and cytoplasmic extensions of the endothelial cells *(EN)*. *EI* marks the nucleus and cytoplasmic flaps of the type I epithelial cell. Collagen fibers *(F)* are evident in the alveolar-capillary membrane.

From Weibel, E.R.: Morphological basis of alveolar-capillary gas exchange, Physiol. Rev. **53:**419, 1973.

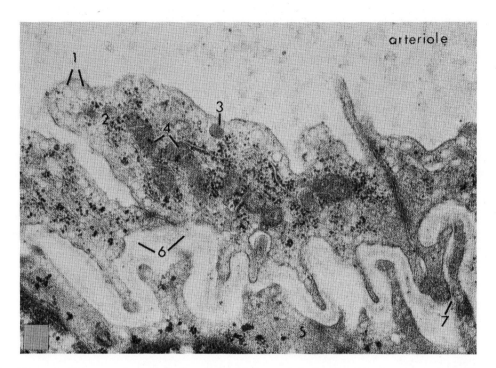

Fig. 7-7. Electron micrograph of a portion of the cytoplasmic flap of a capillary endothelial cell demonstrating the intraluminal projections on the surface of the cell. *1,* Large number of pinocytotic vesicles within the cell; *2,* ribosomes; *3,* endothelial granules; *4,* mitochondria.

From Rhodin, J.: Anatomy of the pulmonary microvascular bed, Microvasc. Res. **15:**169, 1978.

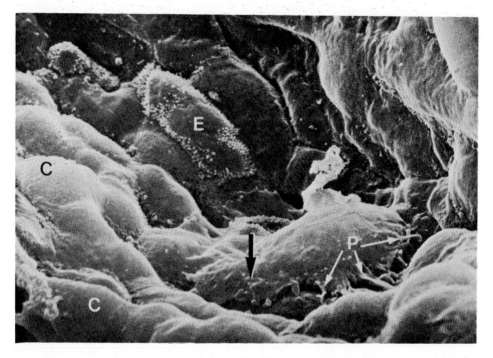

Fig. 7-8. Scanning electron micrograph of the alveolar surface demonstrating an alveolar macrophage. Numerous cytoplasmic extensions *(arrow)* and pseudopods *(P)* attach the cell to the alveolar surface. The bulging capillaries *(C)* and type II cells *(E)* are in the background.

From West, J.B.: Bioengineering aspects of the lung, New York, 1977, Marcel Dekker, Inc.

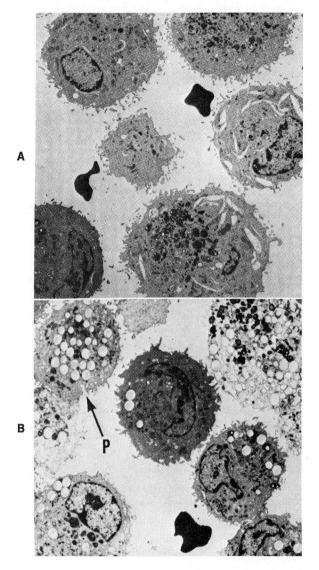

Fig. 7-9. A, Electron microscopy of alveolar macrophages washed from the lung. **B,**Electron microscopy of these cells after incubation with polystyrene latex beads *(P)*, illustrating the phagocytic capability of these cells.

From Sanders, C.L., et al.: Pulmonary macrophage and epithelial cells, Technical Information Center, Springfield, Va., 1977, Energy Research and Development Administration.

Noncellular components of the alveolar wall

Surfactant is an extremely important component of the alveolar wall. As mentioned previously, surfactant is a material that lines the alveolar surface in contact with air. Substantial evidence shows that surfactant is synthesized in type II pneumocytes and stored within the cytoplasmic, lamellar bodies of these cells until released into the alveolar space. Electron microscopy has demonstrated that surfactant is present on the alveolar surface in a number of different morphologic forms. However, tubular myelin structures are characteristically present in the lining material (Fig 7-10).

The exact chemical composition of surfactant has not been defined. However, the material is a unique lipoprotein that is particularly rich in highly saturated lecithins. Approximately 85% of this material is lipid and almost three fourths of the lipid is dipalmitoyl phosphatidylcholine (dipalmitoyl-lecithin). The majority of the remaining composition is protein. Within the protein content, a protein constituent exists that appears to be unique to surfactant.

To understand the function of surfactant, the relationship between the volume of the alveolus and certain physical forces acting at the surface of the alveolus should be understood. For the purpose of this discussion, the alveolus is considered to be an inflatable sphere with a gas phase–water phase (air-tissue) interface. Surface tension is the physical phenomenon that is inherent when an interface exists between matter in two dissimilar phases, such as gas and water. Unbalanced intramolecular forces at such an interface lead to the development of a surface force that acts to decrease the surface area of interface. In a sphere the surface force is inversely proportional to the radius of the sphere and directly proportional to the surface tension. Thus, if surface tension remains unchanged as the sphere becomes progressively smaller, the surface force acting to further decrease the surface area progressively increases. If other factors are not involved, the surface force acting to decrease the surface area will eventually cause collapse of the sphere. Obviously, if this were allowed to happen to alveoli, the gas-exchanging function of the lung would be severely impaired (Fig. 7-11). As a result of its bipolar chemical configuration, surfactant decreases the surface tension at the air-tissue interface of the alveolar wall as the alveolus deflates. As a result, the surface force acting to collapse the alveolus is decreased, allowing the alveolus to be stable at small volumes. Obviously, since the pressure tending to collapse the alveolus is decreased by surfactant, it will also be easier to reinflate the alveolus from a small volume, since less pressure will be required to overcome the existing surface force. Thus surfactant is not only important in stabilizing the alveolus at small volumes but also in determining to a great extent the force necessary to inflate the alveolus.

Surfactant apparently has a relatively short half-life in the lung. Thus surfactant must be continuously produced by type II pneumocytes if the mechanical properties and function of the normal lung are to be maintained. Alveolar wall injury probably disrupts the ability of type II pneumocytes to produce surfactant.

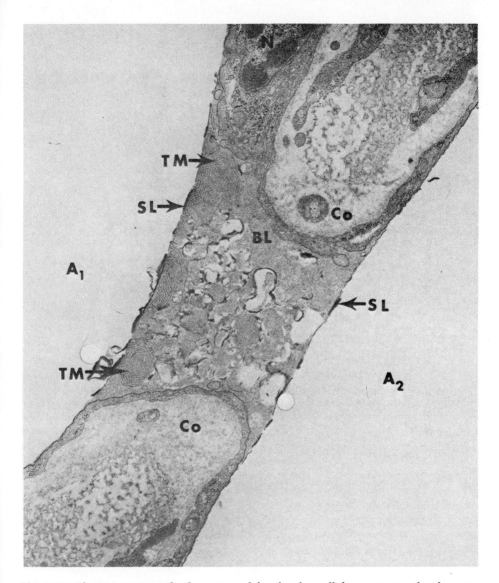

Fig. 7-10. Electron micrograph of a portion of the alveolar wall demonstrating the character-istic tubular myelin structure *(TM)* of surfactant on the surface of the wall. A_1 and A_2, Alveolar spaces *SL*, thin superficial layer of surfactant; *BL*, granular basal layer of surfactant; *Co*, collagen; *N*, nucleus of a type I cell.

From Takaro, T., Price, H.P., and Parra, S.C.: Ultrastructural studies of apertures in the interalveolar septum of the adult human lung, Am. Rev. Respir. Dis. **119:**425, 1979.

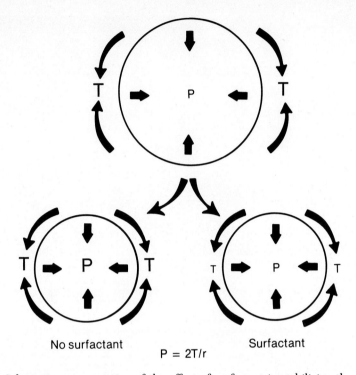

No surfactant

P = 2T/r

Surfactant

Fig. 7-11. Schematic representation of the effect of surfactant in stabilizing the alveolus at low lung volumes. According to the LaPlace relationship (P = 2T/r), the pressure acting to collapse an inflatable sphere is directly related to the surface tension and inversely related to the radius of the sphere. As a sphere decreases in size, the pressure acting to further deflate the sphere is markedly influenced by the effect of surfactant on the surface tension. In the absence of surfactant, surface tension may remain constant, but, since the radius of the sphere has decreased, the pressure must increase *(left)*. In the presence of surfactant, surface tension is decreased; thus the pressure acting to further decrease the size of the sphere may remain constant, stabilizing the sphere at the lower lung volume. The relative size of the symbols in the figure reflects these changes.

Thus collapse of the alveolus caused by surfactant deficiency is a real hazard during the course of acute lung injury.

Collagen and elastin are the major connective tissue proteins in the basement membranes and the interstitial space of the alveolar wall (Fig. 7-12). Approximately three times as much collagen as elastin is in the lung. Under normal circumstances, these proteins, which are probably synthesized by fibroblasts, have a very slow turnover in the lung. However, a marked increase in the synthesis of these proteins may occur after alveolar wall injury.

Four different structural and biochemical types of collagen have been recognized in the human body. The collagen in the interstitial space of the alveolar wall

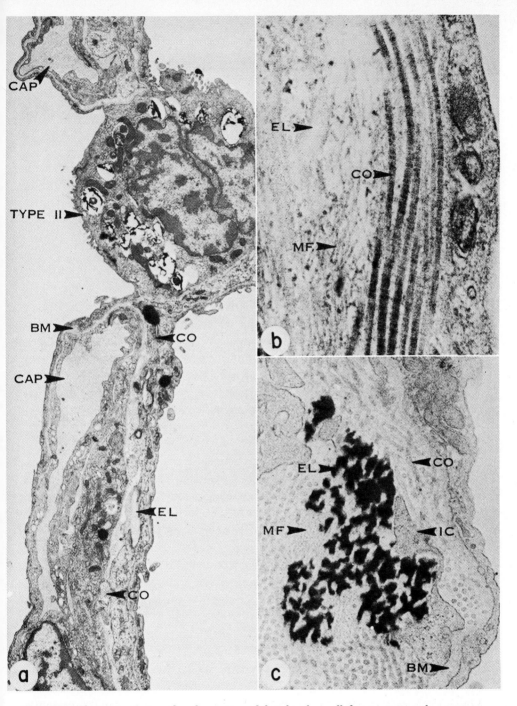

Fig. 7-12. Electron micrographs of a portion of the alveolar wall demonstrating the presence of elastin *(EL)* and collagen *(CO)* in the interstitial space of the alveolar wall. Increasing magnification *(b* and *c)* further defines the structure of these connective tissue proteins. Elastic fibers contain amorphous elastin *(EL)* and microfibrils *(MF)*. *CAP*, Capillaries; *BM*, basement membrane; *E*, type II cell.

From Hance, A.J., and Crystal, R.G.: The connective tissue of the lung, Am. Rev. Respir. Dis. **112:**657, 1975.

is predominantly type I. Collagen is thought to provide the tensil strength of the alveolar wall and thus to be under stretch only at high alveolar volumes. Therefore collagen would limit inflation of the alveolus only when the alveolus reaches a critical volume. In contrast, elastic fibers are presumed to be under stretch at all volumes. Thus elastin is the predominant determinant of the mechanical properties of the alveolar wall at low alveolar volumes.

Collagen and elastin appear to work in concert during inflation and deflation of the alveolus. Their structural relationship is important in determining the mechanical properties of the alveolus. Clearly, biochemical alteration of these proteins or changes in the distribution or interaction of individual fibers may have an effect on the mechanical properties of the alveolus, although the quantity of the proteins is unchanged.

The basement membranes on which the alveolar epithelial and capillary endothelial cells sit are comprised predominantly of type IV collagen. Capillary basement membranes in other organs, particularly the renal glomerulus, are considered to be an integral component of the filtration apparatus of the capillary wall and thus serve as part of the barrier to the movement of certain high molecular weight solutes from the vascular space. However, the alveolar capillary basement membrane does not appear to retard large solutes as effectively as the basement membranes of other capillary beds. Whether this is specifically related to the structure of collagen in the alveolar basement membranes is not known.

FUNCTION

The major function of the lung parenchyma is the exchange of oxygen and carbon dioxide across the alveolar-capillary membrane. Therefore, in a strict sense, a discussion of the function of the lung parenchyma should focus on the physiology of gas exchange. However, measurement of the mechanical properties of the gas-exchanging parenchyma also provides information about the structural integrity of the lung. Clinical studies have clearly demonstrated the value of such tests for identifying the kind of general structural abnormality present in a number of lung diseases. As a basis for understanding the mechanical properties and gas-exchange function of the lung, the mechanical properties and gas function of the individual alveolus will be considered first.

Gas exchange by the parenchyma

Normal gas exchange by the lung requires adequate ventilation and perfusion of individual gas-exchanging units. The factors involved in matching ventilation and perfusion throughout the lung are not entirely related to the mechanical properties of the gas-exchanging parenchyma. Thus this subject will be reviewed in detail later. For the purpose of this discussion, the ventilation and perfusion of individual gas-exchanging units initially will be assumed adequate. The physiology of gas exchange at the alveolar level will be discussed in this section.

Gas exchange across the alveolar-capillary membrane occurs by simple diffusion. Approximately 80% of the alveolar wall surface is in intimate contact with an alveolar capillary and thus available for gas exchange. The minimum barrier between the gases in the alveolar space and the blood is made up of an intercalated layer of fused basement membranes and the cytoplasmic flaps of both an alveolar epithelial cell and a capillary endothelial cell (Fig. 7-13). In the human lung this barrier is only 0.1 to 0.3 μm thick. Approximately a third of the surface area of the alveolar-capillary membrane presents this minimum barrier to gas diffusion. The remaining alveolar-capillary membrane contains variable amounts of connective tissue protein interspersed between the basement membranes.

Bulk diffusion of a gas across a membrane depends on the diffusion and solubility coefficients for the gas in the membrane, the thickness and surface area of the membrane, and the pressure gradient for the gas across the membrane. These factors must be considered in the diffusion of oxygen and carbon dioxide across the alveolar-capillary membrane. The partial pressure of oxygen in the alveolus, the main driving pressure for diffusion of oxygen, is determined by alveolar ventilation, which, for the purpose of this discussion, is presumed to be normal. Although partial pressure determines the driving pressure across the membrane, diffusion is measured as the volume of gas that crosses the membrane per unit of time. Since

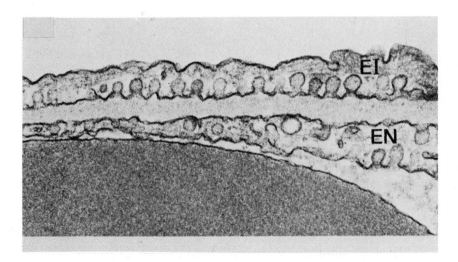

Fig. 7-13. Higher magnification of the alveolar-capillary membrane demonstrating that the thin barrier portion of the membrane is made up of basement membrane and cytoplasmic flaps of the type I epithelial cell *(EI)* and endothelial cell *(EN)*. Numerous pinocytotic vesicles are present in the cytoplasm of both cells.

From West, J.B.: Bioengineering aspects of the lung, New York, 1977, Marcel Dekker, Inc.

the partial pressure and volume of oxygen in the blood at any time are primarily determined by the amount of oxygen that binds to hemoglobin, the chemical reactions in this process must also be considered in the overall diffusion of oxygen.

Thus the major factors that might limit the diffusion of oxygen from the alveolar space into the blood are the actual diffusion of oxygen across the various components of the alveolar-capillary membrane, the chemical reactions involved in the binding of oxygen to hemoglobin, and the surface area of the membrane available for diffusion. Analysis of these factors has shown that diffusion across the membrane has little effect on the normal exchange of oxygen. Thus, even when the membrane is markedly thickened by disease, the diffusion of oxygen is not limited to the degree that total oxygenation of the capillary blood is prevented. When the various components of the diffusion of oxygen are analyzed in the context of the whole lung, the major determinant of the volume of oxygen that can be exchanged from the alveolar space into the blood is the total surface area of the alveolar-capillary membrane.

Distinguishing between abnormalities in the diffusing capacity of the lung and the development of hypoxemia is important. To understand this distinction, it is important to recognize that, in the normal resting person, diffusion of all the oxygen necessary to completely oxygenate the capillary blood occurs in only 20% to 30% of the total time that blood is in the alveolar capillary (Fig. 7-14). This is an extremely important fact, since it means as capillary transit time decreases or as the time required for diffusion increases, oxygen exchange has ample time to take place and fully oxygenate the capillary blood. Thus abnormalities in diffusion do not directly cause hypoxemia.

Carbon dioxide transfer from the capillary blood to the alveolar space also occurs by diffusion. The membrane diffusing capacity for carbon dioxide is approximately twenty times greater than that for oxygen, primarily because carbon dioxide is much more soluble than oxygen in the membrane components. Nevertheless, carbon dioxide actually takes longer to equilibrate across the alveolar-capillary membrane because of the increased affinity of blood for carbon dioxide and the fact that the biochemical reactions involved in carbon dioxide transfer are slower than those of oxygen.

Again, the gas-exchange function of the entire lung is affected little by alterations in the diffusion of gas across the alveolar-capillary membrane. The matching of ventilation and perfusion in individual gas-exchanging units is the principal determinant of pulmonary gas exchange. Alteration of ventilation-perfusion relationships throughout the lung may be caused by diseases involving the airways, vasculature, or gas-exchanging parenchyma. Thus the physiology of these relationships must be considered within the context of the interaction of the various structural components of the entire lung (see Chapter 22).

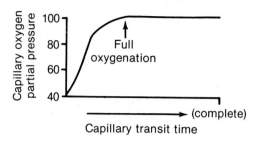

Fig. 7-14. Kinetics of the uptake of oxygen by red cells during their transit through the alveolar capillaries. The cells are fully oxygenated in about a third of the time required for their transit through the capillary.

MECHANICAL PROPERTIES OF THE PARENCHYMA

The lung is passively inflated by the bellows-like action of the chest cage (chest wall and diaphragm). During inspiration, expansion of the intrathoracic space causes the intrapleural pressure to become progressively more negative than atmospheric pressure. This change in intrapleural pressure also causes intra-alveolar pressure to fall. Since pressure at the mouth is atmospheric, a drop in alveolar pressure creates a pressure gradient from mouth to alveolus. If the glottis is open, airflow into the alveolus must occur, resulting in inflation of the lung.

If air is introduced into the alveolar space under pressure, the alveolus will begin to expand. The curve that is constructed in this manner defines the pressure-volume characteristics (or compliance) of the alveolus (Fig. 7-15). The change in volume that occurs for a given change in pressure can be plotted over the entire range of alveolar volume. Careful inspection of the pressure-volume curve demonstrates that the compliance of the alveolus changes over the range of alveolar volume. At low volumes, significant changes in pressure must occur before the alveolus begins to inflate. Similarly, a point is reached during inflation at which changes in pressure again have little effect on increasing volume. Thus the alveolus is not freely distensible. Forces within the alveolar wall initially must resist inflation of the alveolus and eventually limit its maximum volume. Furthermore, when the distending pressure is removed, the alveolus rapidly deflates to its original volume. Thus elastic tissues within the wall are stretched during inflation and provide the force for the alveolus to recoil to its original volume during deflation.

Surface forces generated at the air-tissue interface and tissue forces determine these mechanical properties of the alveolus. The contribution of each of these can be estimated if the alveolus is distended by saline instead of air (Fig. 7-16). When the alveolus is distended by saline, surface forces are eliminated because the air-tissue interface has been eliminated. Thus tissue forces alone determine the pressure-volume characteristics of the saline-filled alveolus. As can be seen by compar-

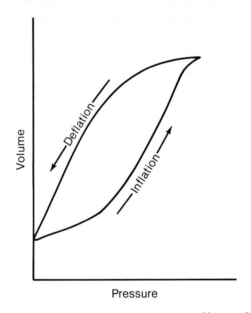

Fig. 7-15. Representative pressure-volume curve of lung inflated with air.

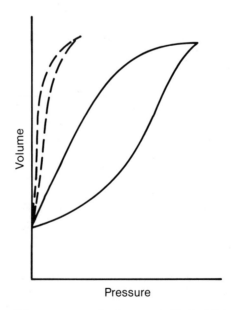

Fig. 7-16. Comparison of the pressure-volume curves of lung inflated with air *(solid line)* or saline *(dashed line)*. The volume of inflation is identical under both circumstances, whereas the pressure required to inflate the lung is markedly decreased when saline is employed.

ing these two curves, 70% to 80% of the pressure needed to inflate the alveolus is required to overcome surface forces. In the absence of adequate surfactant, these surface forces greatly increase, and the pressure required to inflate the alveolus increases substantially. Comparison of the pressure-volume curves of air and saline-filled alveoli also suggest that tissue forces are the major determinant of both the maximum alveolar volume and the recoil pressure of the alveolus, since the maximum and the deflation volumes of the alveolus are similar in both situations. These tissue forces apparently are determined by the connective tissue proteins of the alveolar wall.

The compliance of the lung can simply be considered the sum of the individual compliance of all alveoli. Therefore the forces that determine the compliance of the lung are identical to those described for an individual alveolus. When these relationships are applied to the whole lung, it is important to remember that the intrathoracic lung is usually passively inflated by the bellows-like action of the chest cage. Therefore the ability of the chest cage to generate adequate intrapleural pressure during inspiration is equally important in determining the maximum volume of the lung as it is measured in the clinical laboratory. Thus the maximum volume of the intrathoracic lung is determined by the compliance characteristics of the lung and the ability of the respiratory muscles to generate adequate inspiratory muscle force. Conversely the mechanical properties of the lung influence the pressure the respiratory muscles must generate to change lung volume. For example, as the compliance of the lung decreases, a greater change in pressure is required to inflate the lung to any given volume. Thus in the range of resting tidal volume, more inspiratory muscle force is required to maintain tidal ventilation. The clinical implications of this will be discussed later.

The importance of surfactant in stabilizing alveoli at low alveolar volumes has been discussed. To avoid confusion, it is important to point out that the balance of air remaining in the lung after a maximum expiration is primarily determined by mechanical events that are independent of the action of surfactant. The mechanical properties of the gas-exchanging parenchyma and the small airways influence this volume of residual gas.

Clinical physiologic testing can be placed in proper context if the mechanical properties of the lung, chest cage, and airways are recognized as dynamic determinants of the lung volume measurements routinely performed in clinical laboratories (Fig. 7-17 and definitions on opposite page). With this approach, it is apparent that the total lung capacity is the only volume measurement that directly reflects the compliance of the lung. The residual volume is primarily influenced by airway function. Thus the vital capacity is passively determined by the relationship between the total lung capacity and residual volume (Fig. 7-18). Although traditionally employed as an important index of the mechanical properties of the lung, the vital capacity does not have a direct relationship to the mechanical properties of the lung parenchyma or airways.

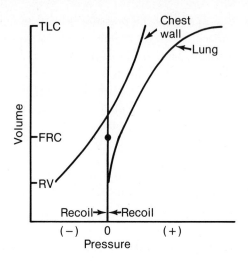

Fig. 7-17. Relationship between the compliances of the lung and chest wall and various lung compartments. To the right of the 0 pressure line the recoil pressures of both the lung and chest wall act to decrease intrathoracic volume and deflate the lung. To the left of the 0 pressure line the recoil pressure of the chest will be outward, tending to increase the intrathoracic volume. The recoil pressures represent changes that occur with muscle relaxation and are overcome by active inspiratory or expiratory muscle activity. Note that the functional residual capacity *(FRC)*, the resting end expiratory volume of the lung, is the volume at which the recoil pressure of the lung inward and the recoil pressure of the chest wall outward are completely balanced in the relaxed state.

DEFINITION OF LUNG VOLUMES

Total lung capacity (TLC): Volume of the lung after a maximum inspiratory effort. At this volume, inspiratory muscle force equals or exceeds the inward recoil pressure of the lung and chest wall combined.

Functional residual capacity (FRC): Volume of the lung at end expiration during quiet, tidal volume breathing. At this volume, the inward recoil pressure of the lung and the outward recoil pressure of the chest are equal.

Residual volume (RV): Volume of the lung after a maximum expiratory effort. This volume is determined either by closure of terminal airways or by maximum compression of the chest wall during a maximum expiratory maneuver.

Vital capacity (VC): Volume of gas that can be voluntarily exhaled from the lung by a maximum expiratory effort begun at total lung capacity. This volume is passively determined by the dynamic determinants of the total lung capacity and residual volume.

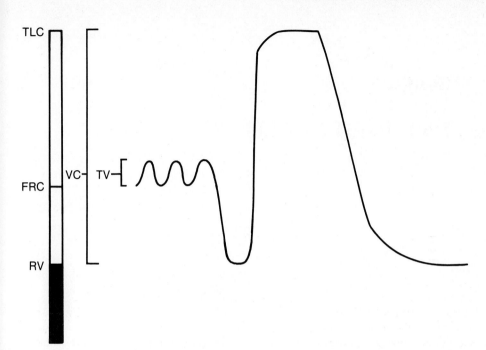

Fig. 7-18. Spirogram depicting tidal volume ventilation and maximum inspiratory and expiratory maneuvers. The spirometric tracing is related to various lung compartments by the bar graph at the left of the figure. This tracing clearly shows that the residual volume, and therefore the total lung capacity, cannot be measured from simple spirometric tracings. In addition, the vital capacity is simply passively determined by the relationship between the total lung capacity and the residual volume as depicted in the bar graph.

Chapter 8

PATHOPHYSIOLOGY

The pathophysiology of lung disease can be best understood when considered in the context of altered lung structure. Therefore a few comments about the general pattern of structural changes that occur in the alveolar wall after injury are appropriate before a discussion of the pathophysiology of diseases involving the gas-exchanging parenchyma of the lung.

Acute alveolar wall injury leads to the development of interstitial and intra-alveolar edema, swelling and sloughing of type I pneumocytes, proliferation of type II pneumocytes, and infiltration of the alveolar wall and alveolar space by inflammatory cells (Figs. 8-1 to 8-3). These changes may not all occur with every form of alveolar wall injury. Furthermore, when the disease is clinically recognized, some of these histologic changes may no longer be apparent.

Damage to type I cells during acute alveolar injury appears to be particularly important in the pathogenesis of some of the other changes just described. Considerable evidence shows that the alveolar epithelial cell is an important component of the barrier to fluid transudation into the alveolar wall. The net forces across the alveolar-capillary wall are such that transudation of fluid into the interstitial space of the alveolar wall occurs continually in the normal lung. However, the fluid is efficiently removed by the action of mechanical forces within the alveolar wall and the pulmonary lymphatic system. Injury to type I pneumocytes leads to increased permeability of the alveolar-capillary membrane. As a result of the increased permeability, increased amounts of fluid containing high molecular weight solutes may enter the alveolar wall and alveolar space. Precipitation of the protein contained in intra-alveolar edema fluid may result in the formation of hyaline membranes on the alveolar wall surface.

As previously mentioned, type I pneumocytes do not appear to have the ability to replicate. Thus, after loss of type I pneumocytes, the alveolar wall epithelial covering can only be replaced by proliferation of type II pneumocytes. Both the loss of the type I cell, which is biochemically and anatomically specialized for gas

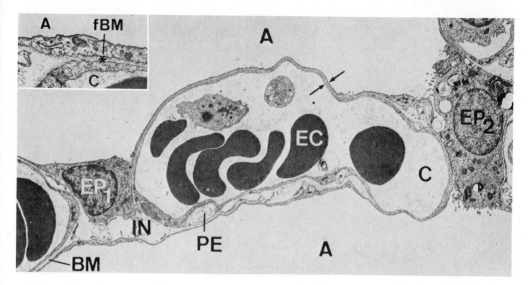

Fig. 8-1. Electron micrograph of a portion of a normal alveolar wall. *A*, Alveolar space; *C*, capillary; *EC*, erythrocyte; *EP₁*, type 1 cell; *EP₂*, type II cell; *IN*, interstitium; *PE*, pericyte; *BM*, basement membrane.

From Bachofen, M., and Weibel, E.R.: Alterations of the gas exchange apparatus in adult respiratory insufficiency associated with septicemia, Am. Rev. Respir. Dis. **116:**589, 1977.

transport, and the formation of hyaline membranes on the alveolar wall surface decrease the rate of diffusion of oxygen across the alveolar wall.

The effect of alveolar wall injury on surfactant production by type II pneumocytes is unknown. Since surfactant is rapidly turned over in the lung, any process that disrupts its production may result in collapse of individual gas-exchanging units.

These acute changes may be variable. Occasionally they may be so severe and widespread that the mechanical properties of the lung become markedly abnormal and gas exchange becomes severely impaired. Acute respiratory failure may result. Because of the special nature of this condition, its clinical and pathophysiologic manifestations will be discussed in Chapter 24.

The pathologic manifestations of acute alveolar wall injury may completely resolve or may evolve into forms of chronic alveolar wall disease. The pathophysiology of two general forms of chronic alveolar wall disease must be considered.

First, type II cell proliferation may persist for long periods of time, and the alveolar wall may be chronically infiltrated by inflammatory cells. In addition, as a result of a marked increase in connective tissue protein synthesis, connective tissue proteins may be deposited in excess in the interstitial space of the alveolar wall.

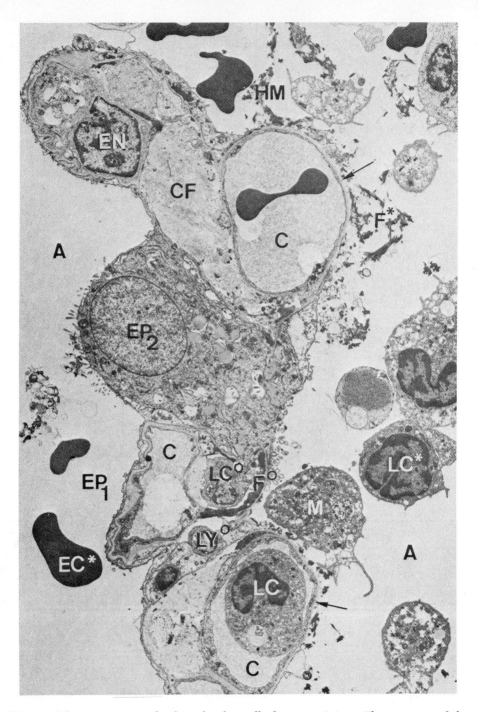

Fig. 8-2. Electron micrograph of an alveolar wall after acute injury. The structure of the alveolar wall is disordered. In addition, inflammatory cells *(IC)*, erythrocytes *(EC)*, and fibrin *(F)* are present in the alveolar space.

From Bachofen, M., and Weibel, E.R.: Alterations of the gas exchange apparatus in adult respiratory insufficiency associated with septicemia, Am. Rev. Respir. Dis. **116:**589, 1977.

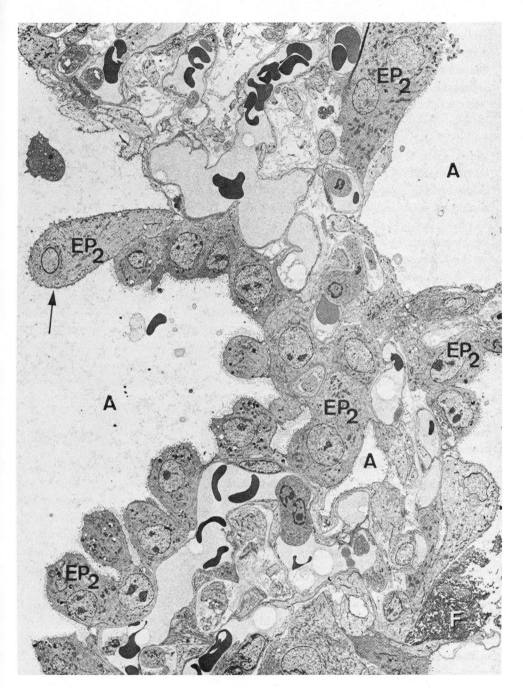

Fig. 8-3. Electron micrograph of an alveolar wall at a later stage during the course of lung injury. The number of type II epithelial cells *(EP₂)* is increased, and they are forming a continuous lining layer on the alveolar surface. The structure of the alveolar-capillary membrane is totally disorganized, and edema fluid is in the alveolar space.

From Bachofen, M., and Weibel, E.R.: Alterations of the gas exchange apparatus in adult respiratory insufficiency associated with septicemia, Am. Rev. Respir. Dis. **116:**589, 1977.

These changes—chronic inflammatory cell infiltration, type II pneumocyte proliferation, and fibrosis of the alveolar wall—combine to produce thickening of the alveolar wall.

Destruction of the alveolar wall may also occur after alveolar wall injury. Acute injury to the alveolar wall may be so severe that the wall is totally destroyed, but this sequence of events is extremely difficult to document. Apparently alveolar wall destruction results from indirect alveolar wall injury occurring over a period of many years caused by the release by both polymorphonuclear leukocytes and alveolar macrophages of lysosomal enzymes, which can degrade the connective tissue proteins of the alveolar wall. With continued release of these proteases, progressive destruction of the connective tissue framework may eventually lead to total loss of the alveolar wall.

From this discussion it should be apparent that alveolar wall injury may result in two major categories of chronic alveolar wall disease, characterized by either thickening or destruction of the alveolar wall. The specific pathologic changes of the diseases in each of these major categories will be described in detail in Chapters 9 through 16. Regardless of the specific pathologic features of individual diseases involving the alveolar wall, these diseases have common pathophysiologic manifestations that can be explained by their production of either thickening or destruction of the alveolar wall.

Thickening of the alveolar wall decreases the compliance of the alveolus. Obviously a greater distending pressure will be required to inflate an alveolus with thickened walls than one with normal walls. The changes in individual alveoli produce a decrease in the compliance of the lung that is reflected by a shift of the pressure-volume curve of the lung downward and to the right.

A decrease in the number of ventilated alveoli produces a similar change in the compliance characteristics of the entire lung. Thus in reality it is not possible to accurately determine whether a low compliance is caused by stiffness of individual ventilated alveoli or simply a decreased number of ventilated alveoli, which have normal compliance.

As a result of a decrease in the compliance of the lung, the total lung capacity (TLC) may decrease. Understanding the relationship between the compliance of the lung and the TLC is important. Theoretically, if identical inspiratory muscle force is generated to inflate a normal and diseased lung, the TLC will be necessarily determined by the compliance of the lung. If compliance is decreased, the volume of the lung must be less than normal. Conversely, if the compliance of the lung is increased, the volume must be greater than normal (Fig. 8-4).

Thickening of the alveolar wall also results in a decrease in the rate of diffusion across the alveolar-capillary membrane. As a result the diffusing capacity of the lung decreases. However, the normal alveolar-capillary membrane provides only a small barrier to the diffusion of oxygen. Since only 20% to 30% of capillary transit

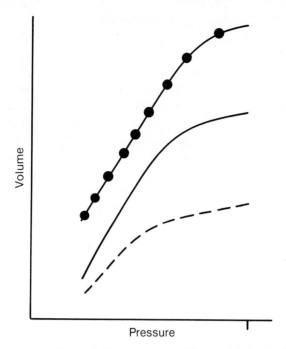

Fig. 8-4. Static, pressure-volume deflation curves of lungs that have normal compliance *(solid line)*, decreased compliance *(dashed line)*, and increased compliance *(dashed and dotted line)*. If the maximum pressure generated with full inspiration is identical in all three instances, the total lung capacities must reflect the compliance characteristics of each lung. The total lung capacity is simply the volume defined by the pressure-volume curve at maximum inspiratory pressure.

time is used in the process of fully oxygenating the blood, it is virtually impossible for thickening of the alveolar-capillary membrane alone to provide a diffusion barrier that prevent full oxygenation of capillary blood. Thus, although the diffusing capacity of the lung is decreased in patients with thickened alveolar walls, this alone does not produce a decrease in the arterial oxygen tension.

In the clinical laboratory the diffusing capacity of the lung is measured with carbon monoxide instead of oxygen. Carbon monoxide is employed because the particular properties of the gas make the measurement of the diffusing capacity far easier. The major problem involved in using oxygen is that the pressure gradient $(P_AO_2\text{-}P_cO_2)$ across the alveolar-capillary membrane cannot be easily or accurately quantitated. Since carbon monoxide is not usually present in blood and only a small amount that is totally taken up by hemoglobin is inhaled in the test period, the P_cCO can be assumed to be zero. Thus the driving pressure (i.e., the gradient across the membrane) is simply the measurable alveolar pressure.

Recent studies have shown that diseases which cause alveolar wall thickening result in mismatching of ventilation and perfusion of the lung. Sophisticated studies of ventilation-perfusion (V/Q) relationships suggest that the major determinant of hypoxemia is the presence of areas of lung that are perfused but not proportionately ventilated (low V/Q areas). This observation suggests that totally or partially collapsed alveoli are present in the lung in these diseases.

Physiologic abnormalities associated with alveolar wall destruction must be considered within the context of the mechanical properties of the entire lung. In areas where alveolar walls are destroyed, the remaining lung consists of large air spaces that are more easily distended than normal alveoli; thus the compliance of the lung is increased. This increase in compliance is reflected by a shift upward and to the left of the pressure-volume curve of the lung and results in an increase in the TLC for the reasons just described.

If the only pathologic abnormality in a lung were the loss of alveolar walls, a decrease in the diffusing capacity would be the only gas-exchange abnormality present. The diffusing capacity would be decreased because the loss of alveolar walls results in a decrease in the total surface area of the alveolar-capillary membrane. As mentioned previously, the alveolar-capillary membrane surface area is the major determinant of the diffusing capacity of the lung. Provided that ventilation and perfusion were matched in the remaining alveoli, significant hypoxemia would not occur.

The abnormalities in the mechanical properties and gas-exchange function of the lung in the diseases that produce diffuse alveolar wall damage can be summarized in the following way: diseases associated with alveolar wall thickening are characterized as having a decreased compliance, decreased TLC, and decreased diffusing capacity. Hypoxemia occurs because areas of lung are perfused but not proportionately ventilated.

Diseases that cause alveolar wall destruction are characterized as having an increased compliance, increased TLC, and decreased diffusing capacity. Arterial blood gas abnormalities also are present if ventilation and perfusion of the lung are mismatched. The arterial blood gas abnormalities are predominantly caused by airway disease.

Chapter 9

EMPHYSEMA

Emphysema is a disease characterized by an increase in the size of the air spaces distal to terminal bronchioles and is partly caused by destruction of the alveolar walls. In a strict sense, emphysema is a pathologic diagnosis. However, certain clinical, physiologic and roentgenographic features of the disease allow a clinical diagnosis to be made with a high degree of accuracy in many cases.

Chronic bronchitis occurs in the majority of patients with emphysema. As a result, for many years little effort has been made to distinguish, for diagnostic purposes, between patients with chronic bronchitis and those with a combination of chronic bronchitis and emphysema. These conditions, along with asthma and bronchiectasis, have simply been grouped in the general diagnostic category of chronic obstructive pulmonary disease, since all of them cause a decrease in expiratory flow rates. Because this term is imprecise and does not focus attention on the patient's specific disease, for diagnostic purposes it should be discouraged. In the appropriate clinical setting, attention should be paid to the clinical, roentgenographic, and physiologic features of the patient's disease so that a diagnosis corresponding to anatomic findings can be made.

PATHOLOGIC CHANGES

Microscopic determination of the severity of emphysema is extraordinarily difficult. Special techniques that are extremely time consuming must be employed for this purpose; thus they are not applicable for routine clinical studies. The severity of emphysema is best recognized by macroscopic inspection of paper-mounted whole lung slices prepared from surgical or autopsy specimens. The severity of the disease can be determined by semiquantitatively grading the extent of lung involvement in these paper-mounted specimens (Figs. 9-1 to 9-3). Clearly, this technique is of no value in the clinical assessment of individual cases. However, these specimens have been used to great advantage in studies of autopsy material and have provided important information about the relationship between various manifestations of the disease and its severity.

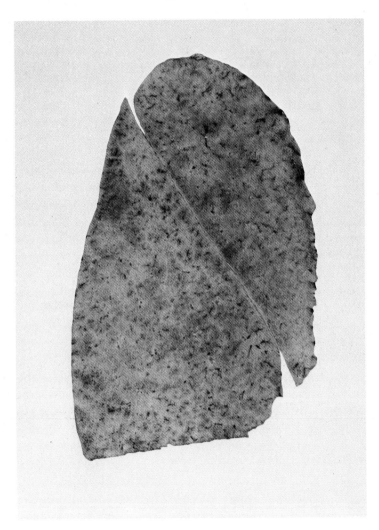

Fig. 9-1. Transverse section of a normal whole lung showing a homogeneous pattern to the cut surface.

From Auerbach, O., et al.: Relation of smoking and age to emphysema: whole lung section study, N. Engl. J. Med. **286:**854, 1972.

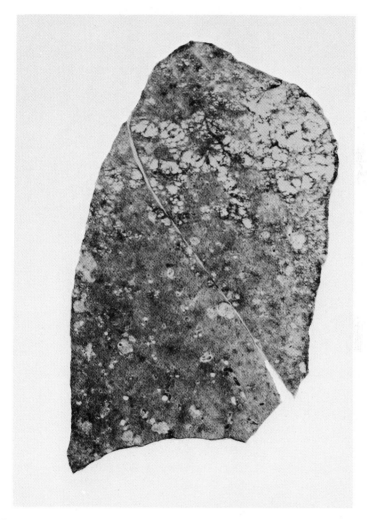

Fig. 9-2. Transverse section of a whole lung showing severe emphysema in the upper lobe and minimum emphysema in the superior portion of the lower lobe.

From Auerbach, O., et al.: Relation of smoking and age to emphysema: whole lung section study, N. Engl. J. Med. **286:**854, 1972.

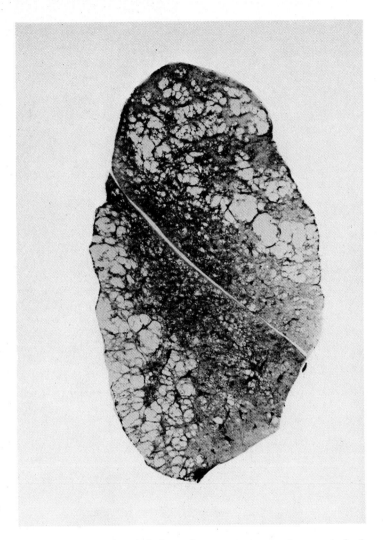

Fig. 9-3. Transverse section of a whole lung showing severe emphysema in both upper and lower lobes.

From Auerbach, O., et al.: Relation of smoking and age to emphysema: whole lung section study, N. Engl. J. Med. **286:**854, 1972.

Microscopically, emphysema is classified by the nature of the involvement of the acinus. The acinus is a cone-shaped–three-dimensional structure that extends from the terminal bronchiole to the periphery of the lung. If air space dilation occurs only in the central region of the acinus, the emphysema is called "centriacinar." If the entire acinus is involved, the term "panacinar" emphysema is employed. Generally these terms correspond respectively with the terms "centrilob-

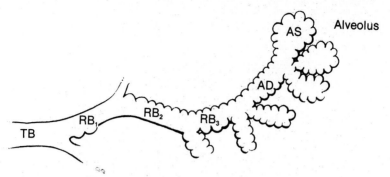

Fig. 9-4. Schematic representation of the component parts of an acinus.

From Thurlbeck, W.M., et al.: Chronic obstructive lung disease, Medicine **49**:81, 1970.

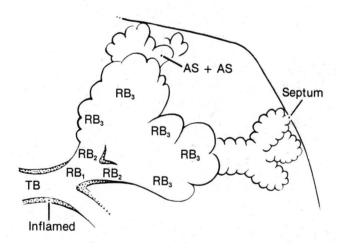

Fig. 9-5. Schematic representation of the changes that occur in centrilobular emphysema.

From Thurlbeck, W.M., et al.: Chronic obstructive lung disease, Medicine **49**:81, 1970.

ular" and "panlobular" emphysema (Figs. 9-4 to 9-9). Lobules are macroscopic structures that are grossly visible on whole lung slices as areas partially outlined by fibrous septa. Thus the lobule is a two-dimensional, macroscopic structure. Panacinar emphysema tends to be distributed diffusely throughout the lung, whereas centriacinar emphysema is usually localized to the lung apices.

Emphysema represents the end stage of a pathologic process in which de-

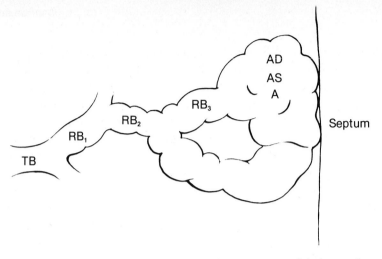

Fig. 9-6. Schematic representation of the changes that occur in panlobular emphysema.

From Thurlbeck, W.M., et al.: Chronic obstructive lung disease, Medicine **49**:81, 1970.

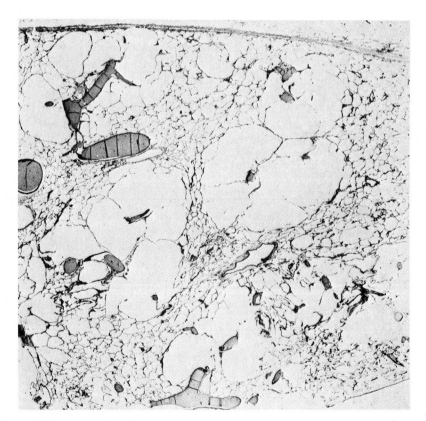

Fig. 9-7. Section of lung showing changes of centrilobular emphysema. The normal alveolar structure surrounds the emphysematous spaces.

From Dunnill, M.S.: The contribution of morphology to the study of chronic obstructive lung disease, Am. J. Med. **57**:506, 1974.

struction of the alveolar wall occurs. The pathologic changes that preceded alveolar wall destruction have not been described. Although inflammation and fibrosis of alveolar walls are occasionally observed in parts of the lung surrounding areas of emphysema, these changes are not related to alveolar wall destruction.

Inflammation of terminal and respiratory bronchioles has frequently been observed in association with centriacinar emphysema. Since most individuals with emphysema also have chronic bronchitis, the significance of these pathologic changes is difficult to determine. However, in some cases, these changes have been observed in lungs with panacinar emphysema and in the absence of other evidence of chronic bronchitis. Nevertheless, at present the bronchiolar pathologic changes cannot be related to the process of alveolar wall destruction that must occur in emphysema.

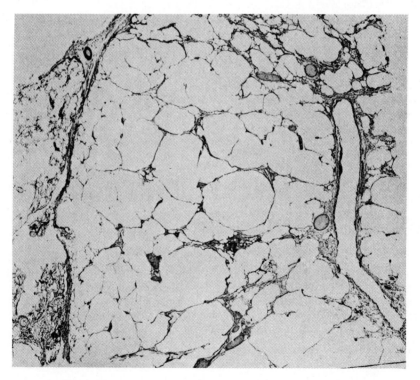

Fig. 9-8. Section of lung showing changes of panlobular emphysema. The architecture of the lung is completely destroyed in this area.

From Dunnill, M.S.: The contribution of morphology to the study of chronic obstructive lung disease, Am. J. Med. **57:**506, 1974.

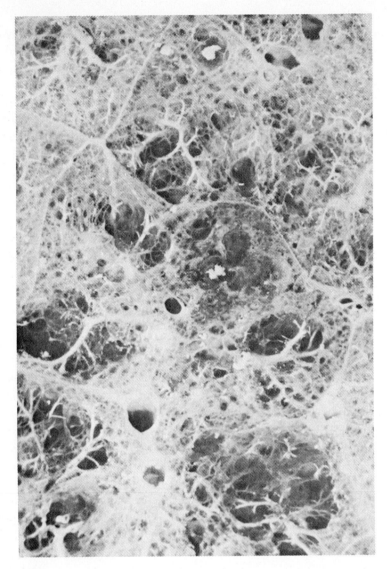

Fig. 9-9. Scanning microscopy of the surface of the lung demonstrating macroscopically the changes of centrilobular emphysema.

From Hugh-Jones, P., and Whimster, W.: The etiology and management of disabling emphysema, Am. Rev. Respir. Dis. **117:**343, 1978.

PATHOGENESIS

The pathogenesis of emphysema is unclear. Multiple factors probably interact to produce this disease. Experimental and epidemiologic studies have suggested at least some of the factors that may be important in this process.

A number of studies have shown that an increased incidence of emphysema occurs in the families of patients documented to have this disease. Although a specific abnormality cannnot be identified in the majority of these individuals, these observations suggest that genetic factors may be involved in the development of the disease.

The possibility that genetically determined abnormalities in the connective tissue proteins in the lung may be important in the development of emphysema must be considered. Nevertheless, no conclusive data support this concept. However, emphysema has been associated with Marfan syndrome and Ehlers-Danlos syndrome, two genetically determined diseases that are characterized by connective tissue abnormalities. In addition, the results of animal studies provide further support for this concept. First, a strain of mice exists that has a genetically determined abnormality in cross-linking of connective tissue proteins. These mice develop physiologic and pathologic abnormalities similar to those observed in human emphysema. Second, if, during the stage of development and maturation of the lung, animals are fed diets containing either penicillamine or beta aminoproprionitrile (BAPN), chemicals that prevent normal connective tissue synthesis, the animals develop changes characteristic of emphysema. As a result of these observations it seems reasonable to speculate that genetically determined abnormalities in the structure or biochemistry of the connective tissue proteins may well be important in the pathogenesis of human emphysema.

A genetically determined deficiency of a serum protease inhibitor has been clearly associated with human emphysema. The major protease inhibitor of human serum is the $alpha_1$-globulin, $alpha_1$-antitrypsin. This protein is an inhibitor of both elastase and collagenase, enzymes with obvious potential to degrade the major connective tissue proteins in the alveolar wall. The concentration of this protease inhibitor in the serum is genetically determined by simple mendelian inheritance, which will be described in more detail later.

As a result of these clinical observations, experimental studies were undertaken to determine the pathogenetic mechanism leading to the development of emphysema in antitrypsin-deficient individuals. These studies have clearly demonstrated that when elastase is instilled into the lungs of experimental animals, the enzyme localizes in the region of the connective tissue protein in the alveolar wall and produces a disease that is pathologically and physiologically similar to human emphysema. This disease can be prevented in these animals by concomitant instillation of normal serum but not by instillation of serum deficient in protease inhibitor. Additional studies have shown that polymorphonuclear leukocytes and alveolar macrophages have the potential to synthesize and release elastase into the extracellular environment. Thus these cells are clearly a potential source for this enzyme in the lung.

Based on these observations, it has been hypothesized that enzymes which may degrade the connective tissue proteins of the alveolar wall are released into the lung from polymorphonuclear leukocytes or alveolar macrophages during inflammatory reactions. Under normal circumstances these enzymes are inhibited, at least in part, by the serum protease inhibitor. In the absence of this protein, enzyme activity proceeds unchecked in the lung and leads to degradation of elastin and other connective tissue proteins. This sequence of events eventually leads to destruction of the alveolar wall.

The relationship between cigarette smoking and emphysema is clear. Epidemiologic studies in several different countries have demonstrated that the frequency and severity of emphysema are greater in smoking individuals. The reason for these differences has not been defined. Although it is possible that constituents of cigarette smoke are in some way directly toxic to the lung, it is more likely that constituents of cigarette smoke stimulate the release of proteolytic enzymes from inflammatory cells. Although smokers' macrophages do not appear to contain higher concentrations of elastolytic enzymes than those obtained from nonsmokers, the number of alveolar macrophages present in the intra-alveolar space of the lung is markedly increased in smokers.

Circumstantial evidence suggests that cigarette smoke influences the interaction of enzyme release and protease inhibitor activity. Clinical studies have shown that individuals with protease inhibitor deficiency who smoke are more likely to develop emphysema than those who do not. Thus the development of emphysema in individuals with normal serum protease inhibitor levels may also be connected to the relationship between the release of enzymes and inhibitor activity in the lung.

ROENTGENOGRAPHIC FEATURES

The roentgenographic manifestations of emphysema are varied. The most common abnormalities are caused by hyperinflation of the lungs or altered distribution of pulmonary blood flow. Four roentgenographic signs of hyperinflation exist. Two of these, increased radiolucency of the lungs and widening of the intercostal spaces, are best appreciated on the posteroanterior view of the chest. These signs actually correlate poorly with the presence of emphysema. An increase in the retrosternal air space and loss of doming of the two hemidiaphragms are the two best roentgenographic signs of hyperinflation. These signs are appreciated best on a lateral view of the chest. On occasion, scalloping of the costophrenic angles may be observed on the posteroanterior view when the diaphragms are depressed to such a degree that the muscular insertions of the diaphragms can be seen. In addition, the cardiac silhouette is usually thin, elongated, and in the midline. These signs are all manifestations of hyperinflation of the lungs and not of emphysema; thus they may be observed during an acute asthmatic episode or acute upper airways obstruction. None of these abnormalities may be present in some patients with marked emphysema (Fig. 9-10).

Two abnormalities of the pulmonary arterial system may be observed on the

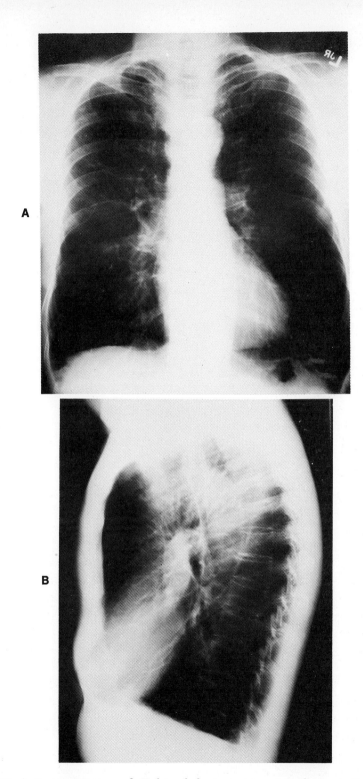

Fig. 9-10. A, Posteroanterior and, **B,** lateral chest roentgenogram demonstrating the roentgenographic abnormalities in emphysema associated with hyperinflation of the lung. Apparent on the lateral view are the marked increase in the retrosternal air space and the flattening of the domes of the diaphragms.

chest roentgenogram of a patient with emphysema. First, if pulmonary hypertension is present, the main pulmonary arteries may be enlarged. Second, branches of the main pulmonary artery may appear as though they are elongated and have lost many of their smaller branches. However, this sign is difficult to interpret accurately and can only be considered useful in the diagnosis of emphysema when clear evidence of hyperinflation is also present.

The anatomy of the smaller pulmonary arteries and the distribution of pulmonary artery blood flow are better evaluated by angiography or perfusion lung scanning. These techniques are far more sensitive than standard chest roentgenograms and may reveal localized regions of emphysema in the lung that are greatly hypoperfused or avascular. However, perfusion defects should not be interpreted as evidence of emphysema, since other diseases, including chronic bronchitis, can cause such defects by physiologically shunting blood away from poorly ventilated regions. Thus perfusion defects are not specific for avascular areas of emphysema. However, in a patient with emphysema the distribution of hypoperfusion within

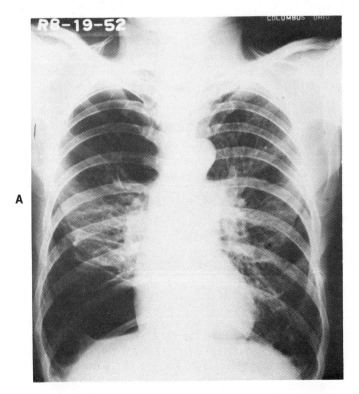

Fig. 9-11. A, Bullous emphysema. Bullous lesions are in both the right upper and right lower lobes.

the lung can suggest the presence of antitrypsin deficiency. In the usual form of emphysema, the disease is most severe in the apex. When associated with antitrypsin deficiency, the disease is usually most severe in the base. In emphysema, perfusion defects detected by scanning techniques usually correspond to the areas of lung that are most severely involved. Thus hypoperfusion of the bases should suggest the presence of antitrypsin deficiency.

Two roentgenographic signs are reasonably specific for emphysema. The presence of bullous lesions on the plain roentgenogram is always highly suggestive of the presence of emphysema. These lesions appear as markedly radiolucent areas demarcated, at least in part, by thin, curvilinear septa (Fig. 9-11). Isolated bullous

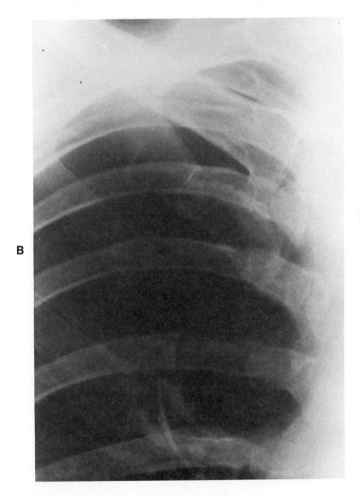

Fig. 9-11, cont'd. B, Close-up of a bullous lesion in the right upper lobe. The thin curvilinear septal lines demarcate the bullous lesion.

lesions may occur in otherwise normal lungs. However, when these lesions are present in patients with symptoms, they are virtually diagnostic of the presence of diffuse emphysema. Second, in the course of pneumonia or pulmonary edema, regions of emphysema may be outlined by the infiltrative process and produce a pattern that has been termed "incomplete consolidation of the lung." Both signs are reasonably specific for the presence of emphysema, since they are based on direct roentgenographic visualization of the pathologic lesions.

PHYSIOLOGIC FEATURES

The physiologic abnormalities associated with emphysema must be clearly distinguished from those caused by chronic bronchitis. As previously mentioned, emphysema and chronic bronchitis often are grouped under the term "chronic obstructive pulmonary disease" because both produce decreased expiratory flow rates. Although emphysema is, in a strict sense, a pathologic diagnosis, the decrease in expiratory flow rates should be documented in the appropriate clinical setting. Physiologic studies are the most accurate way of detecting emphysema, since this disease causes abnormalities in gas exchange and in the mechanical properties of the lung not caused by chronic bronchitis.

The physiologic abnormalities that allow emphysema to be recognized are those which reflect destruction of the alveolar wall. The two major physiologic effects of alveolar wall destruction are an increase in the static compliance (Cst) of the lung and a decrease in the diffusing capacity of the lung. As a result of the increased compliance of the lung, the total lung capacity (TLC) increases. The Cst of the lung is not routinely measured in clinical laboratories. However, the TLC and the diffusing capacity of the lung are easily measured. Studies using autopsy specimens have shown that the results of these physiologic studies tend to correlate with the extent of emphysema present in the lung.

Although emphysema is not a disease of the airways, the disease causes a decrease in expiratory flow rates. Two factors contribute to airflow obstruction in this disease. First, a decrease in the static recoil pressure of the lung results in a decrease in the driving pressure for airflow during expiration. As a result, dynamic compression of airways occurs at higher lung volumes than normal. Second, loss of the elastic properties of the alveolar wall also decreases the tethering effect of the alveolar walls on the airways. As a result, the airway lumen is narrower than normal during expiration. Both of these phenomena contribute to the decreased expiratory flow rates despite the absence of a specific disease of the airways. As a result of these abnormalities in the mechanical properties of the airways, the residual volume of the lung is generally increased. Obviously these abnormalities (decreased flow rates and increased residual values) are not specific for emphysema, and their presence does not aid in distinguishing emphysema from chronic bronchitis.

The combination of alveolar wall destruction and dynamic airways obstruction results in mismatching of ventilation and perfusion in the lung. Resting hypoxemia is almost always present, and the arterial oxygen tension may fall even further after exercise. The abnormalities in gas exchange associated with pure emphysema are not as severe as those observed in patients with chronic bronchitis alone, or patients with a combination of chronic bronchitis and emphysema. Sophisticated studies of ventilation-perfusion (V/Q) relationships in the lung have demonstrated that the major abnormality associated with pure emphysema is an excess of ventilation in areas of little perfusion (high V/Q regions), whereas there is little blood flow to low V/Q regions. In contrast, in chronic bronchitis blood flows excessively to low V/Q regions. Since low V/Q regions contribute most to the development of hypoxemia, these observations explain the differences in the severity of hypoxemia observed in patients with emphysema or chronic bronchitis. Hypercapnia is usually not present until the terminal stage of the disease in patients with emphysema who do not have associated bronchitis.

The following summarizes the physiologic abnormalities produced by emphysema:

Decreased elastic recoil
  Decreased TLC
  Decreased $FEV_1\%$
Decreased diffusing capacity
Ventilation-perfusion mismatching
  Hypoxemia

CLINICAL FEATURES

The clinical features of patients with emphysema are, to a great extent, determined by whether the patient also has chronic bronchitis. Attempts have been made to identify and contrast the clinical characteristics of patients with pure emphysema from those of patients with chronic bronchitis. Although this clinical approach has proved to be of little value, it has served to emphasize the characteristic clinical features that are compatible with clinical diagnosis of emphysema.

The predominant symptom of patients with pure emphysema is dyspnea. Because emphysema evolves slowly, most patients notice progressive dyspnea during exertion over a period of many years, usually beginning in the fifth or sixth decade of life. Eventually dyspnea with only minimum exertion or even at rest develops, severely limiting the patient's ability to perform even the daily activities of living. Cough and sputum production are not a feature of pure emphysema. As the disease progresses, the patient may lose weight. At times weight loss may be so marked that it appears the patient might have a malignant tumor.

An important exception to the slowly progressive course of emphysema is the evolution of the disease in individuals with alpha$_1$-antitrypsin deficiency. The clinical features of this form of emphysema are identical to those observed in other patients, but the disease may be rapidly progressive. Some patients may progress from being asymptomatic to being nearly disabled in a period of several years. In fact, rapid progression of the manifestations of emphysema should suggest the possibility that a patient has antitrypsin deficiency. The absence of a smoking history and the onset of symptoms in the third or fourth decade of life are other features that should suggest the diagnosis of antitrypsin deficiency. Although of no clinical value in an individual case, emphysema associated with antitrypsin deficiency has no sex predilection. As previously mentioned, the majority of patients with the usual form of emphysema are men.

Physical examination reveals hyperresonance to percussion over the lungs and depressed diaphragms. The breath sounds are usually decreased in intensity, and the expiratory phase is prolonged. Rhonchi may be audible. The maximum cardiac impulse is usually displaced medially and can best be palpated in the epigastrium. The heart sounds are also distant. Although gallop sounds may be present, it is usually difficult to appreciate them. Cyanosis is not usually present, even with severe emphysema. Furthermore, manifestations of cor pulmonale, liver enlargement, and peripheral edema are usually absent until the end stage of the disease. Clubbing is extremely unusual in patients with emphysema.

When chronic bronchitis is present, the patient's clinical features are completely different. Although progressive dyspnea is still a prominent complaint, cough and sputum production are also conspicuous. In addition, weight loss is not observed as frequently, and cyanosis and peripheral manifestations of cor pulmonale are common. The disease still progresses slowly over many years. However, in contrast to the course of the disease in patients with pure emphysema, episodes of respiratory decompensation may occur frequently for a number of years preceding death.

DIAGNOSIS

The diagnosis of emphysema can be made with a high degree of accuracy in patients who have progressive dyspnea, roentgenographic evidence of hyperinflation of the lungs, and physiologic studies demonstrating decreased expiratory flow rates, an elevated TLC, and a decreased diffusing capacity. Since the assessment of hyperinflation by standard roentgenographic techniques is somewhat subjective, physiologic studies are essential for accurate diagnosis. The diagnosis cannot be made by routine spirometry alone, since decreased expiratory flow rates are not diagnostic of emphysema. These changes occur with any of the diseases that involve only the airways. Lung volumes must be measured to demonstrate that the TLC is enlarged.

As previously mentioned the majority of patients with emphysema also have chronic bronchitis. Thus the important differential diagnosis is whether the patient has chronic bronchitis alone or a combination of chronic bronchitis and emphysema.

In this situation, careful attention should be paid to the results of physiologic studies to determine if abnormalities caused by alveolar wall destruction are present. The patient who has chronic bronchitis alone should have a normal TLC and a normal diffusing capacity, whereas the presence of emphysema should produce an increase in the TLC and a decrease in the diffusing capacity. In both conditions, expiratory flow rates will be decreased and abnormalities in gas exchange will be present.

Routine laboratory studies are of no value in the diagnosis of emphysema. The serum concentration of the protein alpha$_1$-antitrypsin can be measured. Although the absence of the protein in a patient suspected of having emphysema lends support to the diagnosis, measurement of this protein should not be used as a diagnostic study. However, since the protein is genetically determined, identification of abnormalities in it is important for epidemiologic purposes.

In recent years more than twenty different genotypic expressions of the genetics of this protein have been recognized. For practical purposes only two are of clinical significance. Using standard nomenclature, the normal protein is identified by the letter M, and the most important of the abnormal proteins by the letter Z. Since the protein is determined by simple medelian inheritance with codominant alleles, an individual may be homozygous for either of these proteins (MM or ZZ) or heterozygous (MZ). Normal individuals and the great majority of patients with emphysema have an MM genotype. The ZZ genotype is of particular interest, since it is associated with very low levels of the protein. Individuals with this genotype are likely to develop emphysema. Individuals with the MZ genotype have intermediate serum levels of the protein. Whether such individuals are at increased risk of developing emphysema is controversial.

Although the patient recognized as having emphysema with the ZZ genotype clearly cannot be helped by this information, family members who are ZZ or MZ and who do not yet have emphysema can be identified. These individuals should be counseled not to smoke and to avoid occupations or living situations that result in exposure to high concentrations of pollutants in the air. Although this is not of proven value, some evidence shows that if individuals do not smoke, they may not develop emphysema or may develop a less severe form of the disease.

The presence of antitrypsin deficiency can be suspected in certain clinical situations and has distinguishing features:

No sex predilection

Onset at young age

Rapid progression

Predominant involvement of lung bases

Panacinar involvement

The presence of emphysema in a young individual, a woman, or nonsmoker should alert one to the possibility of antitrypsin deficiency. This does not mean that the disease may not occur in a manner identical to the usual form of emphysema. In addition, the distribution of the disease may suggest the diagnosis. In most cases of emphysema the disease is most marked in the upper lobes. In emphysema associated with antitrypsin deficiency, the disease is often most marked in the lower lobes. This may be recognized by observing bullous changes in the lower lobes on the chest roentgenogram or by demonstrating the presence of areas of marked hypoperfusion in the lower lobes by perfusion scanning. Either of these observations should lead to an evaluation for antitrypsin deficiency.

THERAPY

No specific treatment for emphysema exists. The primary goals of the management of patients with this disease are directed toward the treatment of complications of the disease and establishment of a program to help patients live within the activity limits imposed by the disease.

The therapy of chronic bronchitis is not different in patients with emphysema than in those without emphysema. Antibiotics, bronchodilators, and physical measures of bronchial hygiene should be employed judiciously when indicated. The routine use of these measures in patients with pure emphysema is to be avoided. This form of therapy provides some degree of symptomatic relief in bronchitic patients but does nothing to halt the inexorable, progressive course of emphysema.

Conventional therapy for cor pulmonale should be used when evidence of right heart failure is clinically apparent. An important consideration in such patients is the use of chronic oxygen therapy, which, when administered on a 24-hour basis, seems to improve the patient's psychologic and functional status and may prevent episodes of cardiac decompensation. However, the length of survival may not be significantly affected by this therapy. At present, this form of treatment is prescribed only for patients with marked hypoxemia, most of whom have had an episode of cardiac decompensation. Obviously this therapy must be carefully monitored to maintain the arterial oxygen tension in a safe, acceptable range. Current studies are in progress to determine whether administration of oxygen only at night is of benefit in these patients. This approach to treatment will have obvious advantages if it proves beneficial.

Chapter 10

CHRONIC FIBROSING ALVEOLITIS

Chronic fibrosing alveolitis is a nonspecific disorder of the lung characterized by chronic inflammation and progressive fibrosis of the alveolar wall. Fibrosing alveolitis may occur as a primary, idiopathic lung disease or as part of a systemic connective tissue disorder. In addition, identical pathologic changes may occur in the lung after prolonged inhalation exposure to certain inorganic dusts (asbestos) or during certain forms of drug therapy. This discussion will focus on the idiopathic form of the disease. However, the clinical, roentgenographic, and physiologic manifestations of lung involvement are essentially identical in all forms of the disorder.

Idiopathic fibrosing alveolitis is world-wide in distribution and affects both sexes with nearly equal frequency. Although the disease may have its onset at any age, it is most frequently recognized in patients between 40 and 60 years old. The familial occurrence of the disease has been well documented.

PATHOLOGIC FINDINGS

The pathologic manifestations of fibrosing alveolitis are variable. In fact, because of the widely variable pathologic findings, there is controversy about the classification of the disease. In some patients the predominant finding in biopsy specimens is a marked accumulation of cells in the intra-alveolar space accompanied by inflammatory cell infiltration but little fibrosis in the alveolar wall (Fig. 10-1). Electron microscopic studies have demonstrated that the intra-alveolar cells may be alveolar macrophages or desquamated type II pneumocytes. These pathologic findings are considered by some to be characteristic of a specific entity that has been called desquamative interstitial pneumonitis (DIP). In the majority of patients, biopsy specimens reveal infiltration of the alveolus and alveolar wall by inflammatory cells and variable degrees of alveolar wall fibrosis (Fig. 10-2). These pathologic findings are considered characteristic of usual interstitial pneumonitis (UIP). In some patients the pathologic findings are limited to severe alveolar wall fibrosis without substantial inflammation. This lesion appears to be the end stage in

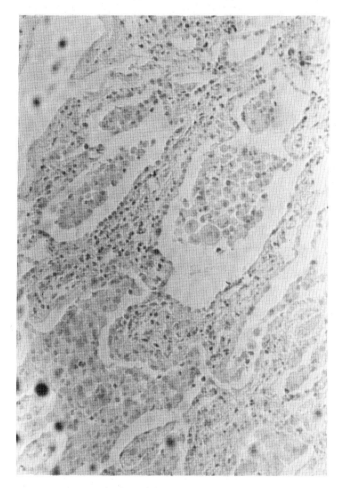

Fig. 10-1. Microscopic section of a lung biopsy specimen demonstrating changes consistent with desquamative interstitial pneumonitis. The cells are accumulated in the interalveolar spaces.

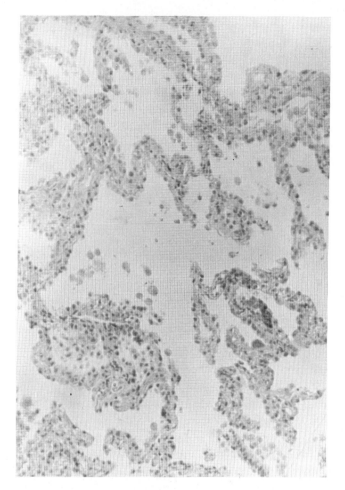

Fig. 10-2. Microscopic section of lung biopsy specimen demonstrating changes consistent with usual interstitial pneumonitis. The inflammatory cells are scattered in the alveolar space and alveolar wall, and the alveolar wall is thickened.

the progression of the disease. In addition to the pathologic changes of the alveolar wall, narrowing of the terminal bronchioles by peribronchiolar inflammation and fibrosis is frequently observed.

As will be discussed later, these different pathologic entities probably have both prognostic and therapeutic significance. These pathologic entities may represent separate diseases, but the prevailing opinion is that they simply represent different stages of the same disease. The observation that different areas of a single biopsy may have findings of both DIP and UIP and that, if untreated, the DIP lesion may progress to the UIP lesion, seem to support this concept. For this reasons the descriptive term "chronic fibrosing alveolitis" seems to be most appropriate for identifying the disease.

PATHOGENESIS

Although the cause of idiopathic fibrosing alveolitis is unknown, immune mechanisms seem to be important in the pathogenesis of the disease. Several lines of evidence support this concept. First, 20% to 30% of patients with fibrosing alveolitis have clinical or laboratory findings that are observed in other diseases which are presumed to be immunologically mediated. Clinical manifestations such as arthralgia and digital ischemia are observed in a small percentage. In addition, abnormalities in specific immunoglobulins, antinuclear antibodies, cryoglobulins, and rheumatoid factor may be present in patients with this disease. Recent studies have also shown that many patients have circulating antigen-antibody complexes. Furthermore, using immunopathologic techniques, antibody has been demonstrated in the alveolar walls of biopsy specimens obtained from patients with this disease. All these observations suggest that humoral immune mechanisms are important in the pathogenesis of the disease. The event that may stimulate inappropriate antibody production is unknown.

CLINICAL MANIFESTATIONS

Dyspnea during exertion is the most common initial complaint of patients with fibrosing alveolitis. This symptom occurs in virtually all patients at some time during the course of the disease. Most patients also complain of a cough, which is characteristically nonproductive.

Although the pathologic features of idiopathic fibrosing alveolitis are limited to the lung, patients may also have systemic symptoms. Approximately 20% of patients have a history of arthralgia. The specific reason for the joint pain has not been defined well but may be related to the presence of circulating immune complexes in these patients. Occasionally a patient will have evidence of digital vascular occlusion manifested by digital pain or skin necrosis over the distal phalanges. As the disease progresses, easy fatigability, anorexia, and weight loss may also develop.

At the time of initial examination, abnormal physical findings are usually localized to the lungs. The majority of patients have fine, end inspiratory rales audible over the bases of the lung posteriorly. Some patients also have clubbing of the digits. As the disease progresses, physical findings compatible with cor pulmonale may also be observed.

ROENTGENOGRAPHIC MANIFESTATIONS

The chest roentgenogram usually reveals diffuse reticulonodular infiltration of the lungs that is most marked at the lung bases (Fig. 10-3). In cases in which DIP is present pathologically, a diffuse, ground glass alveolar filling pattern may be

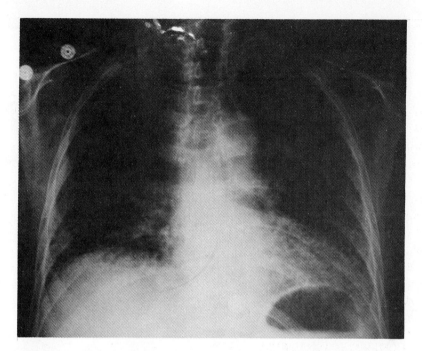

Fig. 10-3. Chronic fibrosing alveolitis. The reticulonodular infiltrates at both bases are predominant.

present in the lung bases. No other consistently observed roentgenographic abnormalities occur in this disease. Between 5% and 10% of patients with fibrosing alveolitis have a normal chest roentgenogram, which is more frequently observed in patients with DIP than in those with UIP.

PHYSIOLOGIC MANIFESTATIONS

The physiologic abnormalities associated with fibrosing alveolitis consist of a decrease in the TLC, Cst, and diffusing capacity of the lung. Patients with moderately advanced disease have resting hypoxemia as a result of ventilation-perfusion abnormalities in the lung. In many patients the arterial oxygen tension decreases during exercise. The arterial carbon dioxide tension is usually decreased. The mechanism for the hyperventilation is unclear. Recent studies have suggested that the degree of fibrosis during pathologic examination of the lung correlates best with the degree of reduction of the Cst of the lung or the magnitude of the alveolar-arterial oxygen gradient during exercise.

DIAGNOSIS

Routine laboratory studies are of little value in making a specific diagnosis. In the majority of patients the sedimentation rate is elevated. About 20% to 30% of

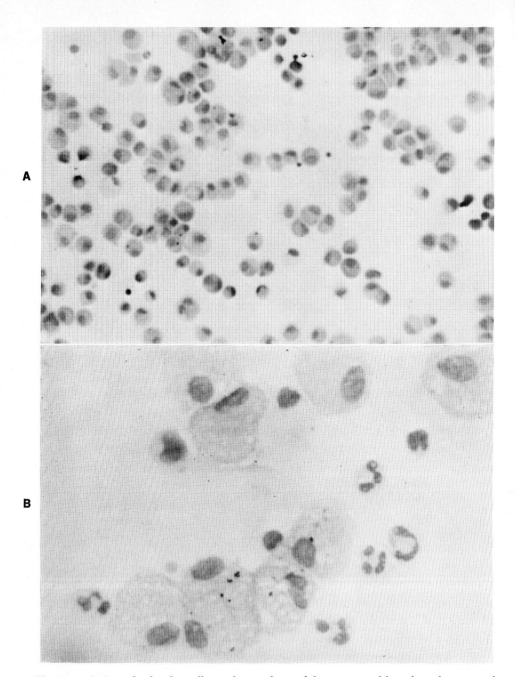

Fig. 10-4. A, Bronchoalveolar cell population obtained from a normal lung by subsegmental lung lavage. Most of the cells are alveolar macrophages. Lymphocytes in small numbers are scattered throughout the cell population. **B,** High-power view of the bronchoalveolar cell population obtained from a patient with fibrosing alveolitis. The number of polymorphonuclear leukocytes, is increased greatly.

patients have nonspecific protein abnormalities in their blood. The C-reactive protein may be elevated, and antinuclear antibodies and rheumatoid factor may be present in the serum. Occasionally a patient may have a circulating cryoglobulin or depression of specific immunoglobulins. These protein abnormalities are nonspecific and do not necessarily indicate a systemic connective tissue disorder.

The diagnosis of idiopathic fibrosing alveolitis is based on the demonstration of compatible pathologic changes in a biopsy specimen obtained from a patient who does not have a systemic connective tissue disorder or who has not been exposed to certain drugs or inorganic dusts. The definitive procedure for obtaining lung tissue for diagnostic purposes is an open lung biopsy. During this procedure, an adequate, representative tissue sample can be obtained for detailed examination.

In recent years, transbronchial biopsy through the fiberoptic bronchoscope has also been advocated for obtaining lung tissue for pathologic examination; however, it has two major drawbacks. First, an extremely small tissue sample is obtained by this procedure. Since a significant sampling error may occur, the biopsy specimen may not be totally representative of the pathologic changes present in the lung. Second, the degree of fibrosis in lung biopsy specimens can only be accurately assessed in biopsies that are fixed in a partially inflated state. If the alveoli are allowed to collapse so that their walls approximate, it becomes difficult, if not impossible, to accurately assess the degree of alveolar wall fibrosis. Obtaining inflated specimens by the transbronchial technique is unusual because of the mechanics of the biopsy procedure. In most biopsy specimens a significant crush artifact further limits the diagnostic value of the procedure. In addition, the size of the specimen precludes to some extent examination of the tissue by special stains or subjecting the tissue to physiochemical analysis.

However, transbronchial biopsy is useful in excluding, with a high degree of certainty, diseases characterized by granulomatous inflammation of the lung. Thus transbronchial biopsy has value if one does not wish to perform an open biopsy but wishes to exclude granulomatous processes.

Recently, differential cell counts of the cells obtained by bronchoalveolar lavage have provided useful diagnostic information in the differential diagnosis of diffuse alveolar wall diseases. In fibrosing alveolitis the bronchoalveolar cell population is characterized by an increased percentage of granulocytes, both neutrophils and eosinophils (Fig. 10-4). These findings clearly differentiate fibrosing alveolitis from the granulomatous disorders that are characterized by an increase in the percentage of lymphocytes.

TREATMENT

Fibrosing alveolitis is a progressive disease if untreated. The duration of the disease cannot be accurately determined in most patients. Many patients apparently have roentgenographic evidence of the disease for a number of years without manifesting symptoms or significant physiologic impairment. For unknown reasons the disease eventually becomes progressive. In some cases it may be rapidly progressive, and patients may actually die within months of their first visit to a physician. This sequence of events probably is what was originally observed by Hammand and Rich and prompted their description of the syndrome of acute, rapidly progressive interstitial fibrosis that bears their name; however, they may have been simply observing the rapidly progressive end stage of a more chronic, progressive disorder. Nevertheless, the 5-year survival rate from the time of diagnosis is approximately 40% for all patients.

However, the prognosis of the disease clearly is related to the pathologic changes in the lung. As a general rule, if inflammatory changes are predominant in the biopsy, the prognosis is more favorable. As fibrosis become predominant, the prognosis decreases. This difference in prognosis is primarily caused by the fact that the disease is more likely to respond to treatment during the inflammatory stage. This has been shown well by studies demonstrating that the majority of patients with the DIP lesion improve or remain stable during treatment, whereas the disease progresses in the majority of patients with the UIP lesion despite therapy. With treatment, the 5-year survival rates of these two groups are approximately 95% and 50% respectively (Fig. 10-5); without treatment both entities progress.

At present, administration of corticosteroids is the accepted form of therapy for fibrosing alveolitis. However, there is great controversy over the dose of corticosteroids and the duration of therapy. A reasonable approach is to administer prednisone, 60 mg/day, for at least 4 to 6 weeks. Most evidence suggests that if the patient's condition is going to respond to corticosteroids, it will show improvement during this time. If the patient has responded, the dose can be tapered to a level

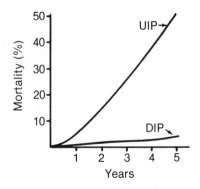

Fig. 10-5. Representative survival curves of patients with the desquamative interstitial pneumonitis or usual interstitial pneumonitis lesion of fibrosing alveolitis. The poor prognosis of patients with the usual interstitial pneumonitis lesion is clearly illustrated.

that maintains the response. If the patient does not respond, the drug should be discontinued or additional drugs should be added to the regimen. No concrete evidence shows that the addition of an immunosuppressive drug will be particularly beneficial, but individual patients have responded to cyclophosphamide or azathioprine. The response to therapy must be monitored by serial physiologic measurements. Symptoms may be misleading, and the chest roentgenogram may not change despite improvement or deterioration in the patient's clinical course.

As the disease progresses, some patients may receive symptomatic relief from continuous oxygen therapy. Although oxygen clearly has no effect on the pathologic lesion, the systemic symptoms of hypoxia and cor pulmonale may be temporarily relieved. Oxygen should be prescribed only after a thorough evaluation of arterial blood gases especially after moderate exercise, since some patients have a substantial drop in arterial oxygen tension afterward.

DIFFERENTIAL DIAGNOSIS

As previously mentioned, chronic fibrosing alveolitis may be associated with several of the connective tissue diseases or may occur after inhalation exposure to certain inorganic dusts or during certain forms of drug therapy. The pneumoconioses and drug-induced lung diseases are discussed in Chapters 13 and 14 respectively, and this discussion will focus on the connective tissue diseases.

Fibrosing alveolitis may occur in rheumatoid arthritis, scleroderma, systemic lupus erythematosus, and dermatomyositis-polymyositis. The clinical, physiologic, and roentgenologic manifestations of fibrosing alveolitis occuring in one of these systemic diseases are indistinguishable from those described for the idiopathic form of the disease. In addition to fibrosing alveolitis, other intrathoracic abnormalities may occur in these connective tissue diseases. Since recognition of these abnormalities in conjunction with fibrosing alveolitis may be useful in differentiating the idiopathic form of the disease from that associated with one of these connective tissue disorders, they will be discussed in this section.

Rheumatoid arthritis

The five intrathoracic manifestations of rheumatoid arthritis are fibrosing alveolitis, rheumatoid nodules, Caplan syndrome, pleuritis (with or without effusion), and pulmonary vasculitis. Although rheumatoid arthritis is predominantly a disease of women, the intrathoracic manifestations occur more often in men. In general the titer of rheumatoid factor in the blood tends to be higher in patients with intrathoracic disease. The major features of Caplan syndrome will be described in Chapter 13.

The most common intrathoracic manifestation of rheumatoid arthritis is pleural involvement. The pleural disease may precede or follow the onset of joint involvement. A higher incidence of pleural involvement appears to occur in pa-

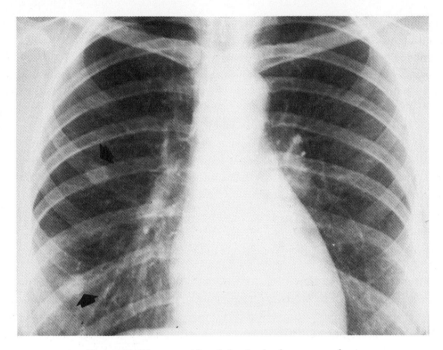

Fig. 10-6. Rheumatoid nodules in the lung parenchyma.

tients with subcutaneous nodules. Pleural effusions are usually unilateral and may be large. The fluid has the characteristics of an exudate with a predominance of lymphocytes. A low glucose concentration is the most characteristic finding of rheumatoid effusions. Although not entirely specific for rheumatoid disease, it is highly suggestive of the diagnosis. In addition, rheumatoid factor and low complement levels may occur in rheumatoid effusions but are not specific for the diagnosis. a pleural biopsy usually reveals nonspecific chronic inflammation, but occasionally rheumatoid nodules are observed. Empyema has been recognized as a complication of a rheumatoid effusion, but its pathogenesis is unclear. Progressive pleural fibrosis without effusion may also occur. Occasionally, a progressive fibrothorax may cause a severe restrictive ventilatory defect necessitating decortication.

Necrobiotic nodules may develop in the lungs or on the pleura (Fig. 10-6) and are pathologically identical to the subcutaneous nodules that occur in rheumatoid arthritis. On the chest roentgenogram the pulmonary parenchymal nodules appear as multiple, well-defined lesions varying from several millimeters to several centimeters in diameter and are usually located in the periphery of the lung. Cavitation of the nodules is common. Although the cavitary lesions are usually thick walled, they may gradually become thin walled and eventually disappear. The nodules may vary in size with variation in joint symptoms. A pleural effusion or a spontaneous pneumothorax may occur if the nodules involve the pleura. No symptoms are associated with the presence of parenchymal nodules.

Inflammation of the pulmonary arteries may occur in patients with rheumatoid arthritis. On occasion the vasculitis may lead to pulmonary hypertension. Rheumatoid pulmonary vasculitis sometimes is associated with eosinophilia and low serum complement levels.

Scleroderma

Parenchymal, pleural, and pulmonary vascular involvement may also occur in scleroderma. In fact, the lung is the second most frequently involved visceral organ in this disease. Only esophageal involvement occurs more often. Although only a fourth of patients have abnormalities on their chest roentgenogram, the results of pulmonary function tests suggest that intrathoracic disease occurs far more frequently. At autopsy more than three fourths of the patients have either lung or pleural involvement or both.

Fibrosing alveolitis is the most common intrathoracic disorder in patients with scleroderma. Patients with this disease who have esophageal involvement may have recurrent bouts of aspiration pneumonia. This possibility should be considered in patients with chronic basilar infiltrates before ascribing the changes to fibrosing alveolitis.

Pleural fibrosis with or without effusion may occur in scleroderma. However, pleural disease is far less prominent in this disease than in rheumatoid arthritis or lupus erythematosus.

Pulmonary vascular involvement also occurs in scleroderma. Intimal and medial proliferation leading to marked lumen narrowing are the characteristic pathologic changes in involved vessels. These vascular changes bear no relationship to the presence of parenchymal fibrosis. In fact, in some patients with vascular involvement, cor pulmonale resulting in death may occur despite little or no parenchymal disease. A decrease in the diffusing capacity with little or no change in lung volumes may suggest the presence of extensive pulmonary vascular involvement.

Systemic lupus erythematosus

The intrathoracic manifestations of systemic lupus erythematosus (SLE) are varied. Pleuritis is an extremely common manifestation of this disease, and pleural effusions are often observed on the chest roentgenogram. In fact, pleural symptoms may be the initial manifestation of the disease. The effusions are usually small and frequently bilateral. The fluid has the characteristics of an exudate and may contain lupus erythematosus cells.

The parenchymal manifestations of SLE are extremely variable. Although not often apparent roentgenographically, pulmonary parenchymal involvement probably occurs in the majority of patients with SLE. Autopsy studies have shown pathologic changes of alveolitis and alveolar wall fibrosis in almost all patients dying with

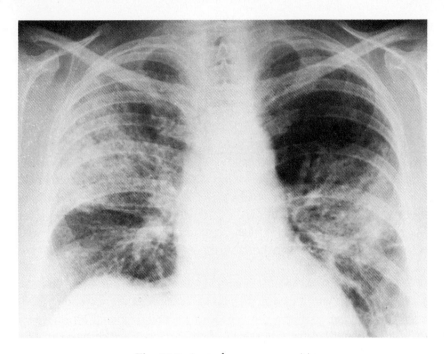

Fig. 10-7. Acute lupus pneumonitis.

the disease. In some patients, decreasing lung size with or without plate-like basilar atelectasis is the only abnormality on the chest roentgenogram. Pulmonary function tests often reveal a decrease in TLC and diffusing capacity despite the normal chest roentgenogram. A small percentage of patients have chronic interstitial infiltrates on the chest roentgenogram. The clinical, physiologic, and roentgenographic manifestations of this entity are indistinguishable from those observed in idiopathic fibrosing alveolitis. No diagnostic pathologic features of either the pleural or parenchymal involvement occur in SLE.

Two forms of acute parenchymal disease are associated with SLE. Diffuse pulmonary hemorrhage has been observed clinically as gross hemoptysis and roentgenographically as diffuse alveolar infiltrates in several patients. This may be confused with pulmonary hemosiderosis, or if renal disease is present, with Goodpasture syndrome. The diagnosis is obvious if other clinical features of SLE are apparent. In the absence of such findings, a correct diagnosis may not be suspected. Examination of lung biopsy specimens by electron microscopy has demonstrated electron-dense deposits consistent with the presence of immune complexes in the subepithelial region of the alveolar capillary implicating immune complex deposition in the pathogenesis of this particular disorder.

Acute lupus pneumonitis is an additional form of acute pulmonary disease observed in SLE (Fig. 10-7). This entity is characterized by the abrupt develop-

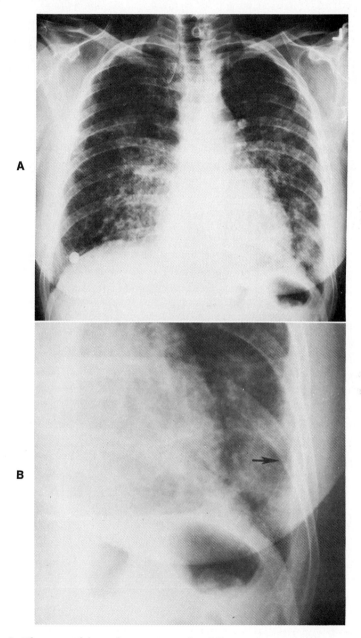

Fig. 10-8. A, Rheumatoid lung disease. Note the diffuse interstitial infiltrates and bilateral pleural thickening. **B,** Close-up illustrating the degree of pleural thickening.

ment of shortness of breath, fever, and a bilateral alveolar filling process on the chest roentgenogram. Cardiomegaly is frequently present. This process often responds rapidly to corticosteroids or immunosuppressive drugs. The chest roentgenogram may clear completely, or chronic interstitial infiltrates may persist. Obviously, acute infectious pneumonitis must be excluded by appropriate blood and sputum cultures in this clinical setting.

Polymyositis-dermatomyositis

Fibrosing alveolitis also occurs in patients with polymyositis-dermatomyositis. The lung involvement may precede skin and muscle disease by many months. The manifestations of the lung disease are identical to those of idiopathic fibrosing alveolitis.

• • •

It should be apparent from this discussion that there are two major intrathoracic processes that, if present in conjunction with fibrosing alveolitis, should suggest a systemic connective tissue disease even if other manifestations of the disease are absent. Pleural involvement and pulmonary hypertension out of proportion to the degree of parenchymal involvement are two findings that should lead to further investigation of the possibility of a systemic disease (Fig. 10-8). About 20% to 30% of patients with idiopathic fibrosing alveolitis have serum protein abnormalities similar to those observed in patients with a connective tissue disease. Thus these studies alone may not be useful for differentiating these conditions.

Chapter 11

SARCOIDOSIS

Sarcoidosis is a systemic disease of undetermined origin that is characterized pathologically by the occurrence of noncaseating granulomas in affected organs (Fig. 11-1). The disease has worldwide distribution. In the United States sarcoidosis appears to be much more common in blacks than whites and slightly more common in women than men. The majority of patients are between 20 and 40 years of age when the diagnosis is first made. However, 30% of the patients are older than 40 years of age at the time of diagnosis, and the disease may first appear in the sixth and seventh decades of life.

The lung is the organ most often involved by disease. However, extrathoracic organs are also frequently involved. Thus patients may initially have clinical manifestations of either pulmonary or extrathoracic organ involvement. In addition, constitutional symptoms of fever, weight loss, and malaise may be present. Almost a third of the patients with sarcoidosis are asymptomatic at the time of diagnosis. In these patients the disease is detected on routine chest roentgenograms. Approximately 20% of the patients initially seek a physician because of respiratory symptoms, and almost 50% have symptoms of extrathoracic involvement. In the majority of patients, pulmonary involvement is ultimately responsible for the predominant manifestations of the disease. However, on occasion involvement of extrathoracic organs may be far more serious than lung involvement.

INTRATHORACIC INVOLVEMENT

The lung is involved in virtually all patients with sarcoidosis. Characteristically the disease produces discrete or coalescent, noncaseating granulomas that are distributed diffusely throughout the gas-exchanging parenchyma of the lung. In a substantial percentage of patients, granulomas are also present in the submucosa of the bronchial wall. In the majority of patients, exertional dyspnea is the only symptom of lung involvement. The severity of the dyspnea is determined by the effect the disease has on the mechanical properties of the parenchyma or airways.

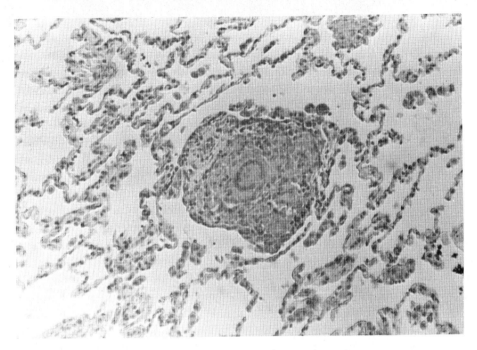

Fig. 11-1. Noncaseating granuloma in lung tissue.

Roentgenographic manifestations

The most common roentgenographic manifestation of pulmonary sarcoidosis is a diffuse interstitial pattern that may be variable. Nodular or linear infiltration may predominate (Fig. 11-2, *A* and *B*). In approximately 20% of patients, large nodular shadows may be seen on the roentgenogram (Fig. 11-2, *C*). These nodular shadows usually appear as ill-defined, coalescent areas of alveolar filling distributed diffusely throughout the lung. However, on occasion the nodules may be discrete. In the majority of patients with these lesions, a diffuse interstitial infiltrate is present in the remaining lung fields. In cases in which the pulmonary involvement progresses to extensive fibrosis, large cystic spaces may develop in the upper lung fields. Sometimes airway involvement may cause partial obstruction of a bronchus leading to roentgenographic evidence of localized atelectasis. The manifestations of parenchymal involvement are entirely nonspecific and therefore have little value in the differential diagnosis of the disease.

Hilar and paratracheal lymph nodes are involved in virtually all patients with sarcoidosis. As a result these nodes frequently enlarge and are visible on the chest roentgenogram. Bilateral hilar adenopathy is the distinguishing feature of sarcoi-

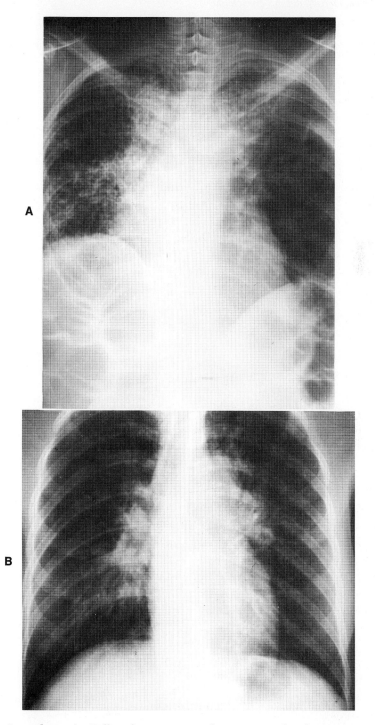

Fig. 11-2. Sarcoidosis. **A,** Diffuse linear interstitial pattern on the chest roentgenogram. Honeycombing is present in the right lung. **B,** Small, ill-defined nodules throughout both lungs. *Continued*.

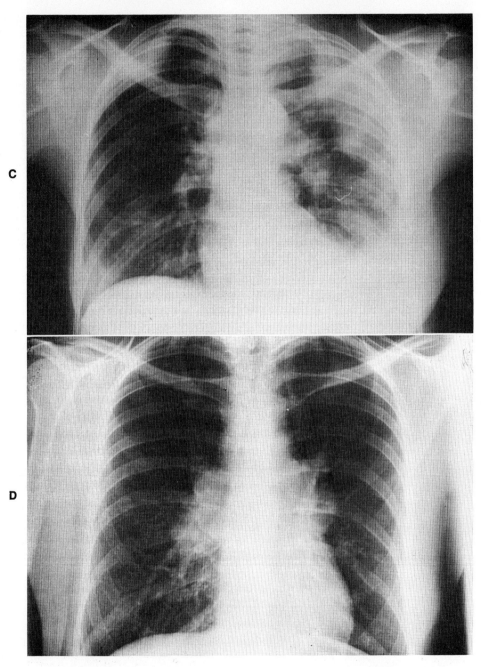

Fig. 11-2, cont'd. C, Large alveolar-filling nodules in both lungs. **D,** Bilateral hilar adeno-pathy. No parenchymal changes have occurred.

dosis (Fig. 11-2, *D*). If present, hilar adenopathy is highly suggestive of the diagnosis in all cases and is virtually diagnostic in appropriate clinical settings. However, the absence of node enlargement does not mean that the nodes are not involved. Also, lymph nodes in the anterior mediastinal chain rarely enlarge in sarcoidosis, a fact that is important in the differential diagnosis of intrathoracic adenopathy.

The pleura is involved in a small percentage of patients. Pleural involvement is rarely associated with symptoms but may produce roentgenographic abnormalities such as pleural thickening or effusion. The pleura is involved pathologically in a much higher percentage of patients than in those who have roentgenographic evidence of pleural disease. The pleural effusions that occur in sarcoidosis are exudative and characterized by a predominance of lymphocytes. A pleural biopsy may reveal noncaseating granulomas.

A classification of the roentgenographic manifestations of intrathoracic sarcoidosis has proved useful for prognostic purposes. However, no direct correlation exists between these roentgenographic manifestations of intrathoracic disease and the extent or severity of extrathoracic disease. Generally patients with evidence of less extensive intrathoracic involvement will also have less severe extrathoracic involvement. However, systemic involvement is probably present in all patients with this disease, and on occasion serious involvement of extrathoracic organs may occur with limited or even unapparent intrathoracic disease.

Despite these exceptions, general conclusions about the course of the lung involvement can be drawn by classifying patients into the following categories:

Stage 0	No roentgenographic abnormalities
Stage I	Bilateral hilar adenopathy alone
Stage II	Bilateral hilar adenopathy accompanied by parenchymal infiltrates
Stage III	Parenchymal infiltrates without hilar adenopathy

Approximately two thirds of the patients with stage I involvement will have complete resolution of their roentgenographic abnormalities. About 50% of patients with stage II involvement and 20% of patients with stage III involvement will have clearing of the abnormalities on the chest roentgenogram. Although not studied well, the abnormalities in pulmonary physiology associated with intrathoracic sarcoidosis generally appear to parallel the roentgenographic stage of the disease. In the majority of patients whose chest roentgenographic abnormalities do not resolve, physiologic abnormalities remain stable. However, some patients have progressive physiologic impairment without any apparent change in the roentgenographic manifestations of their disease. Thus serial physiologic studies are important in monitoring the course of the pulmonary involvement.

There is also a tendency to assign chronology to the disease based on the roentgenographic abnormalities outlined in the classification. In general, patients with evidence of hilar node enlargement are considered to have disease of recent onset, whereas patients without hilar adenopathy are considered to have chronic disease, which is true, since hilar adenopathy usually resolves spontaneously within a 2-year period. However, this can be entirely misleading in individual patients. In some patients hilar adenopathy persists for many years, and disease of recent onset may never exhibit hilar enlargement. Thus caution should be exercised in assigning chronology to the disease simply on the basis of the abnormalities on the chest roentgenogram.

Physiologic abnormalities

In the majority of cases, sarcoidosis involves predominantly the gas-exchanging parenchyma and produces characteristic abnormalities in lung mechanics and gas exchange. Most patients have a decrease in the total lung capacity, static compliance, and carbon monoxide diffusing capacity. Arterial hypoxemia is also invariably present. As discussed previously, the physiologic abnormalities tend to correlate with the roentgenographic classification of the disease. However, the various roentgenographic and physiologic abnormalities are not directly correlated. Occasionally a patient with no obvious parenchymal infiltration on the roentgenogram may have significant physiologic abnormalities. Conversely some patients with extensive roentgenographic abnormalities have minimum physiologic impairment. Furthermore, physiologic abnormalities may progress without changes in the roentgenographic manifestations of the disease. Thus clinical pulmonary function tests should be obtained at the time of original diagnosis to determine the degree of lung involvement and on a serial basis to monitor the course of the disease.

In addition to abnormalities caused by alveolar wall involvement, many patients with sarcoidosis will also have evidence of a mild to moderate decrease in expiratory airflow. The decreased flow is probably caused by direct involvement of the bronchial mucosa or by peribronchiolar infiltration. As a result, clinical pulmonary function tests reveal evidence of a combined restrictive and obstructive ventilatory pattern in some patients.

EXTRATHORACIC INVOLVEMENT

The following approximates the frequency of involvement of various extrathoracic organs:

Site	Approximate incidence (%)
Liver (biopsy)	90
Eye	22
Skin	18
Spleen (palpable)	10
Central nervous system	5
Bone	4

Clinical manifestations of involvement of one or more of these organs may occur either in association with pulmonary symptoms or as the sole manifestation of the disease. Almost 50% of patients with sarcoidosis actually see a physician because of symptoms related to involvement of an extrathoracic organ.

Ocular involvement occurs in approximately 20% of patients. Manifestations of ocular involvement are varied and include iridocyclitis, chorioretinitis, kerato-conjunctivitis, papilledema, cataract formation, and glaucoma. Patients may complain of blurred vision or burning or pain in the eye. However, at times ocular involvement may not be clinically apparent. A slit-lamp examination by an ophthalmologist may be required to detect eye involvement. Recognition and appropriate treatment of ocular involvement is extremely important, since progressive destruction of the eye may cause blindness.

Skin involvement also occurs in approximately 20% of the patients. A variety of skin lesions have been described, but in most cases the lesions are of little clinical significance. However, sometimes the lesions are cosmetically unattractive and may be disfiguring. It is important to recognize the infiltrative skin lesions caused by sarcoidosis, since they are a readily accessible site for biopsy to confirm the diagnosis of the disease. *Erythema nodosum* occurs in 10% to 15% of patients. This skin lesion is usually a manifestation of disease of recent onset and frequently occurs in association with bilateral hilar adenopathy, retinitis, and diffuse joint pain.

Splenomegaly occurs in approximately 10% of patients. In some, abdominal pain caused by enlargement of the spleen is the initial manifestation of disease. Splenomegaly is also associated with hematologic abnormalities such as *anemia, leukopenia, thrombocytopenia,* or any combination. The majority of patients with splenomegaly also have significant liver involvement manifestated by *hepatomegaly* and abnormalities of liver function tests. An occasional patient may have massive hepatosplenomegaly mimicking a lymphoproliferative disorder. Noncaseating granulomas can be found in the spleen and liver in the majority of patients with sarcoidosis, although enlargement of these organs or other manifestations of involvement are not present. In fact, clinical evidence of liver involvement is uncommon. However, cholestatic changes with marked hyperbilirubinemia and an increase in the alkaline phosphatase have been reported in some patients.

Arthritis is an uncommon manifestation of sarcoidosis but when present is often an early complaint. Large, weight-bearing joints are most frequently involved. Although unilateral involvement is common, diffuse arthralgia or arthritis may occur, particularly in patients with erythema nodosum.

Central nervous system involvement occurs in approximately 5% of patients. Most of the central nervous system manifestations are caused by a basal granulomatous meningitis, which infiltrates or compresses adjacent structures. Cranial nerve involvement is the most common central nervous system abnormality. The seventh and second cranial nerves are most often involved. The most common intracranial sites of involvement are the hypothalamus and pituitary gland. Involvement of these structures may cause a variety of endocrine abnormalities including anterior pituitary insufficiency and diabetes insipidus.

LABORATORY STUDIES

Routine laboratory studies are of little value in the diagnosis of sarcoidosis. A number of nonspecific abnormalities occur, and the most important of these will be mentioned.

Hypercalcemia occurs in approximately 15% of patients at some time during the course of the disease. Hypercalciuria is much more common. These calcium metabolism abnormalities appear to be related to excessive calcium absorption by the gastrointestinal tract caused by vitamin D sensitivity. Even in patients who are normocalcemic, parathormone levels are decreased. This observation is consistent with the concept that calcium metabolism is abnormal in most patients.

Recently, an increase in the serum level of angiotensin-converting enzyme has been demonstrated in the majority of patients with sarcoidosis. The reason for this abnormality is unclear. As the assay for the enzyme becomes more readily available, it may prove to be a useful diagnostic tool in selected patients.

Following are a number of immunologic abnormalities that have been recognized in patients with sarcoidosis:

> In vivo
> Anergy
> Lymphopenia
> Decreased circulating T cells
> Hypergammaglobulinemia
> Circulating immune complexes
> In vitro
> Impaired antigen- and mitogen-stimulated lymphocyte blastogenesis and lymphokine production
> Increased suppressor cell activity
> Impaired monocyte and leukocyte chemotaxis

These abnormalities are of interest but have little value in the diagnosis of the disease. A significant percentage of patients have elevated immunoglobulin levels. The specific elevated immunoglobulins appear to vary racially. In conjunction with the increased immunoglobulin levels, there is an increase in the concentration of specifc antibodies against a variety of agents including Epstein-Barr, herpes simplex, rubella, measles, and parainfluenza viruses. These observations appear to have no clinical significance.

Cell-mediated immune responses are depressed in some patients with sarcoidosis. The first evidence of abnormal cellular immunity was the observation that some patients failed to develop skin test reactivity to common recall antigens. However, in recent years, the incidence of anergy is not as widespread among patients with sarcoidosis as formerly believed. In addition, other abnormalities in cell-mediated immunity are only moderately impaired. These abnormalities include a decrease in the absolute number of circulating T cells and a blunted blastogenic response by lymphocytes stimulated with either mitogens or antigens in in vitro cultures. These observations also have little clinical significance.

The Kveim test will be mentioned only briefly, since its diagnostic value is controversial. The Kveim test is performed by injecting a crude extract prepared from the involved spleen of a patient with sarcoidosis into the subcutaneous tissue. From 4 to 6 weeks later the injection site is biopsied and examined histologically. The development of a granuloma at the injection site is considered a positive test. The cellular events involved in this reaction have never been defined. A positive Kveim test is considered by many to be virtually diagnostic of sarcoidosis. However, there is not agreement as to the specificity or sensitivity of the test. Furthermore, with the availability of refined, simple techniques for obtaining tissue for confirmation of the diagnosis of sarcoidosis, such a diagnostic test is not merited. Since the "Kveim antigen" is not commercially available, this test is not in wide use.

DIAGNOSIS

The differential diagnosis of sarcoidosis must be considered within the context of the specific presentation of the disease. For instance, the differential diagnosis of a patient with bilateral hilar adenopathy is entirely different from that of a patient with massive hepatosplenomegaly. A discussion of the differential diagnosis of the varied conditions of this disease is beyond the scope of this chapter. Only cases in which the chest roentgenogram is abnormal will be considered.

Sarcoidosis must always be considered in patients who have bilateral hilar adenopathy with or without parenchymal lung disease. Generally, if the patient is asymptomatic and does not have obvious physical findings compatible with another disease, the diagnosis of sarcoidosis is virtually assured. In this clinical setting, a working clinical diagnosis of sarcoidosis can be made confidently without obtaining tissue for pathologic confirmation of the presence of the disease. However, if atypical clinical features are present, appropriate diagnostic studies must be performed to exclude other diseases, and tissue should be obtained for confirmation of the diagnosis of sarcoidosis. A malignant disorder is the most important type of disease to consider in the differential diagnosis in this clinical setting. Solid tumors rarely exhibit bilateral hilar adenopathy, but lymphoproliferative disorders occasionally do. In addition, tuberculosis, fungal disease, and berylliosis may exhibit bilateral hilar adenopathy.

Approximately 14% of patients with sarcoidosis have parenchymal infiltration without adenopathy during initial examination. The differential diagnosis of diffuse pulmonary infiltration without hilar enlargement is inclusive. Virtually any disease that causes diffuse interstitial infiltrates on a chronic basis must be considered. An appropriate clinical and pathologic evaluation is required to make a specific diagnosis.

In a strict sense the diagnosis of sarcoidosis is based on the presence of non-caseating granulomas in a patient with compatible clinical conditions in whom other causes of a systemic granulomatous inflammatory disease have been excluded by appropriate diagnostic tests. A number of biopsy techniques can be used to obtain tissue for diagnostic purposes. Obviously, easily accessible lesions such as skin lesions or enlarged peripheral lymph nodes should be preferentially biopsied. In the majority of patients such lesions are not present, and a more invasive technique must be employed.

In past years, *liver biopsy* was the most widely used technique for diagnosis because it had a reasonably high yield (60% to 70%) and a low morbidity. However, one of the drawbacks of liver biopsy is that nonspecific granulomatous hepatitis is not an uncommon finding in patients with a variety of other diseases. Thus the specificity of liver granulomas for the diagnosis of sarcoidosis is not as great as the presence of granulomas in other organs.

Within the last decade, biopsy of paratracheal lymph nodes at the time of *mediastinoscopy* has been shown to be diagnostic in virtually all patients with sarcoidosis. Although general anesthesia is required for this procedure, the technique has replaced liver biopsy in most institutions, since the morbidity is acceptably low and the specificity of paratracheal granulomas high.

Most recently, *transbronchial lung biopsy* through the flexible fiberoptic bronchoscope has been of great value in the diagnosis of sarcoidosis. This procedure is easily performed under a variety of clinical situations, since it does not require general anesthesia. In addition, an extremely low complication rate is associated with this procedure. Furthermore, both parenchymal and *bronchial mucosa biopsies* can be performed at the time of bronchoscopy, thus increasing the diagnostic yield. Since the presence of granulomas in these tissues has additional specificity for the diagnosis of sarcoidosis, transbronchial biopsy has become the initial biopsy technique of choice in many institutions. The diagnostic yield of transbronchial biopsy correlates with the roentgenographic manifestations of the disease:

Classification	Positive (%)
Stage I	65
Stage II	80
Stage III	87
All stages	77

Approximately two thirds of the patients with bilateral hilar adenopathy alone (stage I) have a positive transbronchial biopsy, whereas more than 80% of patients with parenchymal infiltrates (stages II and III) have a positive biopsy.

Obviously, *open lung biopsy* yields tissue containing noncaseating granulomas in virtually all patients. However, this procedure is far more invasive and has a higher morbidity than the other procedures. Nonetheless, in an occasional patient, open lung biopsy is required for specific diagnosis.

Analysis of the cells obtained from the lung by subsegmental *bronchoalveolar lavage* is an additional valuable diagnostic technique that is also performed with the fiberoptic bronchoscope. In normal individuals, less than 10% of the cells in the lavage effluent are lymphocytes. More than 90% of the cells are alveolar macro-

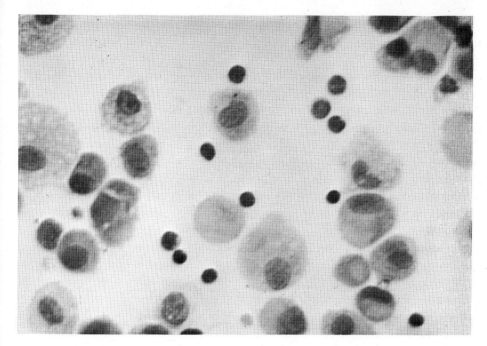

Fig. 11-3. Bronchoalveolar cell population obtained from a patient with sarcoidosis. The number of lymphocytes present in the cell population is increased.

phages (Fig. 11-3). In sarcoidosis several changes are observed in the bronchoalveolar cell population. First, the total number of cells obtained by lavage, and the percentage of lymphocytes in this cell population are significantly increased. Second, lymphocytes that adhere to the surface of macrophages can be easily identified in appropriately prepared smears. These findings are highly diagnostic of sarcoidosis. Bronchoalveolar lavage can be performed at the time of transbronchial biopsy, so that an additional invasive procedure is not required to perform this procedure. The performance of bronchoalveolar lavage and mucosal and transbronchial lung biopsies as part of a single diagnostic procedure has a diagnostic yield in this disease approaching 100%.

TREATMENT

Corticosteroids are the primary drugs used in the treatment of sarcoidosis. Although controversy surrounds the use of these drugs for the treatment of pulmonary involvement, generally they should be used to treat extrathoracic manifestations of sarcoidosis that are considered to be life threatening or that cause significant morbidity. Thus involvement of the eye, central nervous system, and heart are accepted indications for the use of corticosteroids. These drugs are also advocated for use in the treatment of hypercalcemia, disfiguring skin lesions, and severe systemic symptoms.

The major controversy surrounding the use of corticosteroids in the treatment of sarcoidosis focuses on the treatment of patients with pulmonary involvement. To date, corticosteroids have not been clearly shown to reverse or arrest the progression of the pulmonary involvement caused by sarcoidosis. Nevertheless, in most institutions the presence of significant abnormalities in clinical pulmonary function tests is considered an indication for a trial of corticosteroids. The indication for therapy in this situation is based on physiologic abnormalities and not clinical or roentgenographic manifestations of pulmonary involvement.

Patients are usually initially treated with 40 to 60 mg of prednisone daily (or the equivalent of another corticosteroid) for variable periods of time. The duration that a patient should be treated cannot be strictly defined, since clear evidence of superiority of one therapeutic regimen over another has not been demonstrated. The response to corticosteroids must be monitored with serial pulmonary function tests. As has been emphasized repeatedly, the roentgenographic manifestations of pulmonary involvement do not correlate with physiologic abnormalities. If patients fail to improve in a reasonable period of time, the drug should be withdrawn, since continued exposure to the adverse side effects of high-dose corticosteroid therapy is unjustified in the absence of evidence of disease responsiveness.

Chapter 12

ALLERGIC ALVEOLITIS

Allergic alveolitis (chronic hypersensitivity pneumonitis) is an immunologically mediated disease caused by inhalation of antigenic organic dusts. The disease is characterized pathologically by infiltration of the alveolar wall with mononuclear cells and eosinophils and by the presence of noncaseating granulomas.

PATHOLOGIC FINDINGS

The pathologic findings in allergic alveolitis depend on the stage of the disease at which the biopsy is obtained. During the acute stage, diffuse granulomatous inflammation is present. The alveolar wall is infiltrated with mononuclear cells, predominantly lymphocytes and plasma cells. In some patients, eosinophils are prominent. Discrete, poorly formed granulomas are present throughout the lung. Peribronchiolar inflammation and fibrosis and an organizing, endobronchial exudate are occasionally observed. As the disease becomes more chronic, the pathologic changes in lung biopsy specimens may be nonspecific. Marked alveolar wall thickening with fibrosis and lymphocytic and plasma cell infiltration may be present. However, granulomas may no longer be observed. The lung architecture may be severely distorted by massive fibrosis. Cystic changes producing a honeycomb appearance may be found in areas of dense fibrosis.

PATHOGENESIS

Immunologic mechanisms are clearly involved in the pathogenesis of allergic alveolitis. Humoral and cellular immune responses are important in the pathogenesis of this disease. The clinical observations that support this conclusion are described in the following paragraphs. Controlled animal experiments have generally confirmed the validity of these clinical observations.

Most patients with allergic alveolitis have precipitating antibody in their serum directed against the offending antigen. The antibody is predominantly of the IgG class and has the ability to fix complement. If the appropriate antigen is in-

153

jected intradermally into a patient whose serum contains antibody, a typical Arthus type of skin reaction develops at the injection site within 4 to 6 hours, demonstrating the potential for immune complex formation between the antigen and the host's antibody.

Many patients with allergic alveolitis develop acute systemic and pulmonary symptoms 4 to 6 hours after inhalation exposure to the offending antigen, a sequence of events that can be reproduced in selected patients by provocative inhalation testing in the pulmonary physiology laboratory. The similarity in the interval between skin test challenge and the development of the Arthus reaction and inhalation challenge and the onset of clinical manifestations suggests that the pulmonary and systemic symptoms that develop after inhalation of the antigen are caused by immune complex–mediated events.

However, several observations suggest that this type of antibody-mediated reaction cannot be totally responsible for the pathogenesis of the disease. First, many individuals regularly exposed to antigenic, organic dusts have antibodies in their serum similar in nature to those found in patients with clinical disease and yet are asymptomatic and have no manifestations of disease. Second, some patients with allergic alveolitis have only chronic symptoms, rather than the acute symptoms that are most consistent with a systemic antigen-antibody reaction. Third, granulomas are characteristically found in lung biopsy specimens. These lesions are usually considered to be a histologic manifestation of a cell-mediated immune reaction.

These observations can be partially explained by the results of recent studies showing that cellular immune mechanisms are also important in the pathogenesis of this disease. Several lines of evidence support this concept. First, peripheral blood lymphocytes obtained from patients with allergic alveolitis undergo blastogenesis and produce lymphokines when exposed to the offending antigen in in vitro culture. These assays, which are in vitro correlates of cellular immunity, generally discriminate symptomatic, exposed individuals more accurately than does the presence of antibody. Second, studies of the bronchoalveolar cell population obtained from patients with allergic alveolitis by bronchoalveolar lavage have shown that the percentage of lymphocytes is markedly increased (usually greater than 60%) and that the cells are predominantly T-lymphocytes. Furthermore, these cells can produce lymphokines on exposure to antigen. Thus patients do have cellular immunity to the offending antigen, and the inflammatory reaction and pathologic findings in the lung are most compatible with a cellular immune reaction.

On the basis of all these observations, it seems likely that both humoral and cellular immune mechanisms are important in the pathogenesis of allergic alveolitis. The humoral response is probably primarily responsible for the acute pulmonary and systemic symptoms that develop after exposure to the offending antigen. The cellular immune response is probably responsible for the chronic, progressive alveolar wall disease.

Additional, unrecognized factors must also be important in the pathogenesis of the disease, since only a small percentage of persons regularly exposed to potential antigens develop clinical manifestations. This occurs despite the fact that many of these asymptomatic individuals have antibody directed against the offending antigen, and some have evidence of sensitized T-lymphocytes. Local factors may influence the bronchial mucosa and might allow some individuals to become actively sensitized after initial exposure or rechallenge with antigens. In addition, speculation has focused on genetic factors, possibly mediated through immune response genes, which would modulate the immune response of individuals after sensitization to the offending antigen. Additional factors that may modulate the development of clinical manifestations of the disease in individuals who have repeated exposure to antigens known to produce allergic alveolitis have not been defined.

ETIOLOGIC FACTORS

A variety of antigenic agents produce allergic alveolitis. In most instances the antigen is present in the form of organic dusts that consist of molds, fungal spores, or animal proteins. As a result of the small particle size of the antigenic material and the quantity of the material aerosolized in certain environmental settings, large amounts of antigen may be inhaled by exposed individuals.

Specific diseases included under the general classification of allergic alveolitis are, with a few exceptions, named for the occupation or avocation in which the individual comes into contact with the antigen (Table 6). In most patients with clinical manifestations suggesting allergic alveolitis, a careful occupational and avocational history will readily identify the source of the antigen exposure. However, in recent years an increasing number of cases of allergic alveolitis have been shown to be caused by aerosolization of antigenic fungi by the patients' heating and cooling systems. Patients with this form of allergic alveolitis may present a particularly difficult diagnostic problem, since their occupational and avocational exposure histories do not provide any clues to the source of the antigen exposure. Thus the diagnosis of allergic alveolitis may be overlooked unless appropriate diagnostic studies are performed.

Bronchopulmonary aspergillosis is another form of allergic alveolitis in which the environmental history is of little value. This condition is associated with colonization of a bronchus by an *Aspergillus* species. The presence of the fungus in the airway elicits a number of immunologic responses and may lead to the development of allergic alveolitis. In contrast to other forms of allergic alveolitis, the inflammatory reaction may be localized to individual segments or lobes of the lung.

In addition to IgG antibody, patients sensitized to *Aspergillus* species may develop an IgE class antibody. In fact, bronchopulmonary aspergillosis is characterized by markedly elevated IgE levels. The presence of an IgE class antibody may result in the development of classic IgE-mediated bronchospasm. The combination

TABLE 6

Allergic alveolitis

Classification of organic dust	Disease	Source of exposure
Thermophilic actinomycetes	Farmer lung	Hay
	Bagassosis	Sugar cane
	Humidifier lung	Forced air systems
Molds	Maple bark stripper disease	Maple bark
	Malt worker disease	Malt and barley
	Sequiosis	Redwood sawdust
	Suberosis	Cork dust
	Wood pulp worker disease	Logs
	Cheese worker disease	Cheese mold
Animal proteins	Bird fancier disease	Bird (e.g., dove, parakeet) droppings
	Pigeon breeder disease	Pigeon droppings
	Rat handler disease	Rats
	Pituitary snuff-taker disease	Bovine and porcine pituitary

of allergic alveolitis and IgE-mediated asthma is not limited to patients with bronchopulmonary aspergillosis. Patients with all forms of allergic alveolitis may develop acute bronchospasm after antigen exposure if an IgE class antibody directed against the antigen is present. The presence of specific IgE antibody can be demonstrated by appropriate skin testing with the antigen in question. The role of the antigen in the development of acute bronchospasm can be evaluated by provocative inhalation testing in the pulmonary physiology laboratory.

Certain drugs may produce a clinicopathologic syndrome indistinguishable from that observed in allergic alveolitis caused by antigen inhalation. Following are drugs that have been implicated in the development of this kind of hypersensitivity lung disease:

Nitrofurantoin   Procarbazine
Sulfonamides   Bleomycin
Methotrexate   Sulfonoureas
Cromolyn sodium   Penicillin
Gold   Para-aminosalicyclic acid

The drug-induced lung diseases are discussed in detail in Chapter 14.

CLINICAL MANIFESTATIONS

Classically, patients with allergic alveolitis develop pulmonary and systemic symptoms several hours after exposure to an offending antigen. The patient's symptoms usually consist of a nonproductive cough, shortness of breath, fever, chills, myalgia, and anorexia. The syndrome usually resolves spontaneously within 24 to 48 hours after contact with the offending antigen is broken. Most patients are asymptomatic between acute episodes. However, on reexposure to the antigen, the syndrome recurs. Therefore patients usually have a history of recurrent episodes of pulmonary and systemic symptomatology. If the episodes occur frequently, the patient can usually identify the environmental setting in which the syndrome develops.

Some patients either do not have an acute syndrome, or the acute symptoms are so mild they go unrecognized. These patients frequently have persistent or chronic exposure to the offending antigen because the true nature of their disease is not appreciated. If contact with the antigen is not broken, these patients may develop a chronic progressive form of alveolitis. During this stage of the disease, their only complaint may be progressive dyspnea. These patients present a difficult diagnostic problem, since, in the absence of acute symptoms, the possibility of allergic alveolitis is often not considered.

ROENTGENOGRAPHIC MANIFESTATIONS

The roentgenographic manifestations of allergic alveolitis are variable. During acute episodes, the chest roentgenogram is usually normal. However, in some patients a diffuse, micronodular infiltrative process is observed. Patients with persistent symptoms usually have evidence of nodular interstitial disease (Fig. 12-1). As the disease becomes chronic, the interstitial infiltrates become more linear and are indistinguishable from those caused by other progressive alveolar wall diseases. A decrease in lung size with evidence of volume loss predominantly in the upper lobes may be apparent on the chest roentgenogram. Honeycombing may be present in some cases.

PHYSIOLOGIC MANIFESTATIONS

Abnormalities in pulmonary physiology must be considered in relation to the stage of the disease. After acute exposure to an offending antigen, several different abnormalities may occur. In individuals with specific IgE antibody, an abrupt decrease in expiratory flow rates may occur in the first 15 to 60 minutes. The flow rates generally return to normal within several hours. There is usually little change in lung volumes during this period. However, between 6 to 10 hours after acute exposure, a marked decrease in the vital capacity and diffusing capacity occurs. These are the most reproducible changes that develop after provocative testing in a laboratory (Fig. 12-2). These abnormalities usually return to normal by 24 hours.

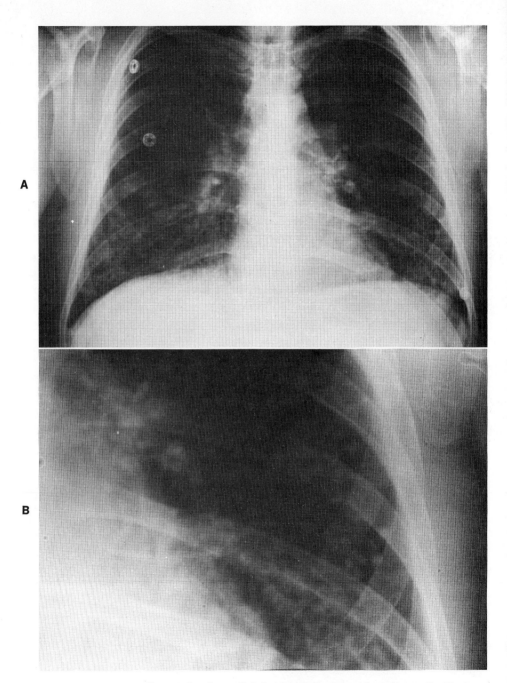

Fig. 12-1. A, Extrinsic allergic alveolitis. Ill-defined nodules are in both lungs. **B,** Close-up demonstrating the nodular lesions.

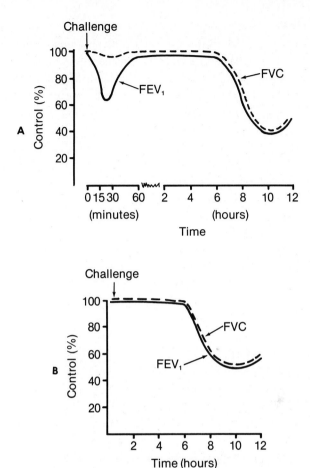

Fig. 12-2. A, Example of the result of a provocative inhalation test demonstrating physiologic changes consistent with both IgE- and IgG-mediated hypersensitivity lung disease. The almost immediate decrease in the forced expiratory volume after the inhalation challenge is characteristic of IgE-mediated bronchospasm. The late decrease in the vital capacity is characteristic of IgE-mediated hypersensitivity pneumonitis. **B,** Example of a provocative inhalation test demonstrating only a late fall in the vital capacity characteristic of IgG-mediated hypersensitivity pneumonitis. This provocative test did not induce IgE-mediated bronchospasm.

Patients with subacute or chronic disease may have persistent physiologic abnormalities consistent with thickening of the alveolar wall. The total lung capacity, static compliance, and diffusing capacity are decreased. Hypoxemia is present as a result of ventilation-perfusion mismatching. Occasionally patients with chronic disease have decreased expiratory flow rates and increased residual volume. Biopsy specimens from these patients generally reveal evidence of bronchiolitis fibrosa obliterans in addition to the more typical pathologic changes of the alveolar wall.

DIAGNOSIS

If a patient has a classic history of recurrent episodes of pulmonary and systemic symptoms after exposure to a well-recognized environmental antigen, a clinical diagnosis of allergic alveolitis can usually be made with a high degree of accuracy. In this situation the demonstration of precipitating antibody against the offending antigen in the patient's serum is all that is needed for confirmation of the diagnosis.

The major diagnostic problems occur either when a patient with compatible acute symptoms does not have an obvious exposure to a known antigen or when a patient has the clinical and roentgenographic manifestations of chronic alveolitis. If the patient with acute disease has been exposed to an antigen not previously recognized to cause allergic alveolitis, serum antibody studies are of little value, since appropriate antigens for diagnostic testing will not be available. If the source of the antigen is suspected, it is possible to perform provocative inhalation testing using the antigen-containing material to determine if physiologic abnormalities characteristic of allergic alveolitis develop after exposure. This diagnostic approach is not without some risk and is limited to special diagnostic centers at present.

Serum antibody studies also have limited value in patients with chronic alveolitis, even in those who have been definitely exposed to antigens that have been implicated in the origin of allergic alveolitis. Since a significant percentage of individuals repetitively exposed to the antigen have serum antibodies without having alveolitis, the demonstration of antibody in a patient with chronic alveolitis simply confirms the possibility that the patient may have the disease. In this clinical situation, in vitro lymphocyte studies of delayed hypersensitivity appear to be more specific. If a patient has evidence of sensitized lymphocytes to the antigen in question by in vitro assay (blastogenesis or migration inhibiting factor production), the alveolitis is probably caused by the antigen in question. The absence of antibody or sensitized lymphocytes would be substantial evidence against the presence of allergic alveolitis.

In many patients with acute or chronic allergic alveolitis, further diagnostic studies are necessary to elucidate the true nature of the disease. Because other routine laboratory studies are of no value, invasive diagnostic studies must be performed. Since few diseases are associated with a granulomatous pneumonitis, the presence of these pathologic findings on biopsy strongly suggests the diagnosis. If the end stage of the disease is present and granulomas are not observed, the biopsy will be of limited value.

Differential cell counts of the bronchoalveolar cells obtained by bronchoalveolar lavage can be useful in making the diagnosis of allergic alveolitis, which is characterized by a marked increase in the percentage of lymphocytes in the bronchoalveolar cell population. The percentage of lymphocytes in documented cases has generally exceeded 60%. Thus bronchoalveolar lavage may be useful in the differential diagnosis and eliminates the necessity for lung biopsy in many cases.

TREATMENT

The most important aspect of the treatment of allergic alveolitis is removal of the individual from contact with the offending antigen. If the disease has not progressed to a state of alveolar wall fibrosis, the disease may then resolve spontaneously. However, corticosteroids may also be of value in reversing the disease process in selected cases. When the disease has advanced to the stage of progressive fibrosis, it is unlikely that any form of therapy will be of value. Nonetheless, all patients should be removed from contact with the antigen in an attempt to at least halt progressive destruction of the lung.

Chapter 13

PNEUMOCONIOSES

The pneumoconioses are lung diseases caused by the inhalation of inorganic dusts. In most circumstances the dust exposure occurs in the course of the patient's daily work. The clinical, roentgenographic, physiologic, and pathologic manifestations of the pneumoconioses are varied but in all cases reflect the effects of the deposition of large quantities of certain inorganic dusts in distal bronchioles and alveolar air spaces. The three major pneumoconioses are silicosis, asbestosis, and coal workers pneumoconiosis. Because of their relative importance, these diseases will be discussed in some detail. The other pneumoconioses are listed in Table 7.

SILICOSIS

Silicosis is the most important of the pneumoconioses. This disease is caused by the inhalation of silicon dioxide, a major component of the earth's crust. Silicon dioxide exists in nature in crystalline forms, the most common of which is quartz, and has certain physical properties that make it desirable for use in industry. Thus exposure to crystalline silica may occur in a wide variety of occupations.

Pathologic findings

Several distinct pathologic manifestations of silicosis exist. Most cases are characterized by the presence of small silicotic nodules (simple silicosis). Histologically the nodules are composed of a central hyalinized zone, a zone of dense cellular connective tissue, and an outer zone of loose connective tissue. With special polarized microscopy, silica particles can be observed in the central and peripheral zones. These nodules are usually unevenly distributed throughout the lungs but have a prediletion for the upper lobes. The nodules are most frequently located in the subpleural connective tissue or the connective tissue framework of respiratory bronchioles and small arterioles. The nodules may also involve the alveolar wall. When this occurs, there is protrusion of nodules into the intra-alveolar space and loss of the epithelial lining layer. In patients with rapidly progressive disease, these

TABLE 7
Less common pneumoconioses

Disease	Inhaled substance
Aluminum lung	Aluminum powder
Antimony pneumoconiosis	Antimony
Baritosis	Barium sulfate
Berylliosis	Beryllium
Carbon and graphite pneumoconioses	Carbon and graphite
Hard metal disease	Tungsten carbide
Shaver disease	Aluminum oxide
Siderosis	Ferric oxide
Stannosis	Tin

nodules tend to be more evenly distributed throughout the lung and involve the alveolar walls more often.

As the disease progresses, massive fibrotic lesions may develop, usually in the upper lobes (e.g., complicated silicosis and progressive massive fibrosis). These lesions are composed of coalescent silicotic nodules that are encompassed by areas of fibrosis. Blood vessels and bronchi in the area may be obliterated by the fibrotic mass. Areas of necrosis may be contained in the center of the mass. These lesions cause distortion of the structure of the lung with contraction in the upper lobes and the formation of large bullae in the adjacent lung.

Acute silicosis is a rare condition caused by exposure to heavy concentrations of free silica. The pathologic changes associated with this condition are distinct from those of chronic silicosis. A predominant feature of this condition is the presence of intra-alveolar acidophilic fluid. The fluid contains lipid, protein, and many alveolar macrophages. The alveolar wall is infiltrated by mononuclear cells and is fibrous. Silicotic nodules are usually few or absent, but silica particles can be identified in the lung.

In addition to the pathologic changes in the lung, silica particles and silicotic nodules may be observed in intrathoracic lymph nodes. As a result, the lymph nodes may become enlarged and calcify. Pleural fibrosis may also be observed, particularly in the presence of massive fibrosis.

An unusual variant of silicosis is found in patients with rheumatoid arthritis. Massive fibrosis appears to occur more frequently in these individuals. In addition, rapidly developing nodules larger than those observed in simple silicosis also occur. Pathologically these nodules are characterized by a central necrotic zone surrounded by a peripheral zone of palisading connective tissue and are thus nearly identical to classic rheumatoid nodules.

Pathogenesis

The results of experimental studies suggest that the pathogenesis of silicosis is related to the cytotoxic effect of silica on alveolar macrophages. The sequence of events that leads to the formation of silica nodules in the lung begins with ingestion of silica particles by intra-alveolar macrophages. The particles are internalized into the cell in a phagosome. The phagosome then fuses with multiple lysosomes to form a phagolysosome that contains silica particles and lysosomal enzymes. The silica causes disruption of the phagolysosome, resulting in the release of the lysosomal enzymes into the cytoplasm of the cell. As a result, the cell dies, and the lysosomal enzymes and other bioactive substances within the cell are released into the lung parenchyma. These substances stimulate an inflammatory and fibrogenic response in the lung.

The mechanism by which silica causes rupture of the phagolysosome is unknown. Current theories suggest that the geometric configuration of silica allows it to react biochemically with the phagolysosomal membrane, thus leading to disruption of the membrane through a biochemical mechanism. This sequence of events not only causes the release of lysosomal enzymes and potentially fibrogenic substances into the lung parenchyma, but also releases the silica particles. As a result, more macrophages accumulate in the area and ingest the silica. Thus the cycle leading to the pathologic changes observed in the lung is perpetuated.

Epidemiologic factors

Obviously, exposure to crystalline silica may occur during mining or quarrying for the material. In addition, silica may be encountered while mining for mineral extraction (e.g., gold, tin, and copper), since silicon dioxide is a component of the residual rock. Potential exposure also exists in a number of nonmining industries in which the hard, heat-resistant properties of crystalline silica are desirable. Thus individuals who work in foundries; who are involved in abrasive blasting, stone cutting, or other masonry work; or who work in areas where glass, pottery, or porcelain are manufactured may be at risk of developing silicosis.

Several environmental factors influence the risk of developing silicosis for individuals working in one of these industries. Obviously the amount of dust production is a critical factor. In this regard, blasting or the use of pneumatic drills or hand tools, particularly in an enclosed space, may lead to heavy exposure to dust clouds containing free silica. The degree of protection from inhalation of the dust by various protective devices also influences the person's risk of developing the disease. If protective hoods and clothing are unavailable because the risk of exposure to silica is not recognized, or if the worker chooses not to conform to requirements for wearing such devices, the risk of silicosis is increased.

In addition to these environmental factors, certain unidentified host factors may influence the response to inhaled silica. Some data suggest that immunologic reactivity may play a role in modulating individual manifestations of the disease.

Clinical manifestations

In the great majority of cases, clinical and roentgenographic manifestations of silicosis do not become apparent until the patient has been exposed to the dust more than 20 years. The initial manifestation of this disease is the development of small nodules on the chest roentgenogram. During this stage of the disease, termed "simple silicosis," the patient is usually asymptomatic.

Simple silicosis has a tendency to progress to complicated silicosis, even if the individual is removed from further dust exposure. As the disease progresses, the individual may develop dyspnea during exertion. This symptom is almost always associated with roentgenographic evidence of complicated disease. Marked dyspnea is usually seen in patients who have significant distortion of the lung architecture and contraction of the upper lobes. Dyspnea may become more severe in patients with progressive bullous formation despite no change in the size of the parenchymal masses.

Patients with silicosis may have cough and sputum production. During the stage of simple silicosis, these symptoms are almost invariably caused by an associated bronchitis related to cigarette smoking. When complicated silicosis develops, the distortion of the bronchial tree impairs airway clearance to a greater extent, and cough and expectoration increase. If cavities are present in the areas of massive fibrosis, cough and expectoration are usually even more significant.

The development of tuberculous or mycotic infection is an important feature of silicosis. These infections are usually associated with complicated or accelerated silicosis. Although *Mycobacterium tuberculosis* is classically associated with this disease, infection with an atypical mycobacterium is frequently present. *M. kansasii* or *M. intracellulare* have been the prevalent atypical organisms identified in patients with silicosis in different parts of the country. In the presence of infection, systemic symptoms of weight loss, anorexia, and fever may occur. In addition, dyspnea, cough, and expectoration may be more marked, and hemoptysis may occur.

As silicosis advances, respiratory failure may develop and clear clinical evidence of cor pulmonale may appear. Relatively few physical findings are apparent until the development of cor pulmonale. Specifically, rales and clubbing, findings associated with other forms of chronic diffuse lung disease, are unusual in patients with silicosis.

Roentgenographic manifestations

The roentgenographic manifestations of parenchymal involvement in silicosis form the basis for classifying the stage of the disease. Distinct roentgenographic manifestations occur in acute, simple, and complicated silicosis.

Diffuse alveolar filling is the characteristic roentgenographic pattern of acute silicosis (Fig. 13-1). Although thickening of alveolar walls is present pathologically, an interstitial pattern is usually not roentgenographically apparent because of the diffuse alveolar filling process. However, occasionally a patient exhibits a diffuse,

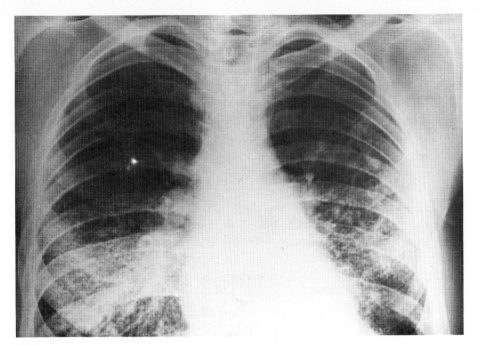

Fig. 13-1. Acute silicosis. A coalescent, alveolar filling pattern is present in both lower lung fields.

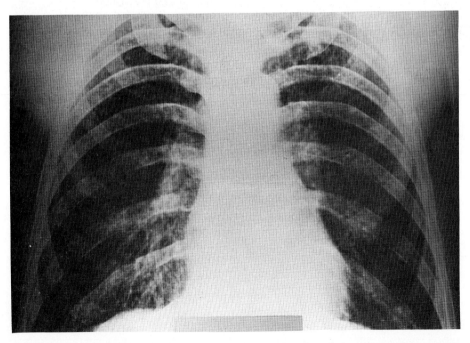

Fig. 13-2. Simple silicosis. Small, discrete nodules are distributed throughout all lung fields.

linear interstitial pattern. Discrete nodules are usually not apparent on the chest roentgenogram during this stage of the disease.

Diffuse, discrete nodules up to 1 cm in size are the characteristic roentgeno-graphic manifestations of simple silicosis (Fig. 13-2). On the basis of the size of the nodular lesions and the extent of parenchymal involvement, simple silicosis can be classified for epidemiologic purposes into a number of subcategories according to internationally accepted criteria, but this classification system provides little addi-tional information about the clinical stage of the disease. On occasion the nodules of simple silicosis may calcify.

Complicated silicosis is characterized by the presence of nodules greater than 1 cm in diameter. Frequently, coalescence of smaller nodules into conglomerate masses can be recognized on serial roentgenograms. The conglomerate masses may reach massive proportions so that they involve large areas of lung (Fig. 13-3). In association with these masses, upper lobe retraction, bullous formation, and distor-tion of the tracheobronchial tree may be present. In addition, cavitation may occur in these lesions as a result of either ischemic necrosis or an associated infection. These lesions are also frequently associated with pleural thickening and adhesions. Spontaneous pneumothorax may occur during this stage of the disease as well.

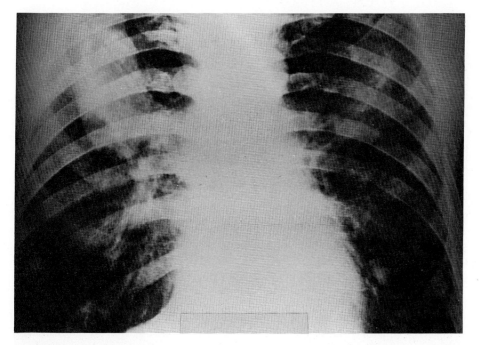

Fig. 13-3. Complicated silicosis. Lesions of progressive massive fibrosis are in both upper lung lobes.

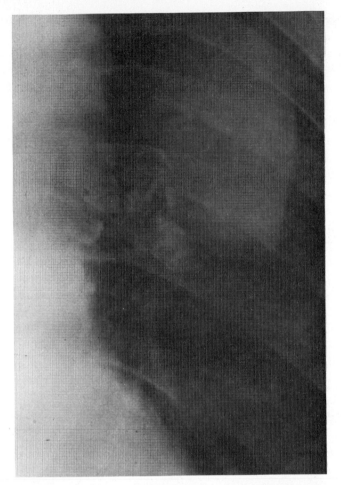

Fig. 13-4. Close-up of the left hilar region in a patient with complicated silicosis. Eggshell calcifications in the lymph nodes are present in the hilar area.

Lymph node enlargement may also be observed on the chest roentgenogram. In addition, calcification of the nodes may occur. Calcification frequently occurs in the periphery of the nodes, giving the pattern of "eggshell calcification" classically associated with silicosis (Fig. 13-4). This form of calcification may be seen in other diseases, but it is highly suggestive of silicosis.

Finally, Caplan syndrome has distinctive roentgenographic features that can be best recognized if serial films are available for review. This syndrome is characterized by the rapid development of rounded opacities. The lesions usually are 1 to 5 cm in size and located in the periphery of the lungs. The lesions usually develop in patients with simple silicosis and can only be clearly distinguished from the development of complicated silicosis by the rapidity with which they appear. Progression from simple to complicated silicosis usually occurs over 5 years, whereas the lesions of Caplan syndrome may appear in crops within a few weeks. The nodules may cavitate or calcify. Occasionally they develop in patients with complicated disease.

Physiologic manifestations

The physiologic abnormalities that occur in patients with silicosis are as varied as the clinical and roentgenographic manifestations of the disease. This variability is caused by the fact that there may be marked differences in the site and distribution of lesions throughout the lung and that patients with silicosis frequently have other lung diseases such as chronic bronchitis, mixed dust exposure, and pulmonary infection. Despite the complexity of the situation, a few general comments about the physiologic manifestations of the disease can be made.

First, routine pulmonary function tests are generally normal in patients with simple silicosis. As the disease progresses, physiologic abnormalities consistent with alveolar wall disease—decreased total lung capacity (TLC), static lung compliance (Cst), and diffusing capacity—are predominant. Hypoxemia, during either rest or exercise, is usually present. As massive fibrosis progresses, severe resting hypoxemia develops. In patients with associated bronchitis, decreased expiratory flow rates may also be observed.

Diagnosis

In most cases the diagnosis of silicosis can be made from clinical information and generally with a high degree of accuracy in patients with a compatible exposure history and roentgenographic manifestations consistent with the disease. Occasionally an adequate exposure history may be absent, or the roentgenographic manifestations of the disease may be atypical. In this setting, biopsy may be required for diagnostic purposes. When lung tissue is necessary, an open lung biopsy provides sufficient tissue for special studies.

Conventional histologic examination is usually adequate for diagnosis, since typical hyaline nodules are almost always present in biopsy specimens. However, since the pathologic findings may not be characteristic, in some cases additional studies may be required. In this situation, examination of the tissue under polarized light may reveal doubly refractile silica particles. X-ray energy spectrometry can also be used to detect excess silica in the lung. These special techniques should be used for patients with an obvious exposure history who have obscure or atypical pathologic changes on routine examination of biopsy specimens.

Therapy

There is no specific therapy for established silicosis. Therefore treatment of patients with the disease is limited to treatment of complications of the disease.

Conventional therapy for infectious complications, associated airways disease, or cor pulmonale should be used when indicated.

Prevention is the most important aspect of the management of silicosis. In industries where the exposure to silica is recognized, appropriate preventive measures that can minimize the amount of respirable silica particles must be instituted. Institution of such measures and compliance with the measures by workers can result in control of the disease. However, silica exposure may occur in previously unrecognized settings. This has recently been documented in several industries. Thus the potential for new industrial sources of exposure to silica must be considered when sporadic cases are documented in patients not thought to have been exposed to the dust.

ASBESTOSIS

Asbestosis is characterized by the development of progressive inflammation and fibrosis of the alveolar wall caused by the chronic inhalation of asbestos.

Pathologic changes

With the exception of the presence of asbestos bodies, the pathologic changes associated with asbestosis are entirely nonspecific. Early changes are characterized by the presence of many macrophages in the alveolar space. The alveolar wall then becomes infiltrated with mononuclear cells and granulocytes. The alveolar wall epithelium becomes hypertrophic and cuboidal, resembling the type II cell proliferation observed in a variety of other diseases. As the disease progresses, varying degrees of thickening of the alveolar wall occur, caused by an increase in connective tissue proteins. Occasionally, marked fibrosis may be the predominant pathologic finding.

The pathologic changes may occur throughout the entire lung but are characteristically more significant in the lung bases. Although the fibrosis may be more apparent in the peribronchiolar regions, the airways are not involved by the disease. Similarly, the tracheobronchial lymph nodes are usually normal. However, asbestos bodies may occasionally be observed in the lymph nodes.

The histopathologic changes and distribution of the disease within the lung do not allow asbestosis to be distinguished from fibrosing alveolitis resulting from other causes. However, the presence of asbestos bodies can be useful in differentiating asbestosis from other forms of fibrosing alveolitis. The asbestos body is an asbestos fiber that has been coated by an iron protein complex. It is yellow-brown and has clubbed ends and a segmented appearance. It appears to initially develop within macrophages. Although asbestos bodies are evidence that an individual has inhaled asbestos, they do not necessarily indicate that the asbestos is related to the underlying lung disease. Asbestos bodies may be observed in otherwise normal lungs and may occasionally be observed in association with diffuse diseases other than asbestosis. However, in asbestosis the number of asbestos bodies is significantly increased, thus allowing a reasonable distinction to be made between asbestosis and the incidental association of asbestos bodies with other lung diseases.

The majority of asbestos fibers in the lung remain uncoated. These fibers can be recognized under polarized microscopy and are far more numerous than suggested by light microscopy. They can be demonstrated in regions of fibrosis where asbestos bodies are not demonstrable. In fact, it is likely that coating of asbestos fibers renders them less likely to stimulate fibrosis.

The core of the asbestos body may not always be asbestos. Since only the iron-containing outer coat can be identified, the term "ferruginous body" has become a more generally accepted description.

Pathogenesis

The pathogenesis of asbestosis is caused by the deposition of small asbestos particles on respiratory bronchioles or alveolar walls where they are ingested by macrophages. The mechanism by which asbestos provokes inflammation and fibrosis of the alveolar wall is unknown. Original theories suggested that physical irritation by the fibers, or the release of silicic acid or metallic ions from the fibers during solubilization, were responsible for the fibrogenic properties of asbestos. Although tissue and cell culture techniques have demonstrated that asbestos has a direct cytotoxic effect on macrophages and other cells found in the lung, these theories have not gained general support.

A more recent theory proposes that immunologic mechanisms are most important in the pathogenesis of the alveolar wall disease. According to this theory, lung tissue becomes antigenic after being damaged, either directly by asbestos or indirectly by macrophages. Thus the progression of the disease occurs through an autoimmune phenomenon. Differences in the immunologic reactivity of individuals would explain the variability in the development of the disease in groups of workers apparently exposed to similar amounts of asbestos. However, no convincing evidence supports this theory.

The cytotoxic effect of asbestos on macrophages may provide the stimulus to alveolar wall inflammation and fibrosis. However, further experimental work is required before the mechanism of the alveolar wall disease can be clearly defined.

Epidemiologic factors

Asbestos, the name given to a number of fibrous silicates, is mined principally in Canada, South Africa, and Russia. The raw asbestos is first processed to release asbestos fibers from the parent rock and then transported for use in a variety of industries. In the United States, most asbestos, because of its fireproofing and insulating properties, is used in the construction industry. Since the material has to be handled in the preparation of these products, workers in these industries may be exposed to asbestos dust. Asbestos is also used in spraying insulation material and in the production of brake and clutch linings, fireproof textiles, and the lining of some furnaces and kilns. Individuals may be exposed during the production of any of those products. In addition, individuals such as plumbers, demolition workers, and shipbuilders, who work in areas where asbestos materials are employed, may be exposed despite not working directly with the material.

Clinical features

The signs and symptoms of asbestosis are identical to those of other forms of diffuse alveolar wall disease. Dyspnea during exertion is the most prominent symptom of the disease. A nonproductive cough is also frequently present. Symptoms do not usually appear until the individual has been exposed to asbestos dust for at least 10 years. However, a heavy exposure to free asbestos fibers may lead to the development of symptoms in a much shorter period of time. In most cases the disease progresses even after the individual has been removed from exposure to asbestos dust. However, some evidence shows that removal from exposure after early detection of the disease may prevent progression to a more advanced stage of the disease.

During physical examination, crackling rales are generally audible over the posterior lungs at the bases. In addition, clubbing of the fingers and toes is often observed.

Roentgenographic features

The roentgenographic manifestations of asbestosis are generally identical to those of other forms of fibrosing alveolitis. The presence of linear infiltrates predominantly in the lung bases is the characteristic findings of the disease. However, several other roentgenographic findings may be present and suggest the diagnosis of asbestosis. First, some patients are also exposed to silica as the result of a mixed dust exposure. Thus nodular lesions characteristic of silicosis may be present on the roentgenogram. Second, pleural fibrosis occurs frequently. Since this is uncommon in the idiopathic form of fibrosing alveolitis it may allow one to distinguish these entities (Fig. 13-5). However, pleural changes may be seen in patients with fibrosing alveolitis associated with systemic connective tissue diseases.

Physiologic features

The physiologic abnormalities of asbestosis are identical to those of other forms of fibrosing alveolitis. The TLC, Cst, and diffusing capacity of the lung are decreased in patients with symptomatic disease. A decrease in the diffusing capacity is one of the earliest abnormalities to develop. Thus this test can be used to detect early disease in exposed individuals. Hypoxemia usually occurs during exercise in patients with early disease and develops at rest as the disease progresses.

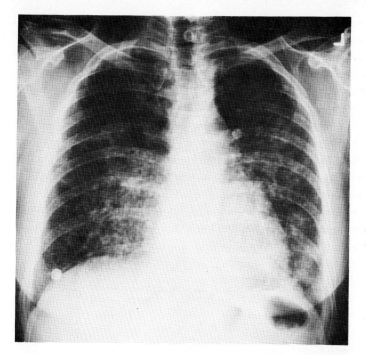

Fig. 13-5. Asbestosis. Both a diffuse interstitial infiltrative process in both lungs and bilateral pleural thickening are present.

Diagnosis

The diagnosis of asbestosis can frequently be made from clinical information. In a patient with an appropriate exposure history, clinical, roentgenographic, and physiologic abnormalities consistent with diffuse alveolar wall disease can be attributed to the asbestos exposure without confirming the diagnosis by lung biopsy. The presence of roentgenographic evidence of pleural disease, or nodular lesions compatible with mixed dust exposure, may help in strengthening the clinical impression. In addition the presence of asbestos bodies in the sputum may add further support to the diagnosis. However, asbestos bodies may be present in the sputum of exposed workers in the absence of lung disease.

If no exposure history exists or the period of exposure is brief, a lung biopsy may be required to make a diagnosis. In this situation, open lung biopsy should be performed so that adequate tissue can be obtained for detailed histopathologic examination. Polarized and electron microscopy may be required to demonstrate asbestos fibers that are not evident by light microscopy. In the absence of an exposure history, the findings of a significant number of asbestos bodies in the biopsy should prompt a search for a source of exposure to asbestos.

Therapy

No treatment for established asbestosis exists. In the early stage of the disease, removal from exposure may halt the progression of the disease. However, in most cases the disease continues to progress. Obviously conventional therapy for lung infections or cor pulmonale should be used when these conditions complicate the underlying disease. As with all the pneumoconioses, prevention is the major thrust of the overall management of the disease. Since asbestos is widely used in a number of industries, the potential for exposure of workers may not always be recognized. If exposure potential is recognized, then accepted methods for minimizing the exposure of the workers to asbestos dust must be instituted.

All workers regularly exposed should periodically undergo pulmonary function tests and chest roentgenograms to detect evidence of early disease. After 10 years of exposure the examination should be performed on a yearly basis. Workers who develop abnormalities consistent with early asbestosis should be removed from further dust exposure.

COAL WORKERS PNEUMOCONIOSIS

Coal workers pneumoconiosis (CWP) is a disease of the lung parenchyma caused by the inhalation of coal dust. Coal miners may develop three different forms of occupational lung disease: CWP, silicosis, and occupational bronchitis. This discussion will be concerned only with CWP.

Pathologic findings

The characteristic pathologic lesion of CWP is the coal macule. The lesion is approximately 5 mm in diameter and appears as a small black nodule in cut sections of lung. Although a propensity for involvement of the upper lobes may exist, the lesion is generally widely and evenly distributed throughout the lung. The lesion is characterized microscopically by the accumulation in peribronchiolar regions of macrophages that have ingested coal dust and variable degrees of reticulin and collagen deposition. With more extensive disease the macule may actually extend into the alveolar walls in the vicinity of the respiratory bronchioles. In association with the coal macule, alveolar ducts become dilated, resulting in a form of centriacinar emphysema.

In a small percentage of cases, lesions of complicated CWP (progressive massive fibrosis) may be present. By definition these lesions must be greater than 1 cm in diameter. Occasionally they may be extremely large and occupy a major portion of an entire lung. These lesions characteristically arise in the posterior portion of the lung and appear as black, irregular, amorphous masses. Blood vessels and airways in the involved lung are simply obliterated by the pathologic process. Special elastin stains are required to identify the presence of the remnants of these structures. As a result of ischemic necrosis, cavitation may occur within these lesions. In addition, these masses may cause gross distortion of major airways.

Microscopically the lesions appear as amorphous fibrous tissue. Coal dust and areas of necrosis are apparent in the tissue. Although collagen may be present on the periphery of the lesion, the bulk of the lesion is comprised of a nonspecific protein structure. It is not unusual to identify mycobacterial organisms in these lesions.

In addition to the classic lesions of CWP, lesions of Caplan syndrome may also be present. These lesions are easily recognized microscopically by their palisading architecture of inflammatory cells and fibroblasts and by the absence of dust particles. Silicotic nodules may also be observed in association with lesions of CWP if silica dust exposure has occurred.

Pathogenesis

After inhalation of coal dust, coal particles are deposited on the mucociliary blanket of the airways or in the alveoli where they are phagocytized by alveolar macrophages. After phagocytosis of coal particles, the macrophages initially appear to migrate to the peribronchiolar area surrounding respiratory bronchioles, where they are removed from the lung by mechanical means. When the amount of coal dust that is inhaled overwhelms this clearance mechanism, the macrophages containing the coal particles accumulate in the peribronchiolar region. The accumulation of these macrophages in the peribronchiolar region results in the deposition of reticulin fibers. In some cases, collagen may also be deposited in the region of the coal macule, leading to more extensive fibrosis in the peribronchiolar regions. The mechanism by which reticulin and collagen are deposited in the coal macule is unknown.

The pathogenesis of progressive massive fibrosis in CWP is a subject of controversy. Although three different theories have been proposed, none has achieved general acceptance. The concept that the development of progressive massive fibrosis is related to tuberculous infection is probably the most popular of these theories. Although infection with *M. tuberculosis* or other mycobacterial species is not uncommon in patients with progressive massive fibrosis, there is no reason to believe that the infection is important in the pathogenesis of these lesions in most cases. In fact, in a majority of patients who develop these lesions, there is no clinical or histopathologic evidence of tuberculous infection. More recently, consideration has been given to the possibility that the lesions represent some type of autoimmune phenomenon. No concrete data support this concept at present. Although miners have varying exposure to silica dust, no evidence supports the concept that the development of complicated CWP is related in any way to mixed dust exposure.

Epidemiologic factors

The development of CWP is related to chronic inhalation of coal dust. Individuals with the heaviest cumulative exposure to coal dust are most likely to develop the disease. A number of different occupations are involved in the mining of coal, and exposure to coal dust varies with each of these occupations. Miners who work at the face of the mine where the extraction of coal is highly mechanized have the greatest exposure to coal dust and the highest incidence of CWP. Maintenance workers and workers involved in the transportation of coal out of the mines are also frequently affected, whereas surface workers are least often affected. The most recent statistics suggest that approximately 10% of miners in the United States have evidence of CWP. The incidence seems to vary markedly in different regions of the country. This is probably related to differences in both the physical and chemical composition of coal and the mining process involved in the extraction of coal from the earth.

Clinical features

The clinical manifestations of CWP are difficult to characterize, since other forms of lung disease are so common in affected miners. Careful epidemiologic studies have shown that the increased morbidity and mortality resulting from the respiratory disorders observed in miners is caused by chronic bronchitis and emphysema. Although smoking is a common habit among miners, the increased incidence of bronchitis cannot be totally attributed to cigarette smoking. Exposure to coal dust alone leads to a form of occupational bronchitis. Dyspnea and cough productive of black sputum are thus frequently observed in patients with CWP but may not be specifically attributed to this disease. In fact, miners with simple CWP are apparently asymptomatic unless they have associated bronchitis.

In miners with complicated CWP, symptoms appear to be directly related to the pneumoconiosis. Patients with lesions of progressive massive fibrosis that are greater than 5 cm in diameter usually have dyspnea and more marked production of black sputum. As the lung disease progresses, manifestations of cor pulmonale may develop. In addition, pulmonary infection with mycobacterial organisms may result in an increase in pulmonary symptoms and the development of systemic symptoms of fever, anorexia, weight loss, and malaise.

Physical findings are usually absent during the stage of simple pneumoconiosis. Findings of cor pulmonale predominate during the late stage of progressive massive fibrosis.

Roentgenographic features

Roentgenographic evidence of CWP does not usually appear until the worker has been exposed to coal dust for approximately 10 years. The progression of roentgenographic abnormalities is also slow. The disease usually does not progress from one subclassification to another in less than 5 years. Although the extent of the roentgenographic abnormalities generally is related to the coal dust content of the involved lung, roentgenographic progression may occur despite the fact that the worker has no further exposure to coal dust.

The characteristic roentgenographic manifestation of CWP is the presence of small opacities in the lung. These lesions are round in almost all cases but may on occasion appear as irregular linear densities like those seen in asbestosis or other fibrosing diseases. The extent of lung involvement is classified on the basis of the size and distribution of the lesions on the chest roentgenogram. Although detailed classification of the small nodular lesions is of value in studying the epidemiologic factors of the disease, it does not have great clinical significance. From a clinical standpoint, it is most important to distinguish simple CWP from complicated CWP.

Complicated CWP is simply defined by the presence of lesions greater than 1 cm in diameter and is classified into stages A, B, and C based on the diameter of the lesions. In stage A the combined diameter of lesions is between 1 cm and 5 cm. In stage B the combined diameter exceeds 5 cm but is less than a third of the total volume of one lung. In stage C the combined diameter of the lesions is greater than the volume of a third of one lung. These roentgenographic stages correlate with the clinical and physiologic manifestations of the disease.

Finally, the lesions of Caplan syndrome must be recognized. These lesions tend to develop on the background of simple CWP, are generally 1 to 5 cm in diameter, and are peripherally located. They can be distinguished from other manifestations of CWP by the rapidity with which they develop. In contrast to the slow progression of lesions of CWP, Caplan syndrome lesions may appear in crops within a few weeks. They obviously may also be recognized by their association with other clinical manifestations of rheumatoid arthritis.

Physiologic features

The physiologic abnormalities that occur in CWP are related to the stage of the disease. As has been mentioned previously, miners have an increased risk of developing chronic bronchitis. Thus abnormalities in gas exchange and the mechanical properties of the lung may be present in miners and have no relationship to CWP. Because of the common association of cigarette smoking and occupational bronchitis, it has been difficult to accurately identify the physiologic abnormalities truly related to CWP. However, several general comments can now be made about these relationships.

Patients with simple CWP generally have normal or nearly normal routine physiologic studies. The only consistent abnormality is an elevation of the residual volume. Special physiologic studies have shown that the increase in residual volume is probably related to increased resistance to airflow at the level of the small airways. The presence of small airways disease in miners with simple CWP has been confirmed by studies showing that dynamic compliance is frequency dependent and the closing volume or closing capacity of the lung is frequently elevated. These findings are not surprising in light of the peribronchiolar location of the coal macule.

Patients with complicated CWP have greater physiologic abnormalities that tend to correlate with the stage of the disease determined roentgenographically. Abnormalities in both gas exchange and the mechanical properties of the lung are present in patients with complicated disease. Resting hypoxemia, which is aggravated by exercise, and a decrease in the diffusing capacity of the lung are usually present in patients with stage B or C. In addition, the Cst of the lung and the forced expired volume to forced vital capacity ratio are decreased. In patients with decreased expiratory flow rates, the residual volume and TLC are generally increased.

Diagnosis

The diagnosis of CWP is based on an appropriate exposure history and the presence of compatible roentgenographic manifestations of the disease. Additional diagnostic studies are of no value. There is no reason to perform lung biopsy to confirm the diagnosis in routine cases. However, infection with *M. tuberculosis* or other mycobacterial species may be difficult to recognize because of the existence of roentgenographic abnormalities of CWP. Thus the patient who develops new pulmonary or systemic symptoms must be carefully evaluated. Additional laboratory studies may be helpful in patients who develop new lesions consistent with Caplan syndrome. The majority of these patients will have a positive test for rheumatoid factor in the serum when the lesions develop. Since the pulmonary nodules may precede the onset of other manifestations of rheumatoid arthritis, serologic studies can be useful.

Therapy

There is no treatment for CWP. Complications of mycobacterial infection or the development of cor pulmonale should be treated by conventional means. Control of the disease is obviously related to preventing miners from being exposed to large quantities of coal dust. The present cases of CWP are related to exposure under conditions existing in the mines 20 to 30 years ago. With changes in the standard for coal dust exposure in the mines now in effect, fewer miners are likely to develop CWP in the future.

Chapter 14

DRUG-INDUCED LUNG DISEASE

A number of drugs may produce diffuse parenchymal lung disease. The clinical, pathologic, and roentgenographic manifestations of these diseases are varied and depend to a great extent on the pathogenesis of the disorder. Before discussing the specific manifestations of the drug-induced diseases, a general discussion of the mechanisms by which drugs produce lung disease is necessary.

PATHOGENESIS

The pathogenesis of most drug-induced lung diseases is not definitely known. However, the clinical, roentgenographic, and laboratory manifestations of these diseases suggest that three major pathogenetic mechanisms are responsible for the development of most drug-induced lung diseases. Following are the drugs that can be associated with each of these mechanisms:

Hypersensitivity pneumonitis	Direct pulmonary toxicity	Increased alveolar-capillary permeability
Nitrofurantoin	Bleomycin	Salicylates
Sulfonamides	Nitrofurantoin	Heroin
Methotrexate	Busulfan	Methadone
Cromolyn sodium	Cyclophosphamide	Ethchlorvynol
Gold	Oxyphenbutazone	Hydrochlorothiazide
Procarbazine	Phenytoin	Colchicine
Bleomycin	Penicillamine	
Sulfonylureas		
Penicillin		
Para-aminosalicylic acid		

Clearly some drugs cause pulmonary infiltration by producing a hypersensitivity reaction in the lung. The acute development of fever, cough, shortness of breath, peripheral eosinophilia, and patchy alveolar infiltrates on the chest roentgenogram are the characteristic features of these reactions. The concept that immunologic mechanisms are important in the pathogenesis of certain drug-induced lung diseases is supported by several clinical and laboratory observations. First, in vitro lymphocyte studies have demonstrated that some patients with this form of drug-induced lung disease have circulating lymphocytes which have been sensitized to the responsible drug. Second, lung biopsies obtained from patients with this form of disease have revealed granulomatous pneumonitis with infiltration of the alveolar wall by eosinophils, lymphocytes, and plasma cells. These pathologic changes are generally considered to be manifestations of a pulmonary immune reaction. Finally, in patients who have recovered, the syndrome has recurred promptly during reexposure to the drug or a related drug. These observations strongly suggest that drugs may produce a hypersensitivity pneumonitis.

Some drugs produce lung disease by directly injuring the alveolar wall, causing progressive alveolar wall inflammation and fibrosis. No experimental evidence conclusively demonstrates that this is the pathogenetic mechanism responsible for the lung disease with all of the drugs included in this category. However, the fact that in all cases the disease seems to appear only after the patient has been receiving the drug for a period of months to years, suggesting that cumulative toxicity is important, tends to support this concept. Progressive dyspnea and interstitial infiltrates on the chest roentgenogram are the characteristic features of this form of drug-induced lung disease. The pathologic changes observed in lung biopsy specimens obtained from such patients are nonspecific and show varying degrees of inflammation and fibrosis of the alveolar wall.

Certain drugs produce acute pulmonary edema. Both experimental and clinical studies have demonstrated that hemodynamics are normal during episodes of drug-induced pulmonary edema. Thus altered permeability of the alveolar-capillary membrane must be responsible for the development of the pulmonary edema. The mechanism by which this occurs is not clear. Some investigators have suggested that central nervous system impulses are somehow involved, whereas others have suggested that the drugs directly affect humoral mediators that control or modulate alveolar-capillary permeability. Regardless, the permeability of the alveolar-capillary membrane may be altered by drugs, leading to the development of acute pulmonary edema. With a rare exception, this particular syndrome has been associated exclusively with drug overdose or drug abuse.

Several drug-induced lung diseases do not clearly fit into one of these categories. However, in these situations the pathogenesis of the reaction is obvious. As an example, intrapulmonary hemorrhage in a patient receiving anticoagulants is clearly explained by the action of the drug on the clotting mechanism.

CLINICAL ENTITIES

For the purpose of this discussion, the drugs that may produce lung disease are grouped under general headings that reflect the clinical context within which they are usually employed. It will be apparent that within each group some drugs produce direct alveolar injury and others produce hypersensitivity reactions. Thus the drugs within each group do not produce disease by common pathogenetic mechanisms.

Antihypertensive agents

Antihypertensives were among the first drugs to be reported to cause diffuse lung injury. However, the specific antihypertensive drugs implicated in the pathogenesis of lung disease are no longer in general clinical use. Both *hexamethonium* and *mecamylamine* were reported to cause progressive interstitial fibrosis. The mechanism by which these drugs caused interstitial fibrosis is unknown. Some investigators believed that the lung disease was, in fact, not caused by these drugs but resulted from the fact that hypertensive patients receiving these drugs survived for a long time with chronic heart failure. As a result these patients had chronic interstitial and intra-alveolar edema that eventually organized and appeared as chronic fibrosis at autopsy.

Although *hydrochlorothiazide* clearly is not employed exclusively for the treatment of hypertension, the lung disease it causes is included in this section because the clinical manifestations of this disease are most likely to be confusing in the hypertensive patient. Several cases have been reported in which acute pulmonary edema developed within 30 minutes of ingesting a single 50 mg tablet of *hydrochlorothiazide*. Since chronic hypertension is associated with left ventricular failure, drug-induced pulmonary edema may be incorrectly attributed to heart failure in this clinical setting. Thus this entity may be much more common than recognized. The pathogenesis of the disease is unknown.

Antineoplastic agents

The development of pulmonary infiltrates in a patient with a malignant disease who is receiving antineoplastic drugs presents an extremely complex clinical problem, since the pulmonary disease may represent progressive malignant disease, a drug reaction, or a superimposed opportunistic infection. Thus it is extremely important to be aware of the antineoplastic agents that have been implicated in the development of drug-induced lung disease. In addition, the interrelationship of certain forms of drug therapy and radiation injury of the lung must be recognized.

Busulfan was the first antineoplastic agent recognized to cause lung disease. Busulfan causes a syndrome characterized by progressive dyspnea and chronic interstitial infiltrates on the chest roentgenogram. Fever may also be a prominent manifestation. The disease usually develops only after the drug has been used for a year. It is not directly dose related and occurs in a sporadic manner. Discontinuation of the drug and the use of corticosteroids has resulted in reversal of the disease in some patients. Pathologic examination of the lung has revealed a mononuclear cell infiltration and fibrosis of the alveolar wall. Proliferation of granular pneumocytes has also been observed. The cells have a bizarre, atypical appearance that can be useful in making the diagnosis by cytologic examination of expectorated cells. The pathogenesis of this disease is not known.

Methotrexate causes an acute, self-limited pulmonary reaction that is characterized clinically by shortness of breath and fever. Eosinophilia occurs in a large percentage of patients, and the chest roentgenogram reveals patchy alveolar or interstitial infiltrates. The disease usually develops within the first 6 months of therapy, and the patient's condition responds rapidly to corticosteroid administration but also resolves with discontinuation of the drug. Pathologic examination of the lung has revealed a mononuclear wall infiltrate with granuloma formation, suggesting a hypersensitivity pneumonitis. However, a chronic infiltrative process has been recognized in several patients, and severe interstitial fibrosis has been documented in patients dying with the disease. The clinical manifestations and pathologic changes suggest that the reaction is immunologically mediated.

The lung disease induced by *bleomycin* has been well characterized. Progressive dyspnea is the major clinical manifestation of the disease. The chest roentgenogram reveals diffuse interstitial infiltrates (Fig. 14-1). Pathologic examination reveals granular pneumocyte proliferation and alveolar wall inflammation and fibrosis. The disease is clearly related to the total dose of drug administered. Clinical manifestations of lung disease are uncommon when patients have received a total dose of less than 300 mg. However, studies have shown that a restrictive ventilatory defect and impaired gas exchange (decreased vital capacity, total lung capacity, and diffusing capacity) may develop during therapy in patients who are asymptomatic and have a normal chest roentgenogram. When the total dose exceeds 450 mg, pulmonary toxicity can be expected in a substantial percentage of patients. Death resulting from progressive alveolar wall disease has been reported.

Several patients have been reported to develop a hypersensitivity pneumonitis while receiving bleomycin. These patients had eosinophilia and an eosinophilic infiltrate in their lungs. Their condition responded to corticosteroid administration.

Cyclophosphamide has also been implicated in the pathogenesis of a chronic interstitial pneumonitis. Because of the paucity of reports, the lung disease may not be truly related to cyclophosphamide therapy. Nevertheless, it is important to be aware that this drug may have the potential to induce lung disease.

Procarbazine also appears to cause a hypersensitivity reaction in the lung. In at least one case, challenge of the patient with the drug after the pulmonary infiltrates had cleared resulted in a recurrence of the lung disease. This observation not only provides evidence that the lung disease was caused by procarbazine, but also suggests that the lung disease was caused by a hypersensitivity reaction. The presence of eosinophilia in several patients further supports the concept that the reaction is immunologically mediated.

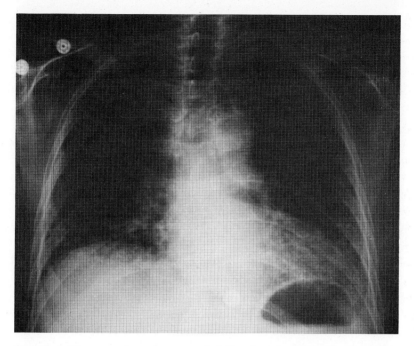

Fig. 14-1. Bleomycin lung disease with diffuse linear infiltrates in both lungs.

Radiation pneumonitis will not be reviewed in this chapter, since it is not a drug-induced disease. However, it is important to be aware of the relationship of drug therapy to radiation pneumonitis so that these forms of lung disease will not be confused. Two clinical situations must be recognized. First, certain forms of chemotherapy appear to increase the potential for radiation injury to the lung. Patients receiving combined chemotherapy and radiation therapy appear to have a higher incidence of radiation pneumonitis than patients receiving comparable doses of radiation alone. In this setting the development of lung disease after exposure to doses of radiation therapy not usually associated with radiation injury may incorrectly be considered to be caused by one of the drugs in the therapeutic regimen. In some situations it may be particularly difficult to differentiate these entities. Second, concommitant corticosteroid administration may suppress the clinical manifestations of radiation injury so that the disease may not become apparent until use of the steroids is tapered or discontinued. Since corticosteroids are frequently included in chemotherapy regimens, the sequence of events leading to clinical manifestations of radiation pneumonitis may incorrectly suggest that the disease results from one of the drugs in the chemotherapy regimen.

Antibiotics

Nitrofurantoin-induced lung disease is the most common drug-induced lung disease recognized. Nitrofurantoin usually produces an acute form of pulmonary disease. The syndrome is characterized by fever, cough, and shortness of breath within hours to days of instituting therapy. Eosinophilia often is present, and the chest roentgenogram reveals diffuse alveolar or interstitial infiltrates (Fig. 14-2). Pleural effusions may also become apparent during the acute illness. The syndrome usually resolves within days after the drug is discontinued. Although the manifestations suggest that the disease is caused by a hypersensitivity reaction, no histologic evidence confirms this. However, several patients with nitrofurantoin reaction have been demonstrated by in vitro lymphocyte assays to have circulating lymphocytes sensitized to the drug. The lymphocytes from at least some patients with an acute reaction undergo blastogenesis or produce lymphokines when exposed to nitrofurantoin in in vitro cultures. Although the results of these in vitro studies do not provide conclusive evidence that the syndrome is immunologically mediated, they at least substantiate the clinical impressions that immune mechanisms are important in the pathogenesis of the syndrome.

Nitrofurantoin may also cause chronic alveolar wall disease. This syndrome is

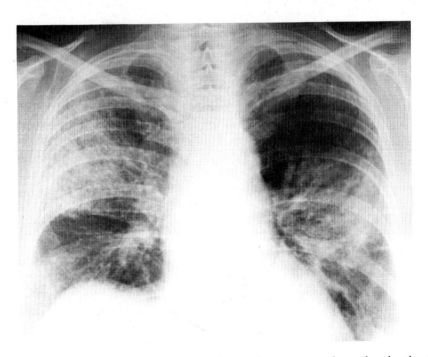

Fig. 14-2. Nitrofurantoin-induced hypersensitivity pneumonitis with patchy alveolar infiltrates in both lungs.

characterized by progressive dyspnea and diffuse interstitial infiltration of the lungs. The reaction usually begins after the patient has been taking the drug for at least 6 months and may appear many years later. In some patients the reaction is reversible when the drug is discontinued or corticosteroids are employed. In most cases the pathologic changes in the lung are those of usual interstitial pneumonitis. However, desquamative interstitial pneumonitis has been documented in two patients receiving chronic nitrofurantoin therapy. The pathogenesis of the chronic alveolar wall disease is unknown.

Penicillin, para-aminosalicylic acid, and the *sulfonamides* have been reported to cause acute drug-induced lung disease. The acute syndrome is characterized by fever, cough, and shortness of breath. Eosinophilia is common, and the chest roentgenogram usually reveals patches of alveolar infiltration. This syndrome usually resolves when drug therapy is discontinued, and the condition may respond rapidly to corticosteroids.

The sulfonamides are pharmacologically related to several other groups of sulfa-containing drugs that are used often in clinical practice. Although these drugs are not antibiotics, they will be included in this section, since cross-reactions between the various sulfa-containing drugs may occur. The clinical and roentgenographic manifestations of the drug reaction are generally similar for each of the drugs. Sulfasalazine is a nonabsorbable sulfonamide used in the treatment of ulcerative colitis. Several cases of a pulmonary reaction to this drug have been reported. A similar reaction has been reported in several patients receiving sulfonylureas for the treatment of diabetes. In one case the pulmonary disease resolved when the sulfonylurea was discontinued and recurred when the patient was placed on sulfamethoxazole for treatment of a urinary tract infection. The drug-induced pulmonary reaction associated with the thiazide diuretics, another group of sulfa-containing drugs, has previously been mentioned in the section on antihypertensives.

Anti-inflammatory agents

One of the most recently recognized drug-induced lung diseases is associated with *gold* therapy. Patients with this syndrome develop cough, dyspnea, and interstitial infiltration several weeks after initiation of gold therapy. Lung biopsies have shown infiltration of the alveolar wall with lymphocytes and plasma cells. The pulmonary disease regresses after discontinuation of therapy. In one of the patients, symptoms recurred on reexposure to gold. Subsequent reports have provided data to suggest that the reaction is probably immunologically mediated.

Several other drugs used in the treatment of arthritis have also been reported to cause lung disease. *Oxyphenylbutazine* and *penicillamine* have been reported to cause chronic interstitial infiltrates after prolonged use. The major clinical feature of these reactions is progressive dyspnea. Spontaneous resolution of the lung disease appears to occur when the drug is discontinued.

Drug abuse and poisoning

Acute pulmonary edema is the most common pulmonary reaction associated with drug abuse or poisoning. Patients with this syndrome usually are in coma with marked respiratory distress. The chest roentgenogram characteristically reveals pulmonary edema with a normal sized heart (Fig. 14-3). This syndrome is most frequently associated with intravenous administration of heroin. However, it has also been reported after nasal heroin, oral methadone, oral salicylates, oral colchicine, and intravenous ethchlorvynol. Cardiac hemodynamics have been documented to be normal during these acute episodes.

Less frequently recognized is the syndrome of angiothrombotic pulmonary hypertension. Patients with this syndrome have gradual onset of dyspnea during exertion associated with progressive linear or nodular infiltrates on the chest roentgenogram. Marked pulmonary hypertension may develop, and the patients may eventually become disabled and die. The pathogenesis of this syndrome has been well defined. Embolization to the pulmonary vessels of the inert filler material used in the preparation of tablets or capsules occurs when these preparations are administered intravenously. Pathologic examination reveals starch or talc granulomas associated with arterial thrombosis and interstitial fibrosis. Tripelennamine has been

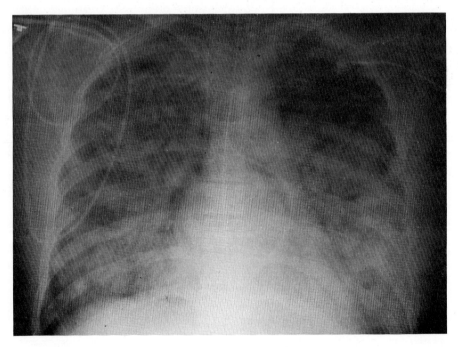

Fig. 14-3. Heroin-induced pulmonary edema with diffuse alveolar infiltrates in both lungs. The heart size is normal.

implicated most frequently in this syndrome, but prolonged intravenous administration of any drug contaminated by an inert substance can be predicted to cause similar pathologic changes.

Miscellaneous

Phenytoin. Conflicting reports have appeared in the literature relating phenytoin therapy to interstitial lung disease. Roentgenographic and physiologic abnormalities consistent with chronic alveolar wall disease have been variably observed in patients taking this drug. In addition, phenytoin has been implicated in the development of acute interstitial process associated with systemic evidence of a drug reaction. These observations suggest that phenytoin may cause alveolar wall disease, although this is rarely clinically apparent. This drug causes generalized adenopathy, and bilateral hilar adenopathy has been documented in several patients.

Cromolyn sodium. Cromolyn sodium has been implicated in the development of lung disease in several patients. In each case the lung disease was associated with eosinophilia and other manifestations, suggesting that immunologic mechanisms were involved in the pathogenesis of the lung reaction. The fact that lymphocytes from patients with clinically apparent adverse reactions to sodium cromolyn undergo blastogenesis and produce lymphokines when exposed to the drug in vitro is evidence supporting this hypothesis. Since this drug is used exclusively in patients with other immunologic lung diseases (asthma and bronchopulmonary aspergillosis), the development of new infiltrates in a patient receiving the drug can cause a great deal of confusion.

Anticoagulants. An uncommon complication of anticoagulants is spontaneous intrapulmonary hemorrhage. Although evidence of bleeding in other parts of the body may be present, hemoptysis may be the only clinical manifestation of this complication. The chest roentgenogram reveals variable pulmonary infiltrates dependent on the degree of intrapulmonary hemorrhage. Examination of alveolar macrophages obtained by bronchoalveolar lavage has recently been demonstrated as useful in substantiating this diagnosis by demonstrating the presence of hemosiderin deposited within these cells.

Chapter 15

EOSINOPHILIC GRANULOMA

Eosinophilic granuloma, Letterer-Siwe disease, and Hand-Schüller-Christian disease have similar clinical and morphologic features that are classified under the category of the pulmonary histiocytic reticuloses. Since Letterer-Siwe disease and Hand-Schüller-Christian disease are extremely rare, the comments in this chapter will be limited to eosinophilic granuloma. However, these diseases share many clinical features, and conversion from one form to another may occur in an individual patient.

Eosinophilic granuloma is an uncommon disease that appears to occur most frequently in adult white persons. Although the disease may be widely disseminated throughout the body, it is most often localized to the lungs and bones. The origin and pathogenesis of the disease are entirely unknown.

PATHOLOGIC CHANGES

The pathologic changes in the lung are variable and depend to a great extent on the stage of the disease when the lung is examined. Early lesions are usually nodular in appearance and microscopically resemble granulomas. These lesions are usually located in peribronchial areas but involve the alveolar walls. Although a variety of cells are present in the lesions, large foamy-appearing histiocytes predominate. In addition, eosinophils usually occur in large numbers. Lymphocytes and plasma cells are also present to a variable degree. Some degree of alveolar wall fibrosis may occur at this stage of the disease.

As the disease progresses, involvement of the alveolar wall becomes more extensive. In addition, the granulomatous inflammation is gradually replaced by fibrosis. As a result, the architecture of the lung may be severely disorganized. Multiple small cysts may develop giving a "honeycomb" appearance during gross examination. As progressive fibrosis develops, the histologic appearance may become totally nonspecific so that it is impossible to make a diagnosis from a biopsy specimen.

CLINICAL MANIFESTATIONS

The clinical manifestations of eosinophilic granuloma are extremely variable. The clinical syndrome depends on the extent of lung involvement and the sites of systemic involvement. Many patients are asymptomatic when the disease is first detected on a routine chest roentgenogram. Cough and dyspnea are the predominant pulmonary symptoms. Spontaneous pneumothoraces occur often and may produce chest pain. Systemic symptoms of fatigue, weight loss, and fever occur in approximately a third of patients. Patients with bone involvement may complain of localized pain over the involved area. Involvement of the posterior pituitary may result in the development of diabetes insipidus.

Physical findings are nonspecific and therefore of little help in diagnosis. Rales may be heard over the lungs, and tenderness may exist over bone lesions. Other physical findings are distinctly uncommon.

ROENTGENOGRAPHIC MANIFESTATIONS

The roentgenographic abnormalities are dependent on the stage of the disease when the roentgenogram is obtained. In the early stage the chest roentgenogram is characterized by the presence of small (1 to 10 mm) nodules that have a predilection for involvement of the upper lobes. As the disease progresses, linear infiltrates predominate. Subsequently multiple cysts become apparent, usually in the upper lobes. The cysts are generally less than 1 cm in diameter but may reach 3 to 5 cm. The presence of diffuse reticulonodular infiltrates with multiple cystic lesions in the upper lobes is highly suggestive of the diagnosis of eosinophilic granuloma. Hilar or mediastinal lymph node enlargement is rarely observed. Spontaneous pneumothoraces are not uncommon. Cystic lesions in the ribs may be observed on the chest roentgenogram.

PHYSIOLOGIC ABNORMALITIES

In the early stage of the disease, routine pulmonary function tests may be normal. As the disease progresses, lung volumes and the diffusing capacity decrease. Expiratory flow rates are normal. Resting hypoxemia occurs in many patients. In some patients the residual volume may increase as the disease progresses, conceivably as a result of the development of cystic structures throughout the lung.

DIAGNOSIS

Lung biopsy is required for diagnosis in most cases. However, in some patients, biopsy of a bone lesion may be diagnostic. The combination of diffuse interstitial infiltrates on the chest roentgenogram and either diabetes insipidus or cystic bone lesions strongly suggests the diagnosis. Lung biopsy may not be diagnostic when progressive fibrosis has replaced the granulomatous lesions. Other laboratory studies are of no diagnostic value.

CLINICAL COURSE

The disease may spontaneously resolve. However, in many patients the pulmonary involvement is slowly progressive over a number of years, and patients may become disabled and eventually die of respiratory failure. No known therapy for the disease exists.

Chapter 16

ALVEOLAR PROTEINOSIS

Alveolar proteinosis is an unusual disease characterized by the accumulation of an amorphous, periodic acid–Schiff (PAS) positive material in the intra-alveolar space.

PATHOLOGIC CHANGES

The pathologic changes observed in the disease are characterized, at least initially, by two predominant features. First, the alveolar air spaces in involved areas of lung are filled with an amorphous PAS positive material (Fig. 16-1). Second, the alveolar walls are normal. Thus, early in the stage of the disease, the pathologic changes are limited to the accumulation of lipid-containing material in the alveolar space.

In some patients with long-standing disease, inflammation and fibrosis of the alveolar walls develop. Indeed, these changes may be observed at a stage when the accumulation of characteristic PAS positive material in the alveolar space is no longer apparent. No specific pathologic changes in the alveolar walls allow diagnosis of the disease during this stage.

PATHOGENESIS

The origin and pathogenesis of alveolar proteinosis are unknown. Analysis of the composition of the material filling the alveolar air spaces has shown that the material has many of the properties of surfactant. The material is high in lipid and protein and has surface active properties. These observations have prompted speculation that the material accumulates in the alveolar space as a result of increased production of surfactant by alveolar type II cells or a decreased clearance of the material, presumably by alveolar macrophages. The results of limited studies suggest that decreased clearance of the material is of primary importance.

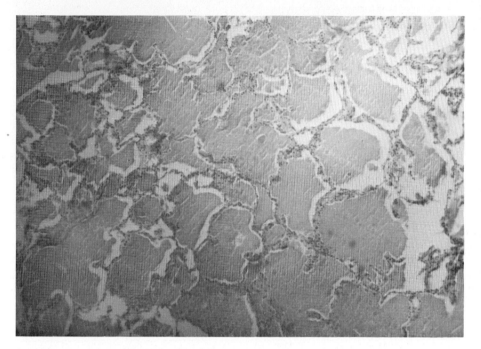

Fig. 16-1. Alveolar proteinosis. Microscopic section of a lung biopsy specimen demonstrating the presence of proteinaceous fluid in the alveolar space. The alveolar walls appear normal.

CLINICAL MANIFESTATIONS

Progressive dyspnea and cough are the predominant symptoms of alveolar proteinosis. These symptoms are nonspecific and provide no clue to the diagnosis. During physical examination, diffuse rales are usually audible over the lungs posteriorly. Digital clubbing and cyanosis are often present. These findings are also present in patients with a variety of different diffuse lung diseases and thus are of little diagnostic importance.

ROENTGENOGRAPHIC MANIFESTATIONS

Alveolar proteinosis is exhibited as classically an alveolar filling pattern on the chest roentgenogram (Fig. 16-2). The alveolar infiltrates tend to be located in the perihilar regions and bases of the lungs. Although other diffuse lung diseases may be manifest by alveolar infiltration, this roentgenographic finding should raise the possiblity that the patient has alveolar proteinosis.

PHYSIOLOGIC MANIFESTATIONS

Routine pulmonary function tests reveal a decrease in the total lung capacity and diffusing capacity but normal expiratory flow rates. Arterial hypoxemia is almost

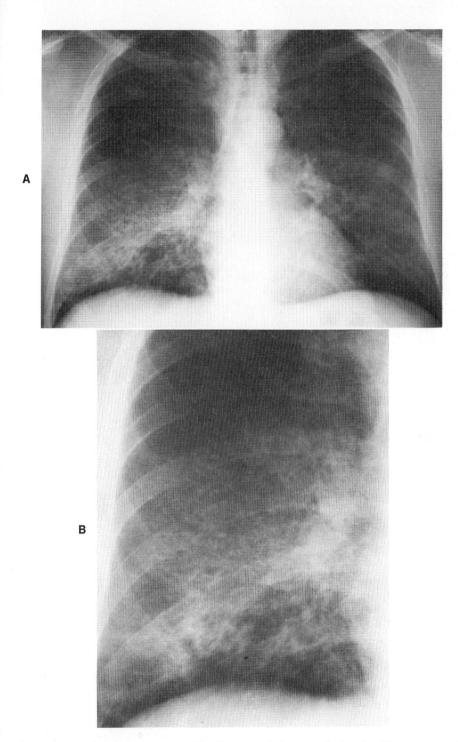

Fig. 16-2. A, Alveolar proteinosis. **B,** Close-up of the typical alveolar filling pattern that characterizes this disease.

always present. These changes are all nonspecific and are observed in most forms of diffuse infiltrative lung disease. However, the specific pathophysiology of the gas-exchange defect causing arterial hypoxemia is highly suggestive of the diagnosis of alveolar proteinosis. This disease is characterized by an increase in the intrapulmonary shunt fraction. In patients with alveolar proteinosis the shunt fraction generally exceeds 10% of the cardiac output and often approaches 15% to 20%. In most other chronic, diffuse lung diseases, the shunt fraction is only minimally elevated and rarely exceeds 10%. Thus analysis of the pathophysiology of gas exchange can be useful in identifying patients with alveolar proteinosis.

DIAGNOSIS

Under most circumstances the diagnosis of alveolar proteinosis is made by lung biopsy. Open lung biopsy is usually performed to obtain tissue for pathologic evaluation. However, transbronchial lung biopsy may also be diagnostic in a high percentage of patients. Although this technique has a substantial sampling error and significant crush artifact of the biopsy specimen, the pathologic changes of alveolar proteinosis are so characteristic that they can usually be identified in transbronchial biopsy specimens.

Recent experience also suggests that the diagnosis can be made by bronchoalveolar lavage. In cases of alveolar proteinosis, the lavage effluent often returns as a creamy-like fluid. In addition, examination of the bronchoalveolar cells obtained by lavage reveals that the alveolar macrophages are filled with PAS positive material. These changes have not been observed in other diseases and thus may be highly specific for the diagnosis of alveolar proteinosis.

Finally, the serum concentration of lactic dehydrogenase (LDH) is elevated in patients with this disease and tends to fluctuate with disease activity. LDH levels may also increase in other forms of diffuse lung disease but usually not with the regularity and to the same degree as that observed in patients with alveolar proteinosis. Although lung biopsy is required for an absolute diagnosis, the combination of diffuse alveolar infiltrates on the chest roentgenogram, an increase in the intrapulmonary shunt fraction, and an increase in the serum concentration of LDH is highly suggestive of the diagnosis.

TREATMENT

The clinical course of alveolar proteinosis is variable. In some patients the disease spontaneously resolves only to reappear at a later date. The disease may remain stable for many years or be progressive. As previously mentioned, interstitial pneumonitis and fibrosis may develop in some patients. These changes are irreversible and generally occur in patients with chronic progressive disease.

No specific treatment for this disease exists. A variety of therapeutic approaches have been used in an attempt to promote resolution of the intra-alveolar material. Corticosteroids, heparin, and trypsin nebulization have all been reported to be successful on occasion. However, because the disease may undergo spontaneous resolution, these sporadic reports must be interpreted with caution.

Physical removal of the intra-alveolar material by whole lung lavage with saline has been employed in a number of patients. There is little doubt that this procedure is beneficial in selected patients. Clearing of the chest roentgenogram and a decrease in the pulmonary shunt fraction in the immediate post-lavage period provide objective evidence of the efficacy of this procedure. Some patients appear to go into a long-term remission after lavage, whereas the material rapidly reaccumulates in others. This procedure should not be undertaken lightly. Because of the complex nature of performing whole lung lavage, the procedure should be performed only in special centers that are experienced in the evaluation and management of patients with this disease.

Patients with alveolar proteinosis have an apparent predilection for infection of the lung by *Nocardia* organisms and various fungi. The reasons for the occurrence of these infections is unknown. It is important to consider the possiblity of such an infectious complication when unusual clinical features develop during the course of the disease so that appropriate treatment can be instituted.

Section three

THE VASCULATURE

Chapter 17

NORMAL STRUCTURE AND FUNCTION

STRUCTURE

The lung is supplied by two arterial systems. The pulmonary artery delivers venous blood to the alveolar-capillary network, whereas the bronchial artery supplies oxygenated blood to the capillaries of the airways, pleura, and major vessels. In addition to these arterial systems, the lung contains an extensive lymphatic network. Each component of the pulmonary vasculature is extremely important in maintaining the overall function of the lung.

Pulmonary arterial system

The main pulmonary artery originates directly from the outflow tract of the right ventricle. The pulmonary arterial system divides in much the same manner as the tracheobronchial tree. Branches of the pulmonary arteries accompany corresponding branches of the airways to the level of the terminal bronchioles. As the main branches of the pulmonary artery enter the hilum of the lung, they become surrounded by sheaths of connective tissue. The vessels remain in these connective tissue sheaths as they course through the lung. This connective tissue layer is perforated only by right-angle branches of the pulmonary arteries that enter each pulmonary lobule to supply the alveolar-capillary system.

Three major types of pulmonary arteries can be identified on the basis of the histologic features of the vessel wall. The vessels accompanying the airways to the level of the terminal bronchioles are the *elastic arteries*. These vessels have distinctive layers of elastic fibers embedded in muscle throughout the thickness of the vessel wall. *Muscular arteries* accompany bronchioles into the lobules of the lung. These vessels have a distinct muscular medium that is well defined by internal and external elastic lamina. Although they are termed "muscular arteries," under normal circumstances the muscular medium comprises less than 5% of the external diameter of the vessel. *Pulmonary arterioles,* the terminal branches of the muscular arteries, are located within the lung lobules. Some of these vessels have incomplete muscle layers, and others have no muscle layer at all. Since the histologic features of these vessels are different from those of systemic arterioles that have well-defined muscular layers, there is some controversy as to whether these vessels should really be considered arterioles. Nevertheless, these vessels directly supply the capillary network of the alveolar wall. In the absence of a muscular layer, it is impossible to distinguish these vessels from venules in histologic sections.

Each arteriole feeds about four to twelve capillary loops, each of which may traverse several alveolar walls before combining to enter a pulmonary venule. Evidence suggests that some arterioles contain contractile cells which allow these vessels to function as sphincters, thus controlling blood flow to the capillary beds. The intermittent perfusion of capillary beds observed under experimental conditions may be related to the sphincter activity of these vessels.

During the stage of growth and development of the lung, a number of important changes occur in the pulmonary vessels. During fetal growth the pulmonary arterial system is perfused by only a small fraction of right ventricular output, the majority being shunted into the aorta through the ductus arteriosus. During this period, the pulmonary arterial system is dominated by small arteries that possess a thick muscular medium and swollen cuboidal epithelial cells, both of which contribute to narrowing the lumen of the vessels. These vessels present a large resistance to blood flow and thus effectively shunt blood into the aorta. At birth the lumen and external diameter of these vessels increase rapidly with thinning of the muscular medium. This is accompanied by a fall in pulmonary vascular resistance and redirection of pulmonary blood flow through the pulmonary arterial system. The muscular pulmonary arteries assume their adult characteristics before 1 year of age.

During fetal development, the large elastic arteries accompany the airways to approximately the level of the bronchioles just as is observed in the mature lung. Changes in these vessels at birth are not nearly so dramatic as those occurring in the muscular arteries. Arterioles are not clearly recognized in the lung until several months after birth. Their development continues as gas-exchanging units develop in the first two decades of life. All the vessels in the lung continue to increase in diameter relative to the thickness of their walls as lung growth continues during the first two decades of life. Other than the development of intimal fibrous thickening, little change occurs in normal pulmonary arteries during adult aging.

In the adult lung, clear evidence suggests that direct communications between pulmonary arterioles and venules occur. The purpose of these communications is unclear. However, they are a potential pathway by which blood may shunt around the capillary network. These anastomoses may provide the pathway for blood flow when perfusion of the capillary bed is limited by contraction of the feeding arteriole.

Certain features of the alveolar-capillary bed have been discussed previously. However, it is worth reemphasizing that this capillary network is not only structured for gas exchange but also to accomplish certain metabolic functions of the lung. The capillary consists of an endothelial cell resting on a continuous basement membrane. Thus, in this sense, it is no different structurally than other capillaries. Ultrastructural examination demonstrates that the margins of adjacent endothelial cells abut bluntly or interdigitate and overlap. Adjacent membranes seem to fuse except for small slits through which the intravascular and extravascular spaces can communicate. The size of the slits apparently is not fixed and is somewhat dependent on the intravascular pressure. The tight nature of the endothelial junctions suggests that the pulmonary capillaries are relatively less permeable than capillaries of many visceral organs such as liver or kidney.

The pulmonary-capillary endothelial cell has numerous surface projections and contains enormous numbers of pinocytotic vesicles. These ultrastructural features are thought to be important in the metabolic function of the lung. The lung is involved in the metabolism of a number of bioactive polypeptides (bradykinin and angiotensin) and biogenic amines (catecholamines and serotonin). The enzymes responsible for some of these activities appear to reside on the plasma membrane of the endothelial cell. Thus the surface projections and pinocytotic vesicles greatly expand the surface area available for metabolic activity.

The pulmonary venous system has no distinctive features. Unlike the pulmonary arteries, veins are remote from the bronchi for much of their course. The pulmonary veins collect blood from the pulmonary capillaries draining gas-exchanging units and also from the capillaries of the pleura and some bronchi. The venous effluent from these latter two capillary beds is deoxygenated venous blood in contrast to the oxygenated blood leaving the alveolar capillaries.

Bronchial artery system

The bronchial arteries arise from the aorta at the level of the first and second intercostal arteries. In addition, one bronchial artery regularly arises from an intercostal artery on the right. A number of anatomic variations occur in the origin of these arteries. Branches may arise from the subclavian, innominate, or internal mammary arteries. Usually two bronchial artery trunks enter the hilum of each lung. These arteries accompany the bronchi to the level of the terminal bronchioles and provide branches that feed the capillary network of the bronchi, pleura, and major vessels. The bronchial veins draining these capillary beds empty into the azygous vein on the right and the hemiazygous or innominate vein on the left.

It has been convincingly demonstrated that precapillary anastomoses exist between the bronchial artery and pulmonary artery. The functional significance of these communications in the normal lung is unclear. However, in disease states these anastomoses may markedly enlarge, resulting in perfusion of the gas exchanging parenchyma by systemic bronchial artery blood that has shunted into the pulmonary artery.

Lymphatic system

The lung possesses an extensive lymphatic network. Lymphatics course across the surface of the lung within the connective tissue of the visceral pleura and

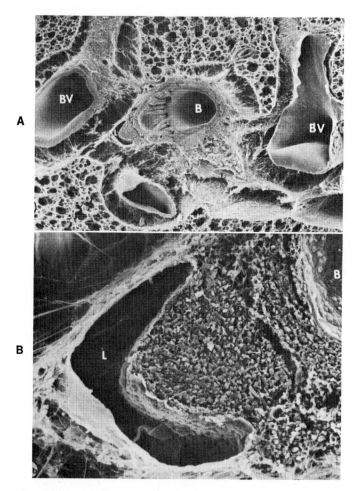

Fig. 17-1. A, Scanning microscopy showing the relationship of the lymphatic channel *(L)* to the airway *(B)* and vasculature *(BV)*. **B,** High-power view of the lymphatic channel demonstrated in **A.**

From Brain, J.D., Proctor, D.F., and Reed, L.M.: Respiratory defense mechanisms, New York, 1977, Marcel Dekker, Inc.

throughout the parenchyma of the lung in the perivascular and peribronchiolar connective tissue. These two lymphatic networks are connected by vessels that penetrate the surface of the lung. Lymph flow is generally separate in each system because of the orientation of valves in the lymphatic vessel. Lymph on the surface of the lung makes its way to the hilum by transversing the surface, whereas interparenchymal lymph is conveyed to the hilum through the perivascular and peribronchial lymph channels (Fig. 17-1). The pulmonary lymph flows into the hilar nodes and then to tracheobronchial and paratracheal nodes. Ultimately lung lymph may drain into either the right lymphatic duct or thoracic duct. Substantial species differences exist in the relative drainage of lung lumph into each of these ducts. In the human the majority of pulmonary lymph empties into the right thoracic duct.

The pulmonary lymphatic vessels consist of endothelial cells that sit on an incomplete basement membrane. In some areas the basement membrane is absent, and the cells are directly in contact with a fine perilymphatic connective tissue. Ultrastructurally, the endothelial cells have numerous luminal cytoplasmic projections (Fig. 17-2). This cell layer is discontinuous with open cell junctions and intercellular gaps. Lymphatic vessels do not extend into the alveolar wall. Terminal branches of the peribronchiolar lymphatics form a juxta-alveolar network that ultimately drain the gas-exchanging tissue (Fig. 17-3). It has been proposed that these lymphatic channels directly communicate with the interstitial space of the alveolar wall.

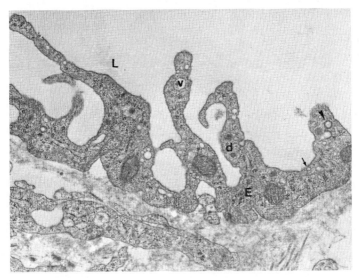

Fig. 17-2. Electron micrograph of a lymphatic endothelial cell. Cytoplasmic protrusions extend into the lumen of the lymphatic channel.

From Lauweryns, J.M., and Baert, J.H.: Alveolar clearance and the role of the pulmonary lymphatics, Am. Rev. Respir. Dis. **115:**625, 1977.

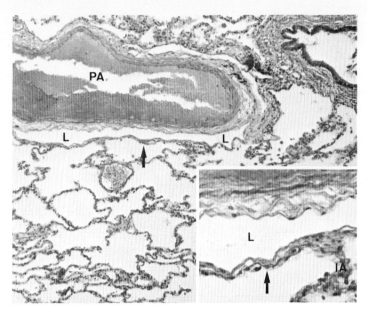

Fig. 17-3. Microscopic section demonstrating the juxta-alveolar channel *(L)* in proximity to the connective tissue sheath of a pulmonary vessel. The insert shows the juxta-alveolar relationship in greater detail.

From Lauweryns, J.M., and Baert, J.H.: Alveolar clearance and the role of the pulmonary lymphatics, Am. Rev. Respir. Dis. 115:625, 1977.

FUNCTION
Pulmonary arterial system

The pulmonary arterial system is characterized by low resistance and high compliance. As a result of these properties, the pressure in the system may remain relatively constant despite marked fluctuations in blood flow. Thus the work the right ventricle must perform to perfuse the pulmonary-capillary bed remains relatively constant despite marked increases in cardiac ouput. Similarly, when cardiac output falls, the perfusing pressure in the pulmonary vascular bed does not decrease proportionately. As a result, capillary perfusion is maintained in all regions of the lung. If the pulmonary arteries were not highly compliant but functioned more like rigid tubes, changes in cardiac ouput would result in marked changes in the perfusing pressure in the vessels.

As pulmonary vascular resistance increases, the right ventricle must perform more work to generate the pressure required to maintain right ventricular output. There is a limit to which the right ventricle may tolerate increased work loads beyond which the structure and function of the right ventricle begin to be altered.

Thus the adverse effects of an increase in pulmonary vascular resistance are manifested primarily by the effects of the increased resistance on right ventricular function. This sequence of changes will be discussed in detail in Chapter 18.

In contrast, a decrease in pulmonary artery pressure may affect the distribution of perfusion in the pulmonary-capillary bed and thus result in abnormalities in pulmonary gas exchange. To appreciate the mechanism by which this occurs, it is necessary to review the factors that influence the distribution of perfusion in the normal lung. Gravity is the most important determinant of the distribution of perfusion in upright humans and will be considered in greatest detail.

Under normal circumstances, the right ventricular systolic pressure transmitted to the pulmonary artery is approximately 25 mm Hg. Although right ventricular diastolic pressure falls to zero, closure of the pulmonary valve maintains a diastolic pressure in the pulmonary artery of approximately 9 mm Hg. Thus mean pressure in the main pulmonary artery is approximately 14 mm Hg. Mean left atrial pressure is 8 mm Hg; thus the pressure drop caused by resistance across the pulmonary vascular bed is only 5 mm Hg.

The effect of gravity on the intravascular pressure at any point in the lung is simple. At the site of measurement the pressure in the pulmonary vessels increases or decreases an amount equal to the height of the blood column above or below the location of the main pulmonary artery. Vascular pressures can be expressed in either mm Hg or cm H_2O (1 cm H_2O is equal to 0.735 mm Hg). Since the effect of gravity on pressure is related to the height of the column of blood in the pulmonary vessels, it is most logical in this context to express pulmonary arterial pressure in cm H_2O. For every centimeter above the level of the main pulmonary artery, pressure in the vascular bed decreases 1 cm H_2O, whereas for every centimeter below this level, the pressure increases 1 cm H_2O. Thus, for purposes of general discussion, if one assumes that mean pressure in the main pulmonary artery is 20 cm H_2O (14 mm Hg), the pressure in a vessel 10 cm above the main pulmonary artery would be 10 cm H_2O, and the pressure in a vessel 10 cm below the main pulmonary artery would be 30 cm H_2O (Fig. 17-4).

These gravity-related pressure changes have several important effects. First, if the height of pulmonary arterial branches above the main pulmonary artery exceeds the perfusing pressure in the main pulmonary artery, blood flow may cease in the apices of the lung. For example, if main pulmonary arterial pressure were 10 cm H_2O and the height of the lung above the main pulmonary artery were 15 cm, the pressure in the pulmonary arterial branch 10 cm above the main pulmonary artery would fall to zero. As a result, no perfusion of capillaries would occur in the top 5 cm of lung. This is a simple analysis that serves to emphasize the effects of gravity on pulmonary artery pressures. It is unlikely that blood flow ever ceases under these conditions in the normal lung.

In the normal lung the gravity-dependent pressure changes are most impor-

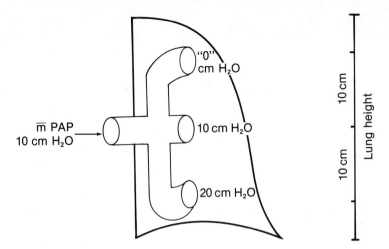

Fig. 17-4. Effect of gravity on the perfusion pressure in the pulmonary arterial system of the upright lung. The mean pressure in intrapulmonary arteries varies from the mean pressure in the main pulmonary artery as it enters the lung by an amount approximately equal to the height of the blood column at the point of measurement above or below the main pulmonary artery.

tant for their effect on regional blood flow. Since the pulmonary arteries are highly compliant, transmural pressure across these vessels has an important influence on blood flow. Larger transmural pressures dilate the vessel, producing a decrease in vascular resistance and an increase in flow. The pressure outside all the pulmonary vessels is identical. However, since intravascular pressure, which is gravity dependent, varies, transmural pressure across vessels also varies throughout the lung. Thus, if the vessels are equally compliant throughout the lung, flow will be greatest in areas with the largest transmural pressure and will change proportionately throughout the lung depending on the relative height of vessels above or below the main pulmonary artery. Although for instructional purposes this explanation is reasonable, it may not be entirely correct, since other factors that influence fluid kinetics have not been considered, and there may well be differences in the compliance of pulmonary arteries at different sites in the lung. Nevertheless, pulmonary blood flow is greatest at the base of the lung in upright individuals and decreases proportionately as the apex of the lung is approached (Fig. 17-5).

Two other factors may affect the distribution of perfusion. Local "autoregulation" of perfusion in capillary beds by constriction of the precapillary arterioles has been mentioned previously. This phenomenon may assume importance in certain pathophysiologic states but probably plays little role in controlling distribution of perfusion in the normal lung. Similarly, alveolar pressure, which is of little importance in the normal lung, may be an important determinant of capillary perfusion

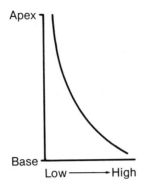

Fig. 17-5. Relative blood flow per unit of lung volume in the upright lung. Blood flow increases per unit of lung volume from the apex to the base.

in certain situations. Because of the potential importance of this phenomenon, it must be reviewed in some detail.

The alveolar capillaries are collapsible vessels that are subject to external pressure. Thus, if alveolar pressure exceeds the arteriolar or capillary pressure, flow through the capillary must cease. In normal humans this probably does not occur. However, if alveolar pressure is increased by positive pressure mechanical ventilation, alveolar pressure may collapse alveolar capillaries and thus alter ventilation/perfusion relationships throughout the lung. Increases in alveolar pressure that are not high enough to produce capillary collapse may still influence capillary blood flow if alveolar pressure exceeds venous pressure. Under normal circumstances, capillary blood flow is determined by the arterial-to-venous pressure gradient across the capillary bed. If alveolar pressure exceeds venous pressure, flow is determined primarily by the transmural pressure gradient across the alveolar-capillary wall. Under these circumstances, flow would continue through the capillary bed but would be determined by the transmural pressure across the capillary wall and the effect of the transmural pressure on the distensibility of the vessels.

Areas within the lung with pressure relationships corresponding to these three conditions have been termed zones I, II, and III respectively by West (Fig. 17-6). Zones II and III are present in the normal lung. Zone II exists in the normal upright lung near the apex. Alveolar pressure exceeds ventricular pressure in these areas, not because alveolar pressure increases near the apex, but because gravity produces a decrease in venous pressure as the apex is approached. If pulmonary venous pressure increases, as might be observed in left ventricular failure, zone II become less extensive. As a result, capillary perfusion becomes more uniform throughout the entire lung.

One final consequence of the effect of gravity on intravascular pressure must be considered. Transmural pressure across capillaries is higher in the base of the

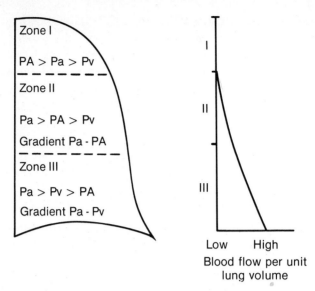

Fig. 17-6. Relationship between alveolar *(PA)*, arterial *(Pa)*, and venous *(Pv)* pressures in various regions of the upright lung and the effect of these relationships on blood flow per unit of lung volume. The zones depicted in the figure are merely representative of potential zones that may exist in the lung.

lung than in other areas. Since the transmural pressure across the alveolar-capillary wall is one of the forces that promotes filtration of fluid from the intravascular compartment to the interstitial space of the alveolar wall, edema fluid is more likely to accumulate in the base of the lung before more cephalad zones are affected.

Pulmonary lymphatics

In recent years the function of the pulmonary lymphatics has been studied in great detail. The lymphatics play an important role in the clearance of particles from the alveolar surface and in the removal of fluid from the interstitial space of the alveolar wall.

Elegant studies using a variety of identifiable tracers have shown convincingly that the pulmonary lymphatics play an important role in the clearance of particulate material inhaled into the alveolus. A number of pathways by which such particles make their way into the lymphatics have been traced. It appears that particulate material, in addition to being ingested by alveolar macrophages that leave the alveolus via the airways, may also be transported into the interstitium of the alveolar wall through type I pneumocytes. The material may then directly enter the lymphatics either through open intercellular junctions or by endocytosis by lymphatic endothelial cells. The material may also be ingested by interstitial macrophages that also enter the lymphatics through the intercellular junctions. Regardless of the pathway, the end result is clearance of the material from the alveolus.

It seems reasonable to conclude that the structure of the lymphatics contributes to its role in particulate clearance. Certainly the discontinuous basement membrane and the open intercellular endothelial junctions suggest that the lymphatics are more permeable than capillary endothelial cells. In addition the lymphatic endothelial cell appears to possess a high endocytic capacity for direct uptake of particles.

It has also been convincingly demonstrated in recent years that the pulmonary lymphatics are critical in controlling the volume of extravascular fluid in the lungs. The pulmonary capillary is freely permeable to water and small solutes. The filtration of fluid across the alveolar-capillary membrane into the interstitium of the alveolar wall is controlled by the same Starling forces that are operative in all capillary beds. This topic will be discussed in detail in Chapter 18.

Chapter 18

PATHOPHYSIOLOGY

The pathogenetic mechanisms involved in pulmonary vascular disease are less well recognized than those involved in diseases of the airways or alveolar walls. Primary pulmonary vascular diseases occur infrequently, and in most situations the origin and pathogenesis of the vascular injury are unknown. However, pathogenetic mechanisms that may be involved in vascular injury can be proposed by extrapolation from certain clinical observations.

The immunologic mechanisms that produce systemic vascular injury may also produce injury to the pulmonary arterial system. Thus the deposition of antibody or antigen-antibody complexes in the vascular wall may elicit an immune reaction that results in infiltration of the vessel and perivascular tissue by inflammatory cells and may result in destruction of the vessel. As will be discussed later, the manifestations of this type of vascular injury are determined to a great extent by the site or sites along the arterial system that such injury occurs. Some immunologically mediated diseases involve primarily the capillary bed, whereas others involve small or large arteries.

The ultrastructure and/or function of the alveolar-capillary bed may be altered by a number of bioactive substances without causing capillary damage that is identifiable with light microscopy. This type of vascular injury generally results in an increase in the permeability of the alveolar-capillary wall so that proteins and other high molecular weight solutes may be filtered into the interstitial space of the alveolar wall. As a result of the increased extravascular lung water and precipitation of proteins on the alveolar wall, the structure and gas-exchange function of the alveolus may be dramatically altered. Certain kinins, prostaglandins, and clotting factors may all be involved in this type of capillary injury. The clinical conditions that are associated with this type of capillary injury are variable and include sepsis, shock, certain drug and toxin exposures, and a variety of other systemic diseases.

Probably the most common disease of the pulmonary arterial system, pulmonary embolic disease, does not truly involve direct injury to the pulmonary vasculature. In this disease the pulmonary vasculature is involved simply because its capillary bed is anatomically imposed between the systemic venous and arterial systems. However, as part of the process involved in clot lysis or recanalization of the vessel, secondary changes may occur in the vessel at the site of impaction of an embolus.

At present, primary diseases of the bronchial artery system or pulmonary lymphatic system have not been identified. Thus discussion of general pathogenetic mechanisms involving these components of the lung vasculature is unnecessary.

Two major pathophysiologic states reflect disease of the pulmonary vasculature. First, an increase in pulmonary vascular resistance may occur if either the compliance or total volume of the vascular bed is decreased. As a result of the increased resistance, pulmonary hypertension may develop. Pulmonary hypertension is important primarily because of its adverse effect on the structure of the right ventricle. Second, an increase in hydrostatic forces or altered permeability of the alveolar capillary leads to increased filtration of fluid across the alveolar-capillary wall into the alveolar interstitial space. In both situations, clearance of the filtered fluid by pulmonary lymphatics is critical in maintaining a relatively normal extravascular lung water volume. If lymphatic function is impaired or the volume of liquid that is filtered overwhelms the clearance mechanism, interstitial and subsequently intra-alveolar pulmonary edema may occur. Thus the discussion of the pathophysiology of pulmonary vascular injury primarily focuses on two clinical conditions: cor pulmonale and pulmonary edema.

COR PULMONALE

"Cor pulmonale" describes abnormalities of right ventricular structure or function associated with pulmonary vascular or pulmonary parenchymal disease. Pulmonary hypertension is the common denominator that leads to the development of right ventricular dilation, hypertrophy, or both. To a great extent the ventricular abnormality in cor pulmonale depends on the degree and duration of pulmonary hypertension. Although there is controversy about the presence of abnormalities of left ventricular function in cor pulmonale, there is no question that the predominant abnormalities in cardiac function are localized to the right ventricle.

Pathogenesis

The pulmonary arterial system is characterized by low resistance and high compliance. In contrast to the systemic arterial system, neural mechanisms appear to play little role in altering the functional characteristics of the pulmonary vascular bed. Thus increased resistance in the pulmonary arterial system usually reflects the presence of diseases that directly affect major pulmonary arteries or obliterate portions of the alveolar-capillary bed. However, alveolar hypoxia and acidemia are powerful stimulants of pulmonary pressor responses.

Under normal circumstances the right ventricle must perform relatively little work to perfuse the pulmonary vascular bed. However, if cardiac ouput remains constant, an increase in resistance in the pulmonary vascular bed results in an increase in pulmonary arterial pressure. In this situation, right ventricular work must increase to maintain constant pulmonary perfusion. As a result the right ventricle may hypertrophy in response to the increased work load. Right ventricular hypertrophy is most likely to develop when the pressure load is increased gradually over an extended period. If pulmonary artery resistance increases abruptly, the right ventricle may not have adequate time to hypertrophy and may simply dilate. Right ventricular failure may ultimately occur under either of these circumstances. When right ventricular failure occurs, systemic venous congestion, salt and water retention, and edema develop rapidly.

The hemodynamic features of cor pulmonale depend on the stage of the disease at the time measurements are obtained. It is instructive to consider the evolution of the hemodynamic changes that occur in this condition. An increase in pulmonary vascular resistance is the first hemodynamic change to occur. At this early stage the pulmonary arterial pressure may remain normal at rest and increase only during exercise in response to an increase in right ventricular output. Eventually sustained pulmonary hypertension develops. Despite the presence of sustained pulmonary hypertension, right ventricular output and right ventricular end diastolic pressures initially remain normal at rest and during exercise. However, to maintain right ventricular output as the disease progresses, right ventricular end diastolic pressure may increase initially only during exercise but eventually also at rest. Finally, as the right ventricle decompensates, right ventricular output fails to increase normally during exercise and eventually becomes decreased at rest. Left ventricular function remains essentially normal throughout this sequence of events.

In patients with pure right ventricular failure, the circulating blood volume is expanded just as it is in left ventricular failure. However, in right ventricular failure the pulmonary blood volume comprises a normal fraction of the total blood volume (approximately 10%). In contrast, in left ventricular failure the pulmonary blood volume may comprise a disproportionately large fraction of the total blood volume. Thus any element of left ventricular failure will tend to exaggerate the hemodynamics of cor pulmonale by increasing the pulmonary blood volume and extravascular lung water. Thus left ventricular function should be carefully evaluated in patients with cor pulmonale, and appropriate treatment should be administered when indicated.

Right ventricular failure may resolve, if factors that contribute to increased pulmonary vascular resistance can be reversed. Primary pulmonary vascular or pulmonary parenchymal diseases are generally chronic in nature and irreversible. Thus structural changes in the pulmonary arterial system caused by these diseases are usually irreversible.

The important role that alveolar hypoxia plays in elevating pulmonary vascular resistance in lung disease is emphasized by the fact that chronic alveolar hypoxia itself, even in the absence of lung disease, may lead to the development of cor pulmonale. Thus it is likely that alveolar hypoxia contributes in an important way to the increased pulmonary vascular resistance associated with pulmonary parenchymal disease. Support for this concept is derived from studies showing that the decrease in the vascular bed is generally insufficient to produce the degree of hemodynamic alteration observed in emphysema and other lung diseases. Thus episodes of right ventricular decompensation may be reversible if alveolar hypoxia can be corrected.

Clinical manifestations

Cor pulmonale is a common cardiac disorder because of its association with chronic bronchitis and emphysema. Nevertheless, the diagnosis is frequently overlooked because the clinical manifestations may be difficult to recognize in patients with extensive lung disease. In addition, there is a tendency to reserve the diagnosis of cor pulmonale for patients with right ventricular failure and to overlook the stage characterized by right ventricular hypertrophy or dilation.

Pulmonary hypertension and right ventricular hypertrophy may be evident during examination of the heart. The second heart sound may be narrowly split and the pulmonic valve closure sound so accentuated that it may be palpable in the second left intercostal space. On occasion, murmurs of pulmonary vascular insufficiency or outlet obstruction may be audible. Finally, a right ventricular lift may be palpable along the sternal border. As right ventricular failure develops, a right ventricular gallop sound and a murmur of tricuspid valve insufficiency may develop. Prominent a and v waves may be identified in the jugular venous pulse.

As the right ventricle fails, venous congestion and peripheral edema rapidly develop. Hepatic enlargement may develop as a result of congestive changes. In addition to lower extremity edema, ascites and hydrothorax may be present. Clinical evidence of decreased cardiac output is frequently present. Cyanosis is often observed during this stage of the disease.

Diagnosis

The physical findings of cor pulmonale are frequently masked by the presence of extensive lung disease. Therefore diagnostic studies must be obtained to make a correct diagnosis. Although the chest roentgenogram is often of little value, severe pulmonary hypertension can be expected if dilated main pulmonary arteries are observed. In the absence of lung disease, attenuation of peripheral vessels may be observed on the chest roentgenogram, but this sign cannot be appreciated when extensive parenchymal disease is present. It is extremely difficult to accurately identify right ventricular enlargement on the chest roentgenogram. However, encroachment on the anterior cardiac border against the sternum on the lateral chest roentgenogram suggests the presence of right ventricular enlargement.

An electrocardiogram may be useful for diagnosis. Right axial deviation and a prominent R wave in lead I are highly suggestive of right ventricular enlargement. In addition, P wave abnormalities may be observed in the limb leads.

Cardiac catheterization is obviously the most specific method for diagnosis. The pulmonary vascular resistance and pulmonary arterial pressure can be directly measured, and the functional state of the right ventricle, at rest and during exercise, can be evaluated. Furthermore, diseases causing an increase in pulmonary-capillary wedge pressure and cardiac shunt lesions can be excluded as causes of pulmonary hypertension at the time of catheterization. Noninvasive techniques for evaluating cardiac function have not yet proved to be highly useful in identifying abnormalities in right ventricular function or the presence of pulmonary hypertension.

Treatment

The treatment of cor pulmonale is directed at decreasing pulmonary arterial pressure. Because of the nature of the diseases that cause pulmonary hypertension, often little can be done to affect the structural changes in the pulmonary vascular bed that develop in the course of these diseases. Thus therapy is primarily directed at correcting alveolar hypoxia by improving ventilation or by the use of oxygen therapy. These principles are most applicable when cor pulmonale is associated with chronic bronchitis and emphysema. Treating exacerbations of bronchitis often results in improvement in ventilation and thus reverses episodes of ventricular decompensation. In addition, the results of clinical studies suggest that chronic use of oxygen by patients with cor pulmonale may affect their long-term survival. Oxygen therapy appears to have little value in the treatment of cor pulmonale without right ventricular failure.

Consistently effective pulmonary vasodilators do not exist. Although tolazoline hydrochloride, isoproterenol, and phentolamine have been reported to be effective in decreasing pulmonary artery pressure occasionally in a patient with primary pulmonary hypertension, these drugs are not recommended for general use in the treatment of cor pulmonale.

When right ventricular decompensation develops, digitalis and diuretics may be effective if employed with caution. Digitalis increases right ventricular output in patients with cor pulmonale and right ventricular failure. However, since the effect is not dramatic, it is difficult at best to estimate a proper dose of the drug. Furthermore, it is unlikely that digitalis is of much benefit unless hypoxia is corrected. In addition, the use of digitalis may be particularly dangerous in the presence of hypoxemia, since arrhythmias tend to occur in this clinical situation.

Diuretics may clearly be of value, since circulating blood volume and extravascular lung water are increased in right ventricular decompensation. However, diuresis must be induced cautiously to avoid volume depletion. If this occurs, right ventricular filling may become impaired, thus producing a decrease in cardiac output. Obviously, serum electrolytes should be closely monitored to avoid metabolic complications of therapy.

PULMONARY EDEMA

The term "pulmonary edema" indicates an increase in extravascular water in the lung. Although pulmonary edema may occur in a number of different clinical conditions, only two major pathogenetic mechanisms are responsible for the development of this state.

Pathogenesis

The alveolar-capillary wall is freely permeable to water and small solutes. As with any capillary, the movement of water from the pulmonary vascular space into lung tissue is governed by Starling forces (Fig. 18-1). The intravascular hydrostatic pressure is the major force that promotes the movement of water out of the intravascular space into tissue. Theoretically, this pressure is opposed to some degree by the tissue hydrostatic pressure. Since this pressure is negligible in the lung, it can, for practical purposes, be ignored. Thus the net pressure across the vascular wall can be considered equal to the intravascular hydrostatic pressure. The oncotic

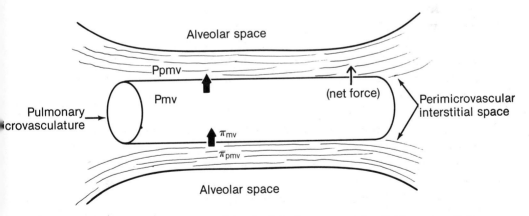

Fig. 18-1. Schematic representation of the Starling forces governing fluid movement from the pulmonary microvasculature into the perimicrovascular interstitial space of the alveolar wall. The hydrostatic pressure gradient (*P*) favors movement of fluid from the intravascular space into the perimicrovascular interstitial space. The oncotic pressure gradient (π) favors movement of fluid from the perimicrovascular interstitial space into the intravascular space. Under normal circumstances the net effect of these forces favors filtration of fluid into the perimicrovascular interstitial space of the alveolar wall.

pressure caused primarily by serum proteins is the major force promoting retention of water in the intravascular space. However, since tissue oncotic pressure is substantial, the net oncotic pressure promoting retention of water in the intravascular space is substantially less than the hydrostatic pressure across the capillary wall. Thus the net Starling forces promote continuous filtration of small volumes of water across the normal alveolar-capillary wall into the interstitial space of the alveolar wall.

Mechanical forces appear to promote the movement of fluid within the interstitial space of the alveolar wall to the lymphatic channels in the peribronchiolar regions. Thus extravascular lung water is continuously being removed from the lung by lymphatic drainage. Obviously the volume of extravascular lung water at any point represents the dynamic balance between the amount being filtered across the capillary wall and the amount being removed by lymphatic drainage.

An increase in extravascular lung water is accompanied by an increase in lung lymph flow. At least for a while the increase in extravascular water is limited to the interstitial space of the alveolar wall and to the lymphatic channels in the peribronchiolar region of the lung. However, eventually alveoli become fluid filled and atelectatic. The exact mechanisms contributing to this sequence of events have not been completely described. Nonetheless, alveolar flooding leads to many of the clinical and roentgenographic manifestations of pulmonary edema. Fluid will continue to be filtered into the lung until the basic pathogenetic mechanism causing the increased fluid filtration is corrected.

Since lung water is drained through the lymphatics, the biochemical composition of lung lymph should reflect in part the composition of the extravascular lung water. In experimental animals and presumably in humans, the concentration of electrolytes and other small solutes in lung lymph is identical to that of plasma, whereas the concentration of protein is substantially lower than that of plasma. The ratio of the protein concentration in lymph to that in plasma is approximately 0.5 under normal circumstances. The importance of this ratio in differentiating the pathogenetic mechanisms that may produce pulmonary edema is discussed in the following paragraphs.

The volume of fluid that is filtered across the alveolar-capillary wall may increase if the hydrostatic pressure gradient across the capillary wall increases or if the permeability characteristics of the membrane are altered. The capillary hydrostatic pressure is primarily determined by pulmonary venous and left atrial pressure. In this form of pulmonary edema, the permeability of the alveolar-capillary membrane does not change. Thus the membrane remains an effective barrier to the movement of high molecular weight solutes into the alveolar wall interstitial space. As a result, the biochemical constituents of lung lymph do not change significantly.

The permeability of the alveolar-capillary membrane may be altered in a variety of clinical conditions. When this occurs, protein and other high molecular weight solutes may accompany fluid into the alveolar wall interstitial space. As a result the protein concentration in lung lymph increases and approximates the value in plasma. Thus, in experimental animals, measurement of the ratio of the protein concentration in lung lymph to that in plasma can be used to differentiate pulmonary edema caused by hydrostatic forces from that caused by alteration in the permeability of the alveolar-capillary membrane.

Etiologic factors

Pulmonary edema may occur in a variety of clinical conditions. The various conditions that cause pulmonary edema may be classified as one of two categories based on the pathogenic mechanism involved in edema formation:

Increased permeability
    Lung infections
    Aspiration pneumonia
    Inhalation of toxins
    Drug overdose
    Sepsis
    Pancreatitis
    Shock
    Drowning and near drowning
    Uremia
Increased hydrostatic pressure
    Left ventricular failure
    Mitral valve obstruction
    Veno-occlusive disease
    Neurogenic pulmonary edema

Hydrostatic pulmonary edema is usually a manifestation of cardiac disease. Left ventricular decompensation and mitral stenosis are the two conditions that most often produce cardiogenic pulmonary edema. In these conditions, elevation of the left atrial pressure is primarily responsible for the increased capillary hydrostatic pressure that promotes fluid filtration into the alveolar wall. The left atrial pressure may drop rapidly after certain forms of drug therapy and may be normal by the time clinical measurements are obtained. Since the clinical and roentgenographic manifestations of pulmonary edema do not resolve as rapidly, the hydrostatic nature of the pulmonary edema may be incorrectly overlooked.

Noncardiogenic, hydrostatic pulmonary edema occurs in several very uncommon conditions such as diffuse veno-occlusive disease and neurogenic pulmonary edema. Diffuse veno-occlusive disease is of unknown origin and occurs primarily in young women. In some patients with veno-occlusive disease, pulmonary edema occurs in a diffuse or patchy distribution throughout the lung. The pulmonary-capillary wedge pressure is normal in this disease. Thus the increased capillary hydrostatic pressure must be caused by an increase in pulmonary venous resistance. The prognosis of this condition is poor.

Recent evidence suggests that neurogenic pulmonary edema is also a form of noncardiogenic, hydrostatic pulmonary edema. The pathogenesis of the pulmonary edema appears to be related to the fact that massive adrenergic neural activity may occur after brain injury and produce dramatic increases in systemic and pulmonary vascular pressures. During periods of transient systemic and pulmonary hypertension, the pulmonary-capillary wedge pressure is elevated, and pulmonary edema develops.

A number of clinical conditions produce pulmonary edema by altering the permeability of the pulmonary-capillary wall. In many of these conditions, the mechanisms by which pulmonary-capillary permeability is altered is unclear. However, increasing evidence shows that bioactive agents such as histamine, kinins, and prostaglandins may directly alter the functional characteristics of the endothelial cell. In some circumstances, infectious agents, inhaled or circulating toxins, or physical agents (e.g., radiation) may directly affect capillary permeability. Thus noncardiogenic pulmonary edema may be seen in a wide variety of clinical conditions including sepsis, shock, pancreatitis, toxic gas or smoke inhalation, aspiration, and pulmonary infections.

Pulmonary edema also occurs in certain drug overdoses. Although the exact mechanisms by which drugs produce pulmonary edema is not defined, it is presumed that alteration of the permeability of the pulmonary-capillary membrane is important. Pulmonary edema may also develop at high altitude. Although the pulmonary arterial pressure is increased in this situation, pulmonary-capillary wedge pressure is normal. Hypoxemia does not appear to increase pulmonary-capillary permeability. Thus the hypoxemia of altitude alone would not be expected to be important in this syndrome. Although a number of theories have been proposed, no single mechanism satisfactorily explains the development of pulmonary edema at high altitude.

Clinical manifestations

Dyspnea is the most prominent complaint of patients with pulmonary edema. Many patients expectorate pink, frothy fluid when extensive intra-alveolar edema is present. In patients with cardiogenic pulmonary edema, dyspnea may initially be apparent only during exertion. However, as extensive edema develops, dyspnea at rest may occur. Initially this may be present only after the patient has been in the supine position for an extended period. During physical examination, diffuse rales are usually audible over the bases but may extend to the apices in some patients. Wheezes and rhonchi may be audible in some patients. Tachypnea and tachycardia are usually present.

The clinical manifestations of pulmonary edema associated with alterations in capillary permeability caused by diffuse capillary wall injury are variable. Patients with this condition usually have acute, profound dyspnea and rapidly develop hypoxemia and respiratory failure. In the initial stage of this condition, surprisingly large volumes of edematous fluid may be coughed or suctioned from the lung. However, as the condition progresses, smaller amounts of edematous fluid can be raised. Patients with this form of pulmonary edema often develop the characteristic clinical, roentgenographic, and physiologic manifestations of the adult respiratory distress syndrome described in Chapter 24.

Physiologic manifestations

Routine clinical pulmonary function tests are not usually obtained during the course of acute pulmonary edema. Thus the extent of the abnormalities that may be seen during this condition have not been adequately documented. However, a restrictive ventilatory defect characterized by a decrease in vital capacity and total lung capacity may occur. In addition, physiologic abnormalities consistent with obstruction in small airways may be seen, presumably because of the increase in peribronchiolar fluid that occurs in this condition. Finally, gas exchange may be grossly abnormal. Hypoxemia is uniformly present as a result of mismatching of ventilation and perfusion throughout the lung. As the degree of alveolar filling progresses, an increase in the intrapulmonary shunt volume may occur and lead to profound hypoxemia. In some patients, alveolar ventilation decreases, causing progressive hypercapnia.

Roentgenographic manifestations

Pulmonary edema produces dramatic abnormalities on the chest roentgenogram. In the earliest stage of this condition, the abnormalities that may be present are an increase in linear markings in the lung fields and the appearance of Kerley B lines at the periphery of the lung bases. These changes probably reflect the increased fluid in the alveolar wall and engorgement of the pulmonary lymphatics. In addition, the vascular markings may be ill defined, and airways viewed in cross sections may be prominent. These changes are probably caused by an increase in fluid in the perivascular and peribronchiolar spaces. If the pulmonary edema is caused by increased hydrostatic pressure, pulmonary vessels in the superior lung fields may be enlarged, presumably as a result of the increased blood flow to these areas.

As the volume of extravascular fluid increases, diffuse alveolar filling becomes apparent and may involve the whole lung. Typically in pulmonary edema associated with cardiac diseases, alveolar filling begins in the perihilar regions and spreads peripherally in a reasonably symmetrical fashion. This may not be the case in pulmonary edema associated with increased capillary permeability.

As previously mentioned, the roentgenographic manifestations of pulmonary edema persist after the pathogenetic mechanism leading to increased filtration of fluid into the lung has been corrected. In fact, intra-alveolar edema may persist for days. The delay in roentgenographic clearing must be caused by a limitation either in lung lymph flow or other mechanisms that are involved in the clearance of extra-vascular water from the lung.

Diagnosis

The diagnosis of pulmonary edema is based on compatible clinical and roentgenographic abnormalities. Obviously at times it may be extremely difficult to differentiate pulmonary edema from a variety of other disorders that may produce dyspnea and rapidly progressive alveolar infiltrates on the chest roentgenogram. Manifestations of cardiac disease help in recognizing cardiogenic pulmonary edema. Noncardiogenic pulmonary edema may be extremely difficult to distinguish from other disorders. The specific conditions associated with increased-permeability pulmonary edema are discussed in Chapter 24.

It may not be possible to distinguish cardiogenic from noncardiogenic pulmonary edema on the basis of the clinical, physiologic, or roentgenographic manifestations of the disease. Measurement of the pulmonary-capillary wedge pressure may be the only method for accurately differentiating these two forms of pulmonary edema. As previously mentioned, if drugs that rapidly decrease pulmonary-capillary wedge pressure have been administered before pressure measurements are made, it may be impossible to initially identify patients with cardiogenic pulmonary edema. However, if the pulmonary-capillary wedge pressure is elevated, the pulmonary edema can be attributed to a cardiac disorder. If the wedge pressure is normal, noncardiogenic causes must be considered.

Although these two forms of pulmonary edema can theoretically be distinguished by measuring the ratio of the protein concentration of lung fluid to that of plasma, it is rarely done in clinical practice. A ratio of less than 0.5 is consistent with hydrostatic pulmonary edema, whereas a ratio approaching 1 is indicative of an alteration in the permeability of the alveolar-capillary membrane. Finally, both conditions may be present in some patients, thus further confusing the diagnostic evaluation. If the pulmonary-capillary wedge pressure is high, this group of patients can be recognized only if the protein concentration of alveolar fluid is measured.

Treatment

Treatment of the underlying cause of the disorder is the main approach to the treatment of pulmonary edema. In hydrostatic pulmonary edema, diuretics, peripheral vasodilators, and inotropic drugs may be employed to decrease left atrial pressure by improving left ventricular function. Detailed description of the specifics of this form of therapy is beyond the scope of this discussion.

The pulmonary edema caused by increased pulmonary-capillary permeability has no specific treatment. There is no known way of reversing the alteration in the pulmonary-capillary permeability that allows the movement of fluid and high molecular weight solutes into the alveolar wall. However, experimental evidence suggests that under some circumstances corticosteroids may be capable of affecting pulmonary-capillary integrity. Little clinical evidence supports this concept. As a result, the management of pulmonary edema in this situation is directed at the therapy of the underlying disease and maintenance of gas exchange by mechanical ventilation if necessary until spontaneous improvement of the underlying lung injury occurs.

In many clinical situations in which direct lung injury alters pulmonary-capillary permeability, pulmonary edema is of critical importance only in the initial stage of the disease. As various components of the lung are injured or destoyed, the effects of the loss of integrity of alveolar structure, the inflammation of the alveolar wall, and the formation of increased fibrous tissue become the important determinants of lung function. Indeed, survival in these conditions is not dictated to any great degree by the continued presence of pulmonary edema but by the degree of lung destruction and fibrosis that occurs during the course of the disorder.

Chapter 19

PRIMARY PULMONARY HYPERTENSION

Primary pulmonary hypertension is a disease of undetermined origin that involves primarily the pulmonary arteries and arterioles. The disease may occur at any age. In children pulmonary hypertension is distributed equally between boys and girls, whereas in the adult age group it predominantly affects young women. Familial cases have been reported.

ORIGIN

The origin of primary pulmonary hypertension is unknown. Although a number of theories about the cause of the disease have been proposed, none has gained wide acceptance. It has been proposed that the disease is the result of vasospastic changes in the pulmonary arterial system. However, neither the pathogenetic mechanism leading to arterial spasm nor the etiologic factors that may cause these events have been defined. Others have suggested that the abnormality responsible for the pulmonary hypertension is the persistence of fetal-type pulmonary arteries possessing a thickened medium and therefore that the disease should be considered a congenital disorder. There is no agreement on this point, but the occurrence of the disease in young children as well as in family members is at least consistent with the possibility that there is a genetically determined abnormality of the pulmonary vasculature. Finally, it is often proposed that this disease is the result of multiple small pulmonary emboli. No evidence supports this concept. Neither the clinical histories of patients with the disease nor the pathologic findings are suggestive of pulmonary embolic disease.

PATHOLOGIC FINDINGS

The pathologic findings of primary pulmonary hypertension are limited to the pulmonary arteries and arterioles. Intimal fibrosis and medial hypertrophy are the most prominent findings. The intimal lesion appears to start as a concentric prolif-

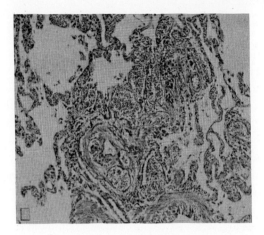

Fig. 19-1. Microscopic section of lung tissue obtained from a patient with primary pulmonary hypertension demonstrating the characteristic plexiform lesions seen in this disease.

From Walcott, G., et al.: Primary pulmonary hypertension, Am. J. Med. **49:**70, 1970.

eration of intimal cells. Fibrosis eventually occurs, and the intima assumes a characteristic, concentric laminar appearance. This particular lesion is infrequently observed in other forms of pulmonary hypertension. In some cases the lumen of the vessel may be totally obliterated. Long segments of vessels may be involved by this process.

Medial hypertrophy occurs in varying degrees of severity and is usually pronounced in infants and young children. In older patients, dilation of pulmonary arteriolar branches occurs, resulting in relative thinning of the arterial walls. Thus the thickness of the medium in these pulmonary arteries may decrease considerably as this process occurs.

Plexiform lesions are the characteristic pathologic finding of primary pulmonary hypertension (Fig. 19-1). These lesions occur in the majority of patients with primary pulmonary hypertension and are rarely seen in other forms of pulmonary hypertension. The exact sequence of events that leads to the development of these lesions is unknown. Fibrinoid necrosis and local vasculitis are also observed regularly.

Patients with long-standing pulmonary hypertension may also have pathologic changes in the heart consistent with cor pulmonale.

CLINICAL MANIFESTATIONS

As previously stated, the majority of adult patients with primary pulmonary hypertension are young women; the female-to-male ratio is approximately 5:1. The median age of patients with this disease is in the early thirties. At the time of diagnosis essentially all patients have exertional dyspnea. Dizziness and syncope are often present and are usually related to exertion. Some patients have precordial chest pain that, although not always related to exertion, may have many of the charactristics of angina.

Raynaud phenomenon is present in approximately a third of the patients with this disease. The occurence of this phenomenon certainly indicates that the vascular abnormalities leading to pulmonary hypertension are not localized to the pulmonary vessels and strengthens the concept that the pathogenesis of pulmonary hypertension may in some way be mediated by spasm of the pulmonary arteries. A small precentage of patients also have joint symptoms. It is clearly important to exclude the presence of a systemic connective tissue disorder in patients with a combination of arthritis and Raynaud phenomenon.

Physical findings are localized to the cardiac examination. The pulmonic valve closure sound may be accentuated. Murmurs of tricuspid insufficiency, pulmonic insufficiency, or pulmonary outflow obstruction may be audible. A right ventricular lift may be present in patients with right ventricular hypertrophy. Systemic manifestations of right heart failure may be observed.

PHYSIOLOGIC CHANGES

The predominant physiologic changes that occur in primary pulmonary hypertension are hemodynamic in nature. However, abnormalities in lung function may occur in some patients with this disease. In the majority of patients, the lung volumes and indices of airflow are normal. However, some patients do have a restrictive ventilatory defect with a decrease in the vital capacity and total lung capacity. The explanation for these changes is unclear.

As would be expected, the major abnormalities involve gas exchange, since perfusion of alveolar capillaries may be markedly altered in this disease. As a result of the loss of perfusion of some alveoli, the ratio of dead space ventilation to total ventilation is increased. Hypoxemia and hypocapnia are usually present. The diffusing capacity is usually decreased in patients with this disease. This abnormality is almost certainly related to obliteration of the pulmonary-capillary bed in conjunction with the large vessel changes that occur in primary pulmonary hypertension.

ROENTGENOGRAPHIC FINDINGS

The roentgenographic manifestations of primary pulmonary hypertension are limited to changes in the pulmonary vessels and heart. The lung parenchyma itself is normal. Enlargement of the main pulmonary arteries is the most obvious roentgenographic finding (Fig. 19-2). In conjunction with this the pulmonary artery branches may taper rapidly, and a general paucity of vascular markings may be apparent in the peripheral third of the lung fields. However, these changes are often subtle and may not be appreciated in many cases.

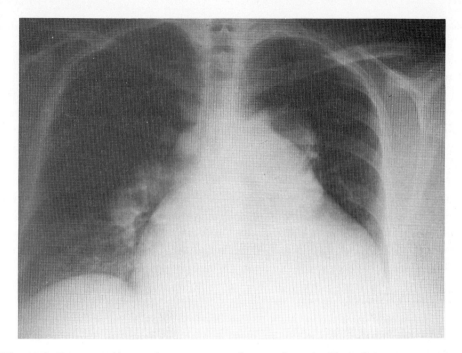

Fig. 19-2. Primary pulmonary hypertension with cor pulmonale. The pulmonary arteries are greatly enlarged, and cardiomegaly is present.

DIAGNOSIS

The diagnosis of primary pulmonary hypertension can be strongly suspected on the basis of the clinical, roentgenographic, and physiologic manifestations previously described. In addition, the electrocardiogram may reveal right axis deviation or evidence of right ventricular hypertrophy.

Cardiac catheterization should be performed in all patients to exclude a potentially treatable cause for pulmonary hypertension. Occasionally mitral stenosis or an atrial septal defect may be overlooked until catheterization studies have been performed. In patients with primary pulmonary hypertension, catheterization studies reveal elevation of the pulmonary arterial systolic and diastolic pressures with a normal capillary wedge pressure. The cardiac output is frequently decreased. A right-to-left shunt at the atrial level may be detected if shunting through a foramen ovale develops as a result of increased pressure in the right side of the heart. Although early reports suggested that patients with this disease tolerated cardiac catherization poorly, more recent experience suggests that the procedure can be performed safely.

On occasion, recognition of other diseases that may mimic primary pulmonary hypertension may be extremely difficult. Patients with a connective tissue disorder occasionally have pulmonary hypertension unaccompanied by other manifestations of the disease. This presentation is most likely to occur in scleroderma. Recurrent pulmonary emboli might conceivably mimic primary pulmonary hypertension. The clinical manifestations of pulmonary embolic disease usually suggest the correct diagnosis. However, foreign body embolization may be overlooked unless a careful history of illicit drug use is obtained. Talc and other inert material injected intravenously may produce obliterative pulmonary vascular disease and lead to pulmonary hypertension.

Several unusual pulmonary vascular diseases may also be confused with primary pulmonary hypertension. Pulmonary veno-occlusive disease is an extremely unusual disease that may not be distinguished from primary pulmonary hypertension in the absence of a lung biopsy. Finally, patients with hereditary hemorrhagic telangiectasia (Osler-Weber-Redu disease) may develop pulmonary hypertension for reasons that are not totally clear. If the cutaneous and mucosal manifestations of his disease are not recognized, the correct diagnosis may be overlooked.

TREATMENT

The natural history of primary pulmonary hypertension is unknown, since the true duration of the disease cannot be accurately documented. The diagnosis is made in most patients when the disease is advanced. The majority of patients die within 3 years of the diagnosis.

There is no effective treatment for this disease. Occasionally reports have suggested that tolazoline (Priscoline), isoproterenol, or phentolamine may decrease the level of pulmonary hypertension and have a beneficial effect in the course of the disease. However, these drugs have been shown to be of value only occasionally. The treatment for the disease is primarily directed at the relief of symptoms and control of right ventricular failure by the use of digitalis and diuretics.

Chapter 20

PULMONARY VASCULITIS

The pulmonary arterial system may be involved by a number of systemic diseases, many of which appear to be immunologically mediated. In some of these diseases, pulmonary vasculitis is a major manifestation, whereas in others vascular involvement occurs only sporadically. Although the clinical and roentgenographic manifestations of pulmonary vasculitis are varied, these diseases will be discussed together in this chapter, since, in a general sense, they share common pathogenetic mechanisms.

GOODPASTURE SYNDROME

Goodpasture syndrome is a disease that occurs predominantly in young men. This syndrome is characterized in its mildest form by recurrent episodes of hemoptysis and dyspnea and in its most severe form by progressive respiratory and renal failure. In most patients, recurrent episodes of intrapulmonary bleeding manifest by bouts of hemoptysis and intermittent infiltrates on the chest roentgenogram precede evidence of renal glomerular involvement. Eventually, however, rapidly progressive glomerulonephritis leading to renal failure develops in the majority of patients. At any time during the course of the disease, profound pulmonary hemorrhage may lead to the development of repiratory failure.

The immunologic mechanism involved in the pathogenesis of this disease has been well defined. For reasons that are unclear, antibody develops against an antigenic determinant of the glomerular basement membrane. This antibody not only binds to the glomerular basement membrane, but also cross-reacts with the basement membrane of the pulmonary capillary. The binding of antibody to the basement membrane provokes an inflammatory response that leads to the loss of integrity of the vessel and progressive organ damage. In the lung this injury is evident by diffuse alveolar hemorrhage and in the kidney by progressive renal failure.

The pathologic changes observed with light microscopy are not diagnostic of this disease. Although characteristic changes of rapidly progressive glomerulone-

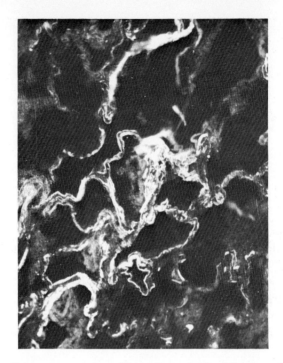

Fig. 20-1. Immunofluorescent staining of lung tissue obtained from a patient with Goodpasture syndrome. The linear immunofluorescence of the alveolar wall is consistent with antibody deposition on the alveolar wall basement membrane.

From Beirne, G.J., et al.: Immunohistology of the lung in Goodpasture's syndrome, Ann. Intern. Med. **69:**1207, 1968.

phritis are present in the kidney, this lesion is nonspecific and may be seen in other forms of renal disease. However, the use of immunopathologic techniques demonstrates antibody to be evenly deposited in a linear fashion along the pulmonary and renal glomerular-capillary basement membranes (Fig. 20-1). These changes are virtually diagnostic of Goodpasture syndrome. In addition, the antiglomerular basement membrane antibody can be detected in serum obtained from patients with this disease.

The diagnosis of Goodpasture syndrome should be considered in patients with evidence of renal disease and pulmonary hemorrhage. Alveolar hemorrhage may not be accompanied by hemoptysis. Focal or diffuse alveolar infiltrates on the roentgenogram may be the only manifestation of intrapulmonary bleeding (Fig. 20-2). The presence of bleeding may be suspected if the hematocrit drops acutely as the infiltrates develop. The presence of alveolar bleeding can be confirmed by performing segmental bronchoalveolar lavage of an area observed to be abnormal on the chest roentgenogram. Since alveolar macrophages ingest red cell fragments

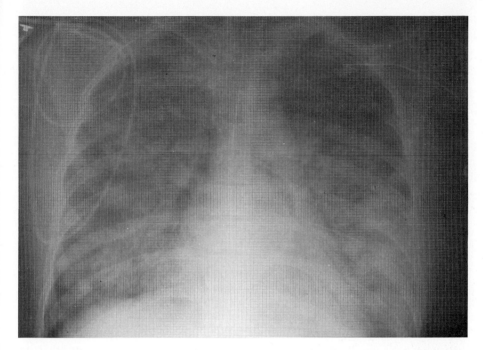

Fig. 20-2. Goodpasture syndrome with acute intrapulmonary hemorrhage.

and hemoglobin in the alveolar space, microscopic examination of an iron stain of the alveolar macrophages obtained by this technique will confirm the fact that bleeding has occurred. As mentioned previously, the diagnosis can be documented by immunofluorescent staining of either lung or renal biopsy specimens. Circulating antibody and the deposition of antibody in the alveolar-capillary wall can be detected before the onset of any evidence of renal glomerular involvement. Thus the diagnosis of this disease can be made during the initial stage, which is characterized solely by alveolar hemorrhage.

It is important to make a specific immunopathologic diagnosis of Goodpasture syndrome, since other diseases may also cause alveolar hemorrhage with or without glomerular involvement. Pulmonary alveolar hemorrhage is the only manifestation of idiopathic pulmonary hemosiderosis, whereas alveolar hemorrhage and progressive glomerulonephritis may occur in diseases mediated by immune complex injury.

The treatment of Goodpasture syndrome is controversial. The goal of therapy should be to prevent continued antibody production to halt the progressive renal damage. High-dose, intermittent pulse therapy with corticosteroids alone or corticosteroids in conjunction with cyclophosphamide have been recommended as the most effective form of therapy. In addition, in acutely ill individuals with life-threatening alveolar hemorrhage, plasmaphoresis has occasionally been employed to rapidly decrease the concentration of circulating, preformed antibody. Based on the rationale that the removal of the kidney could, by removing the source of antigen, halt antibody production, bilateral nephrectomy has been employed as therapy for this disease in the past. There is no role for this approach to therapy at present.

The clinical course of the disease is extremely variable. A high percentage of patients die regardless of the therapy employed. However, there is no doubt that some patients have a relatively mild form of the disease which does not appear to be progressive in nature. Although no conclusive evidence shows that early treatment of the disease is more likely to be successful, recent experience suggests that this prognosis is the case. Thus an attempt should be made to diagnose the disease at its earliest stage. It appears that following the course of the disease during therapy by assaying the titer of antiglomerular basement membrane is useful.

IDIOPATHIC PULMONARY HEMOSIDEROSIS

Idiopathic pulmonary hemosiderosis (IPH) is a disease primarily of infants and children characterized by recurrent alveolar hemorrhage. The pathogenesis of the disease is unknown. Since IPH is characterized by recurrent episodes of diffuse alveolar hemorrhage, it may be confused with Goodpasture syndrome or other immunologically mediated diseases that produce alveolar bleeding.

The clinical features of IPH are usually subtle. In many children, weakness and lassitude related to chronic iron deficiency anemia are the major symptoms that bring the patients to medical attention. The iron deficiency state is simply related to blood loss caused by recurrent hemorrhage into the lung. During the bleeding episodes, cough, fever, and shortness of breath may be present. Hemoptysis is variable. The chest roentgenogram may reveal localized or diffuse alveolar infiltrates. In the absence of hemoptysis, the diagnosis is often overlooked, and the patient's symptoms are attributed to recurrent infections of the lung. The interval between episodes varies and may be several years. In this case, iron deficiency anemia may not be present, and the diagnosis may be particularly difficult to make.

The diagnosis of IPH is best made by lung biopsy during or shortly after an acute episode of bleeding. The biopsy generally reveals diffuse alveolar bleeding with little abnormality in the alveolar wall or architecture (Fig. 20-3). However, in severe cases fibrosis of the alveolar wall may also be apparent. In the few cases in which immunologic studies have been employed for studying this disease, they have not detected abnormalities attributable to immunologic injury of the alveolar capillary. Ultrastructure studies have suggested the existence of an abnormality in the capillary epithelial cells. However, more studies need to be done to confirm the presence of this lesion in other patients. Although the cause of the lesion is unclear, the occurrence of the disease in infants and young children suggests that it may be a developmental defect.

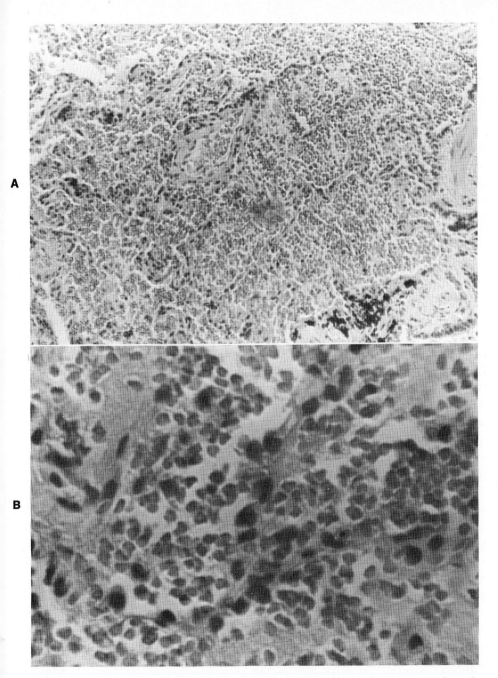

Fig. 20-3. A, Microscopic section of lung tissue obtained from a patient with idiopathic pulmonary hemosiderosis. The architecture of the lung is barely recognizable because of the red cells filling the interalveolar spaces. **B,** Higher-power view showing in greater detail the erythrocytes in the alveolar space.

There is no specific therapy for IPH. However, corticosteroids appear to be useful in controlling the episodes of bleeding in some patients. Because of the extreme variability in the course of the disease, it is difficult to truly assess the effect of any form of therapy.

COLLAGEN VASCULAR DISEASES

The pulmonary vascular bed may be involved in the systemic connective tissue disorders. The pathologic condition of the pulmonary vessels in these diseases is extremely varied. Changes characteristic of an inflammatory vasculitis may be present in some cases, whereas in others intimal proliferation and medial thickening are the only findings. Nevertheless, because these systemic diseases are thought to be immunologically mediated, it is reasonable to assume that the changes in the pulmonary vessels have a similar pathogenesis.

The clinical and roentgenographic manifestations of pulmonary vascular involvement in collagen vascular diseases is also extremely varied. If the site of involvement is predominantly the small arterioles and arteries, pulmonary hypertension may be the dominant clinical finding. This manifestation is particularly characteristic of scleroderma and has also been observed in systemic lupus erythematosis, rheumatoid arthritis, and polymyositis.

If the site of the involvement is the capillary bed, diffuse alveolar hemorrhage may occur. This manifestation of pulmonary vascular involvement in the connective tissue diseases has been best documented in systemic lupus erythematosis. In these documented cases, electron microscopic examination of lung tissue has demonstrated immune complex deposition in the basement membrane of the alveolar capillaries (Fig. 20-4).

Polyarteritis nodosa and Takayusu arteritis are systemic diseases that involve predominantly medium sized and, in the case of Takayusu arteritis, large arteries. The pulmonary arteries may be involved in both diseases. Because the site of involvement is in larger vessels, the manifestations are far different from those observed with other vascular diseases. Similar to involvement in other organs, polyarteritis nodosa may produce multiple aneurysms of the pulmonary arteries. These lesions may appear as small nodules on the chest roentgenogram. However, pulmonary angiography clearly demonstrates that the lesions are, in fact, aneurysms. Takayusu arteritis is characterized pathologically by granulomatous vasculitis involving medium and large arteries. Although this disease is most often associated with involvement of the aortic arch, other sites are also frequently involved. Pulmonary artery involvement usually occurs clinically as pulmonary hypertension. However, the distinguishing feature is that pulmonary angiograms may demonstrate stenosis or total obstruction of major branches of the pulmonary artery. Progressive dyspnea and cor pulmonale leading to death may develop in patients with this disease.

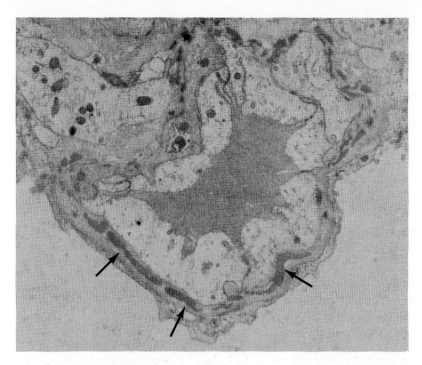

Fig. 20-4. Electron micrograph of an alveolar-capillary wall in the lung of a patient with lupus erythematosis. The electron-dense deposits *(arrows)* in the alveolar-capillary membrane are consistent with immune complex deposition.

Modified from Elliott, M.L., and Kuhn, C.: Idiopathic pulmonary hemosiderosis: ultrastructural abnormalities in the capillary wall, Am. Rev. Respir. Dis. **102:**895, 1970.

WEGENER GRANULOMATOSIS

Wegener granulomatosis is a systemic disease characterized by necrotizing granulomatous vasculitis of the upper and lower respiratory tract and necrotizing glomerulonephritis. The disease is presumed to be mediated by immunologic mechanisms. The pathologic changes produced by the disease are distinctive. Necrotizing granulomatous lesions with inflammation of small arteries and veins are almost always present in the lung and respiratory tract. In addition, focal and segmental glomerulonephritis progressing to necrotizing glomerulonephritis occurs in the kidney in the great majority of patients. Granulomatous inflammation and vasculitis are variably observed in others.

The clinical manifestations of Wegener granulomatosis are extremely varied. Systemic symptoms of weight loss, fever, anorexia, and malaise are frequently present. In addition, local symptoms related to specific sites of involvement may also occur. Cough with sputum production, nasal discharge, arthralgia, skin lesions, and symptoms of peripheral neuropathy may be observed. Symptoms attributable to involvement of other organs are observed far less often.

The chest roentgenogram is almost uniformly abnormal. Mass lesions are the most common abnormalities observed. These lesions may be single or multiple and frequently cavitate (Fig. 20-5). In addition, localized or diffuse patchy infiltrates may be present. Adenopathy and pleural effusion are distinctly uncommon. Sinus films frequently demonstrate opacification or air fluid levels in the sinuses. Examination of the urine sediment may reveal erythrocytes and red blood cell casts. As the disease progresses, azotemia may develop and lead to marked renal failure.

The diagnosis of Wegener granulomatosis is made by demonstrating the characteristic pathologic features in biopsy specimens. Lesions in the upper respiratory tract, if present, lend themselves most easily to biopsy. However, lung or kidney biopsy may be required for diagnosis.

The treatment of the disease has been well defined in recent years. The disease is responsive to cyclophosphamide. Untreated Wegener granulomatosis pursues a rapidly fatal course with a mean survival time of 5 months. More than 90% of untreated patients die within two years. Corticosteroids alone usually prolong the mean survival time, but the long-term prognosis is not appreciably altered. In

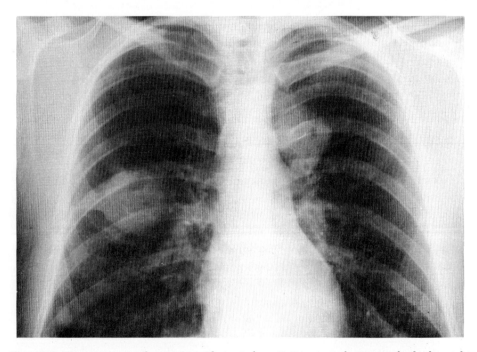

Fig. 20-5. Wegener granulomatosis with typical cavitating mass lesions in both the right upper and left upper lobes.

contrast, cyclophosphamide regularly induces long-term remissions of the disease. In patients with fulminant disease, corticosteroids should initially be used in conjunction with cyclophosphamide, but eventually corticosteroids can be discontinued, and the patient can be treated with maintenance doses of cyclophophamide alone. In patients with less fulminant disease, corticosteroids are not necessary.

Lymphomatoid granulomatosis is an unusual form of vasculitis that also regularly involves the lung. The histopathologic features of this disease differ from those of Wegener granulomatosis in that granulomas are less common and the cellular infiltrates are characterized by the presence of atypical lymphocytoid and plasmacytoid cells.

The roentgenographic manifestations of lung involvement are essentially identical to those seen in Wegener granulomatosis, although skin and central nervous system involvement occur more often. In addition, this disease involves the kidney less frequently and does not produce necrotizing glomerulonephritis. The renal lesion is characterized by nodular infiltration of the parenchyma by the characteristic cellular infiltrate.

Untreated lymphomatoid granulomatosis is usually rapidly fatal. Although patients with severe disease may not respond to therapy, remission can be induced by cyclophosphamide and corticosteroids if therapy is instituted early in the course of the disease.

Chapter 21

PULMONARY EMBOLIC DISEASE

The term "pulmonary embolus" is used to describe the impaction of a segment of a venous thrombus or other particulate material in a branch of the pulmonary artery. The clinical, roentgenographic, and physiologic manifestations of pulmonary embolic disease are determined by the site and extent of pulmonary vascular occlusion and by the patient's underlying cardiopulmonary status. Although this chapter will focus on pulmonary emboli that arise from a thrombus in the systemic venous system, many of the comments may be applied equally to other forms of pulmonary emboli.

PATHOLOGIC CHANGES

The primary pathologic feature of pulmonary embolic disease is reflected by changes that occur in the pulmonary arteries at the site of impaction of the emboli and by changes that occur in lung tissue distal to the site of obstruction. The changes in the pulmonary arteries depend on the interval between the embolus and the pathologic examination. With a fresh embolus, there may be no changes in the pulmonary artery other than the presence of the intraluminal embolus. In the majority of cases, emboli undergo complete lysis in a period of several weeks to months, leaving no abnormalities in the involved artery. However, on occasion an embolus may undergo organization within the lumen of the artery. During this process, endothelium may grow over the surface of the clot. This organized embolus may eventually recanalize, resulting in the formation of sinusoidal channels or multiple, thin-walled bands that span the lumen of the vessel. Intimal plaques may develop proximal to and at the site of the embolus. Occasionally inflammation and necrosis occur in involved vessels. Intimal plaques and bands are usually the only changes in pulmonary arteries examined several months or longer after an embolic episode.

Lung tissue distal to the obstructed vessel may undergo infarction. However, because of the dual blood supply to the lung, infarction appears to be a relatively uncommon event. After obstruction to a pulmonary artery, the associated capillary bed may be perfused by blood flowing from an adjacent pulmonary arteriole or from the bronchial arterial system. Although edema and hemorrhage may occur in these areas, these changes will resolve spontaneously if the collateral circulation is adequate to prevent actual infarction. However, if collateral circulation is inadequate, infarction may develop. Hemorrhage and necrosis may eventually occur in the area of infarcted lung, resulting in complete disruption of the normal alveolar architecture. Subsequently, organization of this area may result in the formation of a scar. It is usually impossible to determine the true origin of a scar formed as a result of pulmonary infarction, unless vascular changes of a pulmonary embolus can be identified in a nearby artery.

PATHOGENESIS

Although pulmonary emboli may arise from a venous thrombus in any major systemic vein, the great majority arise from a thrombus in a pelvic vein or the deep venous system of the lower extremities. Only a small percentage of patients who develop a deep venous thrombus in the lower extremities develop clinical evidence of pulmonary embolic disease. It seems likely that small emboli which lodge in small peripheral branches of the pulmonary artery go unrecognized. Nevertheless, is seems reasonable to conclude that emboli do not occur in the great majority of patients with venous thrombosis. The factors leading to fragmentation of the venous thrombus that allow a segment of the clot to circulate and impact in a pulmonary artery are unknown.

Despite a lack of total understanding of the sequence of events that lead to the development of a pulmonary embolus, certain conditions that predispose to venous thrombus formation have been identified. Lower extremity venous thrombosis is often associated with trauma or infection of the extremity, prolonged immobility, venous variocosities, obesity, or chronic heart failure. Direct injury to a vein or stasis of venous blood flow are the important factors that appear to promote local thrombus formation in these conditions. Although somewhat controversial, compelling evidence suggests that deep venous thrombosis and pulmonary emboli also occur more frequently in women taking oral contraceptives. The mechanism by which these drugs promote thrombus formation is unknown.

Superficial thrombophlebitis may lead to the development of deep venous thrombosis. Without specific treatment, a clot will propagate into the deep venous system in a small percentage of patients with superficial phlebitis. This sequence of events should be prevented, since pulmonary emboli do not arise from a thrombus in a superficial vein. In the majority of patients, specific factors that may contribute to the formation of a venous thrombus cannot be identified. Although it has been proposed that a hypercoagulate state exists in many of these patients, little objective evidence supports this theory.

CLINICAL MANIFESTATIONS

The clinical manifestations of pulmonary embolic disease are extremely varied. Both the physical signs and symptoms of the disease depend on the site of the embolus and the extent to which the pulmonary vascular bed is occluded. For clinical purposes, two separate clinical syndromes caused by pulmonary emboli should be considered. It is instructive to consider the manifestations of emboli that lodge in peripheral branches of the pulmonary arteries as being distinct from those caused by larger emboli that lodge in the main pulmonary arteries or their major branches. However, this approach is based somewhat on an artificial distinction, and a great deal of overlap in the syndromes may occur.

The signs and symptoms of peripherally located emboli are usually considered manifestations of pulmonary infarction. Pleuritic chest pain and shortness of breath are the most common initial complaints. Although hemoptysis and fever are also frequently observed, it is not unusual for these symptoms to occur 1 to 2 days after the onset of chest pain. A single embolus to only one area of lung probably occurs infrequently. Thus patients may complain of recurrent episodes of chest pain or hemoptysis before the incident that prompted them to visit a physician. Similarly they may have bilateral chest symptoms when first seen.

Physical examination early in the course of the syndrome often reveals tachypnea and tachycardia. Localized rales or a pleural friction rub may be audible over the involved area. If a pleural effusion has developed by the time the patient is first examined, dullness to percussion and decreased breath sounds may be observed. Although emboli most frequently arise from clots in the lower extremities, the majority of patients with pulmonary embolic disease do not have clinical evidence of deep venous thrombi.

The signs and symptoms of emboli that lodge in the proximal pulmonary arteries are primarily related to the hemodynamic events resulting from major obstruction of the blood flow in the pulmonary vascular bed. Acute shortness of breath, syncope, dizziness, weakness, and substernal chest pain are the most common symptoms observed in these patients.

Tachypnea and tachycardia are frequently present during physical examination. However, localized signs over peripheral areas of the lung are usually not present. Hypotension and findings of acute pulmonary hypertension or cor pulmonale are not uncommon. Thus a loud pulmonic valve closure sound, a right ventricular lift, distended neck veins, or a murmur of tricuspid valve or pulmonic valve insufficiency may be present.

ROENTGENOGRAPHIC MANIFESTATIONS

Although the chest roentgenogram is abnormal in the majority of patients with documented pulmonary emboli, the abnormalities are usually nonspecific and certainly not diagnostic of the disease. A localized parenchymal infiltrate or a pleural effusion are the most important abnormalities. In most cases the parenchymal infiltrate is somewhat ill defined and peripherally located. Characteristically the process extends to a pleural surface. As the process evolves, it may assume a convex border and take on the appearance of what has been described as a "Hampton hump". Volume loss and areas of linear atelectasis may also be observed. Pleural effusions occur frequently.

In cases in which the embolus is centrally located, the only roentgenographic abnormalities are those directly related to vascular obstruction. Areas of relative hypoperfusion of the parenchyma may be observed on a plain roentgenogram. Rarely an abrupt cutoff of the vascular shadow leading to this area can also be seen. If a large embolus lodges in a main pulmonary artery, the hilar shadow on the involved side may be small, and hypoperfusion of the entire lung on the side of the embolus may be apparent. In addition, the contralateral hilar shadow may be enlarged because of dilation of the pulmonary artery that is receiving the majority of right ventricular output.

PHYSIOLOGIC MANIFESTATIONS

Pulmonary emboli produce a number of physiologic abnormalities. In an attempt to approach these physiologic abnormalities in an organized manner, it is useful to clearly differentiate events that occur downstream from the site of impaction from those occurring proximal to the embolus. The major downstream events are caused by cessation of blood flow in the pulmonary-capillary bed usually perfused by the occluded vessel. Two major events may take place in these areas. First, an immediate alteration in local ventilation-perfusion (V/Q) relationships occurs. Alveoli that continue to be ventilated cannot contribute to gas exchange, since their alveolar capillaries are no longer perfused. Since gas exchange does not occur in these alveoli, the ventilation of these areas is "wasted," and therefore these alveoli represent areas of dead space ventilation. The overall effect of such areas on total gas exchange by the lung depends on their magnitude. If a large number of alveoli are transformed into areas of dead space ventilation by occlusion of their pulmonary artery blood supply, gas exchange by the lung may become grossly abnormal.

In addition to the increase in dead space ventilation, other events associated with pulmonary emboli also affect gas exchange by the lung. It has been proposed that a number of bioactive agents such as histamine, bradykinin, or prostaglandins are released locally into the lung after a pulmonary embolus. These agents may have a marked effect on V/Q relationships by influencing the distribution of perfusion throughout the entire lung. Although the exact mechanism by which this occurs has not been clearly defined, substantial evidence shows that the gas-exchange abnormalities which occur in pulmonary embolic disease cannot simply be explained by the mechanical interruption of perfusion distal to impaction of an embolus. Thus the abnormalities in gas exchange may well result from both an increase in dead space ventilation caused by mechanical obstruction to blood flow and a more generalized abnormality in V/Q relationship, presumably caused by vasoactive mediators released during the embolic episode.

The major physiologic effects that occur proximal to the site of a pulmonary embolus are related to obstruction to pulmonary artery blood flow. There are several consequences of this event. First, if right ventricular output is maintained, the blood flow that would normally perfuse areas distal to the site of obstruction must be diverted to other regions of the lung. This redistribution of pulmonary blood flow may have an effect on pulmonary gas exchange. If the major portion of pulmonary blood flow is diverted to relatively underventilated regions, the V/Q ratios in these areas may decrease further, leading to the development of progressive hypoxemia. In addition, if substantial obstruction of the pulmonary vascular bed results from multiple small emboli or several large centrally located emboli, pulmonary artery pressure may increase substantially. Under some circumstances, the right ventricle may not tolerate the increase in pressure, and thus the right ventricle may fail, resulting in the development of acute cor pulmonale. Obviously, left ventricular output also decreases substantially in this situation, producing hypotension or other evidence of decreased systemic perfusion.

DIAGNOSIS

The clinical, roentgenographic, and physiologic manifestations of pulmonary embolic disease are extremely varied and may be observed in a variety of other diseases. Thus a logical diagnostic evaluation must be undertaken to diagnose this disease correctly.

To make a diagnosis of pulmonary embolic disease, various imaging techniques must be employed to demonstrate a specific abnormality in pulmonary perfusion. As previously mentioned, although roentgenographic abnormalities occur in a large percentage of patients with a pulmonary embolus, they are nonspecific and cannot be considered diagnostic. Similarly, electrocardiographic abnormalities and other routine laboratory studies are of little value in confirming the diagnosis of this disease.

Clearly, a pulmonary angiogram is the most sensitive and specific technique for making the diagnosis of a pulmonary embolus. The demonstration of either an intraluminal filling defect or an abrupt cutoff of a branch of a pulmonary artery is virtually diagnostic of pulmonary embolic disease (Fig. 21-1). There is no question that pulmonary emboli can be missed by routine angiography. An injection of contrast material into a suspicious vessel detected by a routine main pulmonary artery injection combined with multiple views of the suspicious vessel may be required to demonstrate a diagnostic abnormality. However, if careful attention is paid to these technical details, a normal pulmonary angiogram excludes the diagnosis of pulmonary embolic disease. Neither delayed filling nor hypoperfusion of areas of lung distal to an embolus alone can be considered diagnostic of an embolus.

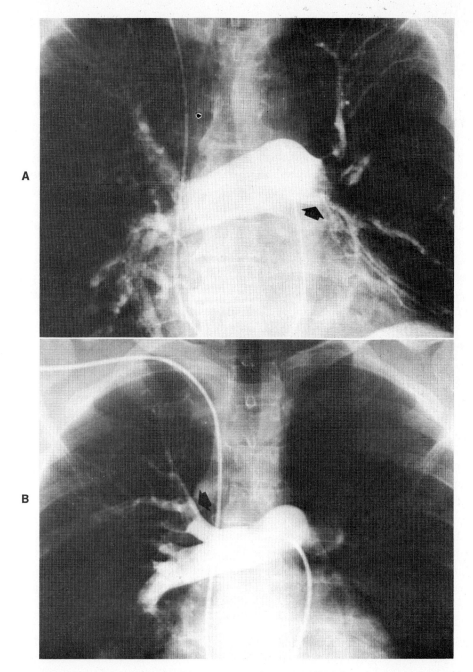

Fig. 21-1. Pulmonary angiogram demonstrating abrupt cutoff of dye caused by an embolus in the, **A,** left main pulmonary artery at the takeoff of the branch to the left upper lobe and, **B,** pulmonary artery to the right upper lobe.

Perfusion lung scanning is a less direct way of assessing the presence of an obstruction to pulmonary vascular blood flow. With this technique, particulate material labeled with a radioactive isotope is injected into a systemic vein. The particles are of a predetermined size that allows them to be trapped in the precapillary pulmonary arterioles. The distribution of pulmonary blood flow can then be determined by measuring the radioactivity in the various lung fields. Although the amount of radioactivity in any area of lung can be quantitated in a relative fashion, a visual representation of the distribution of radioactivity has proved to be of most value in the evaluation of individuals suspected of having a pulmonary embolus. Underperfused regions of lung appear as relatively cold areas on the lung scan. As with any study, special consideration must be paid to the technical aspects of the procedure to ensure that reliable data are collected. As with pulmonary angiography, the diagnostic accuracy of lung scanning is increased if multiple views of the lungs are obtained.

Perfusion lung scans are extremely useful in the evaluation of patients suspected of having a pulmonary embolus. However, the perfusion abnormalities demonstrated by this technique may be caused by a number of different conditions. Specifically, underlying pulmonary parenchymal disease will produce perfusion defects on a lung scan. Thus making the diagnosis of pulmonary emboli based on scan abnormalities without first performing a pulmonary angiogram is controversial.

Despite certain limitations in interpretation of scan abnormalities, there is general agreement about the role of the scan in certain patients suspected of having pulmonary embolic disease. A normal lung scan excludes the diagnosis of pulmonary embolus. This is an extremely important point. It means that the lung scan can be used to effectively screen out a substantial percentage of the patients in whom the diagnosis of pulmonary embolic disease is being considered. Patients with unexplained episodes of shortness of breath, recurrent chest pain or near syncope usually fall into this category. If a normal lung scan is obtained in such patients, further evaluation for pulmonary embolic disease is unnecessary.

Abnormal perfusion scans can be divided into two major categories: those which reveal defects that are segmental in size and distribution and those which do not. In interpreting the significance of these perfusion defects, it is important that the defects coincide with areas that are normal on the chest roentgenogram. If the area with the perfusion defect is normal on the chest roentgenogram, segmental defects have a high probability of being caused by an embolus. Conversely, nonsegmental defects are unlikely to be caused by emboli. Approximately 75% of patients with documented pulmonary emboli have high-probability scan defects, whereas less than 25% have low-probability scans.

The question in applying these data as an absolute diagnostic test is whether this degree of specificity and sensitivity can be accepted when the complications and therapy of disease may be life threatening. Regardless, it seems reasonable to consider the results of the perfusion scan within the context of the clinical presentation when making a decision as to whether a pulmonary angiogram should be performed. Some authorities would argue that a pulmonary angiogram is always required to absolutely exclude or confirm the diagnosis, whereas others would argue that the angiogram can be used selectively. Obviously a reiteration of the arguments that have been mounted on both sides of this tissue is beyond the scope of this discussion.

The use of ventilation scanning in conjunction with perfusion scanning has proved to be of value in further defining the specificity of perfusion defects. Ventilation scans are obtained by having the patient inhale an inert radioactive gas and determining the distribution of ventilation in much the same way that blood flow is assessed by the perfusion scan. The rationale for the value of this technique in pulmonary embolic disease is based on the fact that perfusion defects attributable solely to parenchymal processes or airways diseases should be accompanied by matched ventilation defects, whereas perfusion defects in areas in which ventilation has been maintained have a high probability of being caused by a pulmonary embolus (Fig. 21-2). In fact, with good technique most authorities agree that such abnormalities have such a high probability of being a pulmonary embolus that pulmonary angiography is not required to confirm the diagnosis.

Arterial blood analyses are frequently obtained in evaluating patients suspected of having a pulmonary embolus. However, the results of arterial blood gas analysis are of little diagnostic value. As discussed previously, V/Q abnormalities are uniformly present in this disease. As a result, hypoxemia occurs in the majority of patients during the acute stage of the disease. However, hypoxemia is present in the majority of patients with any form of pulmonary disease and in patients with acute myocardial infarction or congestive heart failure. Thus a low arterial oxygen tension (P_aO_2) is a nonspecific finding and of no diagnostic value. A small percentage of patients with pulmonary embolic disease have a normal P_aO_2. In many of these patients a more sophisticated analysis of gas exchange would probably reveal a defect in oxygen exchange across the lung even when the P_aO_2 itself is normal. Nevertheless, this does not change the fact that a normal P_aO_2 does not exclude the presence of a pulmonary embolus.

In recent years interest has increased in the use of techniques to detect the presence of thrombosis of the deep venous system of the lower extremity in patients suspected of having a pulmonary embolus. Venograms, Doppler techniques and lower extremity plethysmography to assess blood flow, and scanning techniques to detect incorporation of fibrinogen labeled with a radioactive isotope into a thrombus have all been advocated for use in this clinical setting. The rationale for this approach is based on the concept that, since the majority of emboli arise from deep venous thrombosis of the lower extremity, normal venous studies would disprove the presence of a pulmonary embolus. Although this is generally true, emboli will

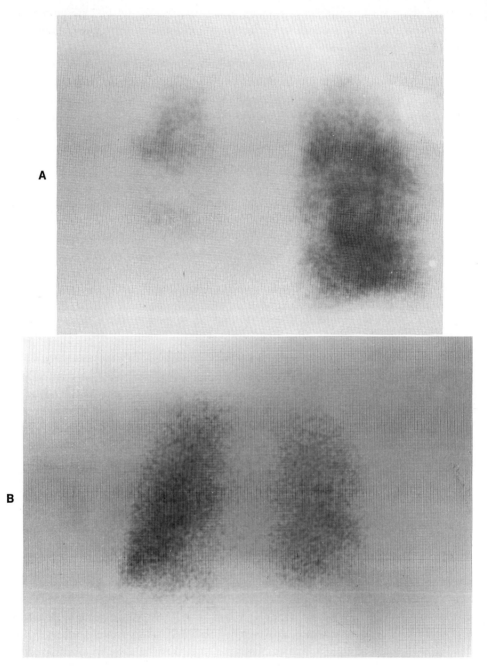

Fig. 21-2. A, Perfusion lung scan (posterior view) demonstrating large perfusion defects in the left lung. **B,** Ventilation lung scan (posterior view) obtained simultaneously showing normal ventilation in the areas of impaired perfusion.

occasionally arise from other sites and thus be overlooked by this diagnostic approach. In general, therapeutic decisions should be based on studies that directly assess pulmonary perfusion abnormalities.

TREATMENT

The primary goal of treatment in pulmonary embolic disease is to prevent additional embolic episodes. Heparin is the drug of choice for this purpose, and it can be administered by a variety of techniques. However, continuous intravenous infusion is generally agreed to be the best method for administering the drug to achieve a relatively constant level of anticoagulant activity. Heparin should be administered at a dose that maintains the partial thromboplastin time in the range of two and one half to three times normal. The incidence of bleeding complications is higher when the drug is administered intermittently by intravenous or subcutaneous routes, since extremely high levels of anticoagulant activity may be present immediately after administration of each dose.

The duration of heparin therapy required to prevent recurrent emboli is unclear. Although 5 days would appear to be adequate, most patients are treated for a period of 7 to 10 days. Oral agents are frequently employed to provide chronic anticoagulant therapy after heparin is discontinued, although no clear data indicate that chronic anticoagulation for weeks to months after an embolus has any effect on preventing recurrent emboli. However, chronic anticoagulant therapy carries a significant risk of producing bleeding complications; thus it should not be instituted without careful consideration of the risks involved.

Other approaches to therapy may be required in certain clinical situations. Heparin obviously cannot be employed in patients who have an absolute or a relative contraindication to anticoagulant therapy. In this situation, mechanical blockade of the inferior vena cava may be necessary to prevent embolic episodes. Inferior vena caval blood flow can be surgically interrupted by plicating or externally clipping the vessel. The same effect can be achieved by passing an expandable "umbrella" into the vena cava from the jugular vein. Each technique employed to interrupt vena caval blood flow has certain risks and complications. Obviously a major surgical procedure is required with external approaches, and infection or vena caval perforation may occur with the "umbrella" technique. The relative risks of heparin therapy must be weighed against these complications.

Generally a patient who reembolizes or who bleeds while receiving adequate anticoagulation by heparin should be considered a candidate for vena caval interruption. The goal of this therapy clearly is to prevent further embolization to the lung, despite the fact that the patient cannot continue heparin therapy. The specific techniques used in this situation depend on a number of clinical variables. However, application of the vena cava clip is probably the most frequently used procedure in this situation.

The primary effect of heparin is the prevention of further embolization from the site of the venous thrombus. There is little evidence that heparin has any significant effect on emboli lodged in the pulmonary vascular bed. These emboli appear to undergo spontaneous lysis. In some situations, rapid lysis of an embolus may be desirable. Patients with centrally located emboli that have produced major obstruction to pulmonary blood flow resulting in substantial adverse hemodynamic effects might benefit from such therapy. In addition, patients with central emboli without adverse hemodynamic effects might also be considered candidates for such therapy on the assumption that the occurrence of even a small additional embolus might result in hemodynamic instability.

Urokinase and streptokinase are thrombolytic agents that can be administered by continuous intravenous infusion. These agents have been shown to promote lysis of pulmonary emboli over a period of hours. A national study of the value of urokinase in patients with pulmonary emboli has demonstrated that it has limited usefulness, since it is unusual to encounter a patient who has substantial obstruction to the pulmonary vascular bed accompanied by hemodynamic instability. Most patients have peripheral emboli and respond appropriately to heparin therapy. Thus urokinase is of potential value in only a small percentage of patients with pulmonary embolic disease.

Centrally located emboli can be removed surgically. Embolectomy is not performed often, not only because few patients are expected to benefit from such a procedure, but also because the mortality and morbidity associated with the procedure are high.

Finally, prevention of deep venous thrombosis in high-risk situations should be beneficial in reducing the incidence of pulmonary embolic disease acquired in the hospital. Low-dose heparin therapy (1500 units subcutaneously/12 hours) has been shown to effectively prevent venous thrombosis in certain clinical situations. Because of the relative safety of this therapy, it is used in a variety of patients requiring prolonged bed rest. In low doses, heparin prevents venous thrombosis by an antithrombin activity that is not reflected in standard tests of anticoagulant activity. Thus the partial thromboplastin time remains normal during this form of therapy.

CLINICAL COURSE

The majority of patients with pulmonary emboli who receive prompt and effective therapy experience an uneventful clinical course. However, in a small percentage of patients, the clinical course is complicated despite adequate therapy.

First, persistent hypotension and acute cor pulmonale develop in some patients with major occlusion of their pulmonary vascular bed and may lead to death. This sequence of events occurs in less than 5% of patients with pulmonary emboli.

Second, reembolization occurs in some patients. The greatest concern for this group of patients is that progressive obstruction of their pulmonary vascular bed by multiple emboli may lead to hemodynamic instability. For this reason, an aggressive approach to prevent further emboli by interruption of vena caval blood flow must be undertaken. Embolization should be adequately documented before these techniques are employed. In some circumstances, documentation of reembolization may be difficult, particularly if the original diagnosis was based solely on a perfusion scan defect. Changes in defects on perfusion scans may occur during the uncomplicated resolution of an embolus. Thus a change on serial scans cannot be interpreted as being indicative of recurrent emboli. Obviously the development of new defects in an area of lung not involved initially is highly suggestive of a new embolus. Less dramatic changes may not be interpretable. Obviously it would be useful to be able to compare serial pulmonary angiograms in this clinical setting. New defects on the angiogram can be explained as evidence of new emboli. This is one argument for obtaining pulmonary angiograms in the majority of patients with embolic episodes at the time of initial evaluation.

An additional complication is bleeding attributable to heparin. Frequently the bleeding is minor and of little significance. However, on occasion major life-threatening hemorrhage may occur. Profuse bleeding is particularly serious not only because the bleeding may be life threatening, but also because interruption of vena caval flow may be necessary if heparin must be discontinued.

As stated previously, the majority of emboli undergo spontaneous lysis. Serial perfusion scans and angiograms have demonstrated that this process occurs over weeks to months. It is extremely unusual for a scan or angiogram to revert to normal within 1 to 2 weeks after diagnosis. In a small percentage of patients, perfusion defects persist for at least a year. The significance of these defects is unclear. Rarely a major central embolus may fail to undergo lysis. Persistent dyspnea may be the only clinical manifestation of this complication. In this clinical setting, serial scans and angiograms should be performed to document the persistence of vascular obstruction. If a major central lesion fails to resove in 3 to 4 months, consideration should be given to embolectomy. Occasionally a patient may have multiple emboli that fail to undergo lysis in the major branches of the pulmonary artery. The location and extent of these emboli may make surgical removal impossible. In this situation, chronic pulmonary hypertension and cor pulmonale may develop and lead to death.

Finally, patients who have received adequate therapy may reembolize after leaving the hospital. The reasons for this are unclear, but patients who have recurrent embolic episodes should probably be maintained on chronic anticoagulant therapy if this is feasible. It is also important to point out that some patients with multiple recurrent emboli in small peripheral pulmonary artery branches may have manifestations of pulmonary hypertension without clinical evidence of previous episodes of an acute embolus. At this stage of the disease, it is virtually impossible to make the diagnosis clinically. However, a lung biopsy may reveal intraluminal webs or bands indicating prior embolization.

Section four

RESPIRATORY FAILURE

Chapter 22

VENTILATION AND GAS EXCHANGE

Gas exchange (oxygen and carbon dioxide) is the primary function of the lung. For normal gas exchange to occur, the various components of the respiratory system must function in a highly integrated fashion. First, the respiratory control mechanisms and the respiratory muscles must act in concert to provide a level of alveolar ventilation that is appropriate for the level of metabolic activity. Second, perfusion must be closely matched to ventilation for efficient gas exchange to occur by bulk diffusion across the alveolar-capillary membrane. For ventilation and perfusion to be closely matched, the mechanical properties of both the airways and alveoli and the hemodynamics of the pulmonary vascular system must be normal. Diseases that involve any of these components of the respiratory system produce abnormalities in gas exchange resulting in hypoxemia alone or a combination of hypoxemia and hypercapnia.

Minor abnormalities in gas exchange occur in all lung diseases and in most diseases that affect the neuromuscular components of the chest cage. Mild to moderate derangements in arterial oxygen and carbon dioxide tensions are not usually of great significance. However, severe, life-threatening hypoxemia and/or hypercapnia may develop during the course of a number of diseases and produce a condition referred to as "respiratory failure." This pathophysiologic state is arbitrarily defined as the presence of an arterial oxygen tension (P_aO_2) of less than 60 mm Hg or an arterial carbon dioxide tension (P_aCO_2) greater than 50 mm Hg. Respiratory failure may be acute or chronic and may be caused by a large variety of diseases. Nevertheless, all cases of respiratory failure can be classified into one of three major categories. Each of these categories is characterized by a predominant pathophysiologic abnormality in gas exchange. Since management of each of these forms of respiratory failure is markedly different, it is extremely important to correctly classify each case of respiratory failure on the basis of the underlying gas-exchange abnormality.

Before the clinical features of the different forms of respiratory failure are discussed, it is important to understand the way in which the components of the respiratory system are integrated to maintain normal gas exchange. A few comments about oxygen and carbon dioxide are initially in order so that the consequences of abnormal gas exchange can be placed in proper context.

Oxygen

Oxygen is essential for cellular metabolism. In resting humans, the total volume of oxygen necessary to meet the metabolic requirement of the body is approximately 150 to 250 ml/minute. In a maximally exercising, trained athlete, the oxygen requirements may exceed 3 L/minute. To meet these demands, oxygen is transported to the cells in the blood. Inadequate delivery of oxygen to cells results in cellular dysfunction that may eventually lead to organ failure. To understand the relationship between hypoxemia and cell dysfunction, it is important to understand the relationship between the P_aO_2 and delivery of oxygen.

The volume of oxygen delivered to each organ is determined by the volume of oxygen contained in a given volume of blood and the volume of blood perfusing the capillary bed of the organ per unit of time. If both these factors are known, the volume of oxygen delivered to the organ per unit of time can be calculated. Perfusion of the body as a whole is determined primarily by the cardiac output and is for the most part independent of gas exchange. The volume of oxygen contained in blood is determined by the concentration of hemoglobin and the partial pressure of oxygen (PO_2).

The majority of oxygen in blood is bound to hemoglobin. When fully saturated, 1 gm of hemoglobin binds approximately 1.34 ml of oxygen. The degree of saturation of hemoglobin is directly related to the PO_2 in the blood. A plot of the relationship of the PO_2 to the percent saturation of hemoglobin is known as the "oxyhemoglobin dissociation curve" (Fig. 22-1). From this curve, the percent saturation of hemoglobin can be ascertained for any P_aO_2. This relationship can be influenced by temperature, pH, and physical characteristics of the hemoglobin molecule.

Two aspects of the oxyhemoglobin dissociation curve are very important. First, the curve reaches a plateau of 100% saturation when the PO_2 is approximately 100 mm Hg. As a result, increasing the PO_2 above this level has virtually no effect on the volume of oxygen bound to hemoglobin. Second, the curve is steep between a PO_2 of 20 and 50 mm Hg. Thus small changes in PO_2 in this range result in relatively large changes in the volume of oxygen bound to hemoglobin. The clinical significance of these relationships will become clear later.

In addition to the oxygen bound to hemoglobin, a small volume of oxygen is dissolved directly in cells and plasma. This volume (in milliliters) is also determined by the PO_2 in blood. Approximately 0.003 ml of oxygen is dissolved in 1 dl of blood for every millimeter of mercury, PO_2.

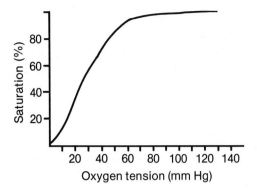

Fig. 22-1. Oxyhemoglobin dissociation curve. A curvilinear relationship exists between oxygen tension and hemoglobin saturation.

The total oxygen content of blood is the sum of the volume of oxygen bound to hemoglobin and the volume of oxygen dissolved in plasma. At a normal hemoglobin concentration of approximately 15 gm/dl, the volume of oxygen bound to hemoglobin is approximately sixty-five times greater than the volume of oxygen dissolved in plasma. This fact clearly illustrates the importance of hemoglobin in the process of tissue oxygenation, since it is the volume of oxygen in blood (arterial oxygen content) that primarily determines the adequacy of this process. However, because of the characteristics of oxygen binding by hemoglobin (illustrated by the shape of the oxyhemoglobin dissociation curve), the relationship between the P_aO_2 and arterial oxygen content is not linear. The effect on gas exchange by the lung will be discussed later.

Carbon dioxide

Carbon dioxide is a by-product of aerobic cellular metabolism, and thus the body continuously produces it. The primary pathway for elimination of carbon dioxide from the body is by diffusion across the alveolar-capillary membrane into the alveolar gas to be expired into the environment. The major effect of an alteration in carbon dioxide excretion by the lung is on the acid-base balance of blood. To understand this effect, it is important to understand the way in which carbon dioxide is transported in the blood.

Carbon dioxide diffuses from the tissue into capillary blood in response to a partial pressure gradient across the capillary wall. The majority of the carbon dioxide diffuses into erythrocytes, whereas a small fraction remains dissolved in plasma. Within the red cell, most of the carbon dioxide is hydrated to form carbonic acid (H_2CO_3). This biochemical reaction may be driven in either direction and is accelerated by carbonic anhydrase. The H_2CO_3 formed by this reaction is rapidly ionized to hydrogen ion (H^+) and bicarbonate (HCO_3^-). These ionic constituents may remain in the cell or diffuse into plasma. A small amount of the carbon dioxide that enters

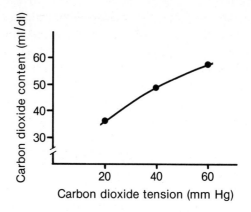

Fig. 22-2. Relationship between carbon dioxide tension and carbon dioxide content. This relationship is nearly linear over the physiologic range of carbon dioxide tensions encountered in almost all clinical situations.

the erythrocyte combines with hemoglobin to form carbaminohemoglobin. In contrast with oxygen, the total carbon dioxide content of blood is related to the partial pressure of carbon dioxide (PCO_2) in blood in an almost linear fashion. The P_aCO_2 varies in direct proportion to changes in the carbon dioxide content of arterial blood (Fig. 22-2).

Changes in arterial carbon dioxide tension (P_aCO_2) are extremely important in acid-base balance, since the concentration of H_2CO_3 in blood is determined by the PCO_2 according to the following relationship:

$$H_2CO_3 = PCO_2 \times 0.0301$$

where 0.0301 is the solubility coefficient of carbon dioxide in plasma at body temperature. In turn, the pH of blood is in part determined by the concentration of H_2CO_3 according to the relationship defined by the Henderson-Hasselbalch equation:

$$pH = 6.3 + \log \frac{HCO_3^-}{H_2CO_3}$$

Thus an increase in PCO_2 increases the concentration of H_2CO_3, which results in a decrease in pH (acidemia). Conversely a decrease in PCO_2 decreases the concentration of H_2CO_3 and results in an increase in pH (alkalemia).

The pH of blood is also influenced by a number of metabolic factors that are independent of changes in the PCO_2. The concentration of HCO_3^- is primarily determined by renal tubular function. In addition, complex interactions of various buffer systems act to keep the pH in a normal range. All these processes are critical for acid-base balance. However, for the purpose of this discussion, it is essential to understand only that the P_{CO_2} directly determines the concentration of H_2CO_3 in blood and therefore is an important determinant of systemic acid-base balance.

In the alveolar capillary, carbon dioxide diffuses into the alveolar air space to be expired. In resting humans, approximately 300 L of carbon dioxide are expired each day. Alterations in alveolar ventilation by affecting the total carbon dioxide content of blood influence the P_{CO_2} of arterial blood. It is extremely important to appreciate the linear nature of the relationship between P_{CO_2} and carbon dioxide content. As will be discussed later, this relationship allows a normal P_{CO_2} to be maintained by the lung despite marked inhomogeneity in regional gas exchange.

In summary, blood gas derangements are significant because of their metabolic effects. Hypoxemia decreases the oxygen content of arterial blood. As a result, cellular hypoxia may occur, unless compensatory increases in hemoglobin concentration or cardiac output occur. Hypocapnia or hypercapnia produce respectively respiratory alkalosis or acidosis that results in alterations in blood pH unless appropriate metabolic compensatory mechanisms become effective. Systemic acidemia or alkalemia interferes with optimal cell function and when severe may actually be life threatening. In addition to these metabolic effects, the level of P_{O_2} and P_{CO_2} may directly produce certain clinically significant physiologic responses. For example, a high P_{CO_2} may directly depress mental function independent of changes in pH. Similarly, a low P_{O_2} may stimulate catecholamine secretion by the adrenal medulla, leading to tachycardia and hypertension.

PHYSIOLOGY OF GAS EXCHANGE

To maintain normal arterial oxygen and carbon dioxide tensions, alveolar ventilation must be adequate to excrete the carbon dioxide produced over a wide range of metabolic demands, and ventilation and perfusion must be closely matched to facilitate oxygenation of blood flowing through the pulmonary capillaries.

Ventilation

When gas is inspired into the lungs, only a portion is distributed to the alveoli in the gas-exchanging parenchyma of the lung. The remainder of the inspired gas simply fills the conducting airways and does not come into contact with alveolar-capillary membranes. The volume of inspired gas that does influence gas exchange within the alveoli is referred to as "alveolar ventilation." The volume of inspired gas that simply fills conducting airways is referred to as "anatomic dead space ventilation." In certain pathologic conditions, the perfusion of some alveoli may be completely interrupted. As a result, ventilation of these alveoli cannot contribute to gas exchange. The portion of inspired gas distributed to these alveoli is referred to as "physiologic dead space ventilation." Thus total dead space ventilation includes ventilation of conducting airways (anatomic dead space) and unperfused alveoli (physiologic dead space). Total ventilation is the sum of the alveolar ventilation and the total dead space ventilation.

Carbon dioxide excretion by the lung is directly related to the alveolar ventilation. Thus the P_aCO_2 is also directly related to alveolar ventilation. This relationship can be expressed by the following:

$$P_aCO_2 = K \frac{\dot{V}CO_2}{V_A}$$

where $\dot{V}CO_2$ represents carbon dioxide production, V_A represents alveolar ventilation, and K is a constant. This equation simply states that the P_aCO_2 is directly proportional to carbon dioxide production and inversely proportional to alveolar ventilation. Thus if carbon dioxide production is constant, a decrease of alveolar ventilation to half of normal would result in a doubling of the P_aCO_2. Similarly, if carbon dioxide production increases as a result of exercise or other metabolic conditions, the P_aCO_2 will increase unless alveolar ventilation increases proportional to the increase in carbon dioxide production.

Several points about this relationship must be emphasized. First, total ventilation is not directly determined by this relationship. For instance, if dead space ventilation increases for any reason, total ventilation must increase to maintain alveolar ventilation constant. Thus simply measuring minute ventilation will not provide information about the adequacy of alveolar ventilation. Second, the adequacy of alveolar ventilation under any condition can be determined simply by measuring the P_aCO_2. Thus hypoventilation and hyperventilation are by definition present when the P_aCO_2 increases or decreases respectively, regardless of the total ventilation.

Under most circumstances, the P_aCO_2 is carefully maintained in a narrow range by continued adjustments in the level of alveolar ventilation. The adjustment of alveolar ventilation is primarily achieved by the integrated activity of neural centers that sense small changes in the PCO_2 in arterial blood and stimulate appropriate respiratory muscle activity. Thus the level of total ventilation is such that alveolar ventilation remains appropriate for any level of carbon dioxide production. The organization of the various components of the nervous system involved in the control of ventilation has been extensively investigated for a number of years. Detailed description of all neural structures involved in this process is beyond the scope of this discussion. However, within the central nervous system a number of pathways function in an integrated manner to maintain adequate alveolar ventilation and a normal breathing pattern. Experiments have shown that some areas of the cerebral cortex, midbrain, thalmus, hypothalamus, and medulla influence breathing. Although the specific function of these areas is of considerable interest to neurophysiologists investigating breathing, it is not necessary to be completely knowledgeable of each of these regions and their function to develop a functional concept about ventilatory control mechanisms.

However, there is no doubt that the medulla is the site of the principal neural components that control spontaneous breathing. Both inspiratory and expiratory neurons can be identified in the dorsolateral portion of the medulla surrounding the nucleus ambiguous, the motor nucleus of the vagus, and glossopharyngeal nerves. These neurons are self-reexciting and mutually inhibitory, thus providing a mechanism for the rhythmic pattern of normal breathing. Certainly these neurons may be influenced by other neural stimuli; however, little is known about connecting networks within the brain that would link these various regions. The integrated central impulses descend in the anterolateral portion of the spinal cord to segmental levels where synapses with motor neurons of various respiratory muscles occur. It is very likely that these impulses are also influenced by afferent proprioceptive activity arising from the respiratory muscles themselves.

A change in the pH of the extracellular environment of the central chemoreceptor neurons appears to be the major stimulus for the medullary center to stimulate motor neuron activity in respiratory muscle. The central nervous system extracellular pH is directly influenced by the P_aCO_2, thus providing the necessary link between P_aCO_2 and $\dot{V}_A$. The exact nature and location of these chemosensitive structures within the medulla is unknown. It would appear that they are located near the surface where they can be influenced by the cerebrospinal fluid (CSF). The connecting pathways that might link these structures with efferent neurons of the medulla have not been defined.

Changes in the extracellular fluid of the brain can be monitored by studying the CSF, which is formed mainly by the plexi of the lateral cerebral ventricles. The CSF is not simply an ultrafiltrate of plasma. Active transport is required to move certain substances into the fluid. This transport is extremely important when considering acid-base changes in the CSF. The pH of CSF is lower than that of arterial blood. The CSF P_{CO_2} is approximately 7 to 9 mm Hg higher than that of blood, whereas the concentration of HCO_3^- is approximately the same in CSF and blood. Since bicarbonate is the only buffer in the CSF, pH changes are entirely related to the relationship between P_{CO_2} and HCO_3^-. This relationship can be expressed using an appropriate Henderson-Hasselbalch equation.

Carbon dioxide diffuses into the CSF, but $H+$ and HCO_3^- do not. Thus changes in alveolar ventilation that alter the P_aCO_2 have a rapid effect on CSF pH. An increase in CSF P_{CO_2} decreases the pH in the CSF, thus stimulating ventilation. A decrease in P_{CO_2} increases pH and depresses ventilation. Since the concentration of HCO_3^- changes only slowly, metabolic (nonrespiratory) acid-base abnormalities do not rapidly alter CSF pH and thus stimulate rapid changes in ventilation. In summary, changes in P_aCO_2 by mediating changes in CSF pH stimulate the medullary respiratory center to alter its neural discharge to the respiratory muscles in such a way that alveolar ventilation remains appropriate for any $\dot{V}_{CO_2}$. For this physiologic response to be effective, the neural pathways involved must be intact, and the respiratory muscles must be capable of responding to generate the required level of ventilation.

During normal resting ventilation, the diaphragm accounts for the majority of the muscle activity required for adequate ventilation. As minute ventilation increases, either because of an increase in alveolar ventilation, an increase in dead space ventilation, or both, respiratory muscle activity must increase to provide the work required to generate the increase in ventilation. In this situation, the intercostal muscles, abdominal muscles, and other accessory muscles of respiration may be used.

Although the central chemoreceptors of the medulla provide the predominant mechanism for the control of ventilation, it is important to recognize that peripheral chemoreceptors also influence ventilation. The peripheral chemoreceptors are located in the carotid and aortic bodies and communicate their impulses to the brain via afferent fibers of the vagus and glossopharyngeal nerves. The carotid bodies are located in the bifurcation of the common carotid artery, whereas the aortic bodies have been poorly localized. Although these chemoreceptors are primarily stimulated by a fall in the P_aO_2, they also respond to changes in arterial pH. It is clear that the carotid bodies are far more important than the aortic bodies in controlling ventilation in response to hypoxemia.

Under normal circumstances, hypoxemia is not a potent stimulus to increase ventilation. Substantial increases in alveolar ventilation are observed only when the P_aO_2 falls below 50 mm Hg. Furthermore, conflicting ventilatory responses occur during hypoxemia-induced hyperventilation because the decrease in PCO_2 that occurs during hyperventilation depresses ventilation through central receptor activity. The peripheral chemoreceptors appear to stimulate respiratory muscle activity through the same central neurons and efferent fibers as those stimulated by the central chemoreceptor impulses.

Ventilation-perfusion relationships

Although the P_aO_2 is influenced by changes in alveolar ventilation, the P_aO_2 is most dependent on close matching of the distribution of ventilation and perfusion throughout the lung. The mechanical properties that influence ventilation and perfusion of individual gas-exchanging units have been discussed previously. The factors that influence matching of ventilation and perfusion throughout the entire lung will be considered at this time.

The distribution of perfusion throughout the lung depends primarily on the gravitational effects described in Chapter 17. Therefore in upright humans, perfusion per unit of lung volume is lowest at the apex of the lung and progressively increases as the base is approached. Perfusion may begin to decrease again at the extreme base as the result of a decrease in capillary diameter. This alteration in capillary lumen size has been attributed to increased perivascular pressure caused by increased fluid accumulation in the perivascular space. The relative distribution of perfusion in the upright lung is represented in Fig. 22-3.

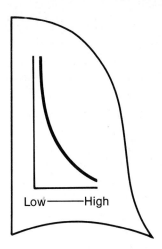

Low————High

Fig. 22-3. Distribution of blood flow per unit of lung volume in the upright lung. Blood flow per unit of lung volume is highest in the base and decreases progressively as the apex is approached.

Because regional perfusion is simply gravity dependent, changes in position greatly influence the distribution of perfusion throughout the lung. In the supine individual the effects of gravity are markedly diminished, since the anteroposterior distance of the lung is less than the base-to-apex distance. As a result, the range of transmural pressures in the pulmonary vascular bed is narrowed in the supine lung, and perfusion per unit of lung volume is more homogeneous. These observations are based on relative values for the perfusion of relatively large areas of lung. At any given time, perfusion of individual capillary beds may vary widely in such regions of lung because of local homeostatic mechanisms.

Ventilation per unit of lung volume also varies in different regions of the lung. In upright humans, ventilation is lowest in the apex and highest at the base. Gravity does not directly influence the distribution of ventilation throughout the lung in the same manner that it influences perfusion. However, the differences in ventilation are indirectly related to gravity through the effect of gravity on pleural pressure.

The pleural space is usually thought of as a freely communicating space with a single pressure. In fact, there are regional differences in pleural pressure that are thought to be caused by variations in chest cage movement over different regions of the lung. The greater the outward recoil of a region of chest wall, the more negative the pressure in the pleural space underlying that region of chest wall. In addition, the weight of the lung as it is suspended from the hilum is greater at the base because of the effect of gravity. This effect may also influence regional differences in pleural pressure.

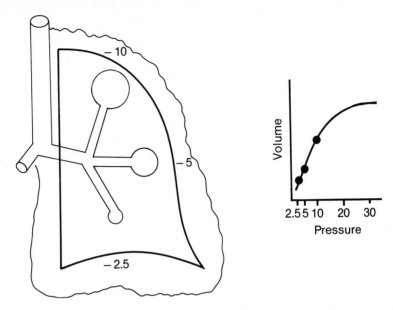

Fig. 22-4. Effect of gravity on interpleural pressure at functional residual capacity is depicted in the lung schematic. The pressure is more negative over the top of the lung when compared with the base. The effect of these differences in pleural pressure on resting alveolar size is depicted in the lung schematic and can be explained by reference to the static, deflation pressure-volume curve for the lung depicted on the right side of the figure. Assuming that the compliance of individual alveoli is constant throughout the lung, the resting volume of alveoli is determined by the transpulmonary pressure. The three points represented on the pressure-volume curve correspond to the transpulmonary pressure for the three alveolar units represented in the lung schematic. The differences in the size of each alveolar unit is apparent by reference to the volume axis of the pressure-volume plot.

Regardless of the exact cause, pleural pressure is most negative at the apex and increases progressively as the base is approached. The differences in pleural pressure mean that at any lung volume, alveoli in different zones of the lung are exposed to different transpulmonary pressures. Since the compliance of all alveoli throughout the lung is thought to be essentially identical, the resting volume of alveoli will vary in direct relationship to the transpulmonary pressure to which they are exposed. Since the transpulmonary pressure is greatest at the apex, the alveoli in the apex will be larger than those at the base at any lung volume below total lung capacity (TLC) (Fig. 22-4). At TLC all alveoli will be of equal size. Therefore, during a maximum inspiratory effort, smaller alveoli at the base must receive a greater volume than those at the apex to reach an identical volume at TLC. The differences in alveolar volume are responsible for the differences in distribution of ventilation per unit of lung volume in the normal upright lung.

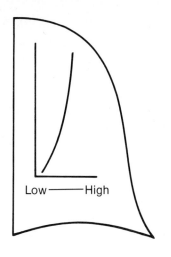

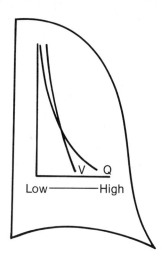

Fig. 22-5. *Right,* Distribution of ventilation (V) and perfusion (Q) per unit of lung volume in the upright lung. *Left,* Ratio of ventilation to perfusion in the upright lung. V/Q ratios are lowest in the base of the lung and increase progressively as the apex is approached.

For normal gas exchange, matching of ventilation and perfusion is essential. Although both ventilation and perfusion are lowest in the apex and increase progressively toward the base, the relative changes that occur from apex to base are different. Relatively speaking, perfusion is lower than ventilation at the apex and increases at a much greater rate than does ventilation as the base is approached. As a result, perfusion is relatively greater than ventilation at the base. In simple terms this means that the ratio of effective ventilation to perfusion is high at the apex (greater than 1) and low at the base (less than 1) (Fig. 22-5).

The importance of ventilation-perfusion (V/Q) ratios to normal gas exchange can be analyzed in the following way. Oxygen is continuously added to the alveolar space by ventilation and removed by blood flow. Thus the concentration of oxygen in the alveolar space and in the pulmonary venous blood, assuming complete equilibration across the alveolar-capillary membrane, will be determined by the ratio of the rate that oxygen is added to the rate at which it is removed. In other words, the $P_{A}O_{2}$ and $P_{a}O_{2}$ will be determined by the V/Q ratio. A V/Q of 1 represents normal gas exchange in the lung, whereas a V/Q greater than 1 results in an increase in $P_{A}O_{2}$ and $P_{a}O_{2}$, and a V/Q less than 1 results in a decrease in $P_{A}O_{2}$ and $P_{a}O_{2}$.

In the normal lung V/Q ratios range between 0.3 and 3.0; however, most alveoli have V/Q ratios of approximately 1. Obviously, an abnormality in the neuromuscular mechanisms responsible for effective ventilation, an abnormality in either the mechanical properties of the airways and alveoli, or the distribution of pulmonary blood flow may change the V/Q ratios of alveoli throughout the lung and decrease the proportion of alveoli with normal ratios. As a result of any of these pathophysiologic states, gas exchange across the lung may become abnormal, leading to hypoxemia alone or a combination of hypoxemia and hypercapnia.

It is important to consider at this point the relationship between alterations in individual V/Q ratios and overall gas exchange by the lung. To grasp these concepts it is essential to understand that the PCO_2 and PO_2 in the systemic arterial circulation is the result of mixing of blood from individual gas-exchanging units. Blood leaving these units may have a wide range of oxygen and carbon dioxide partial pressures. The resultant partial pressure when all of these units are mixed is not the mean of the individual partial pressures. When the various blood samples are mixed, the mixture will have a gas content that is the mean of the content of all of the individual samples. The PO_2 and PCO_2 are then simply determined passively on the basis of the mean content of oxygen and carbon dioxide in the mixed blood.

Recall that in the physiologic range there is a linear relationship between carbon dioxide content and PCO_2 and a sigmoid-shaped relationship between oxygen content and PO_2. The differences in these relationships are extremely impor-

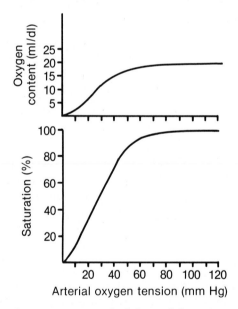

Fig. 22-6. Relationship of oxygen tension to both hemoglobin saturation and oxygen content. Because of the sigmoid shape of the oxyhemoglobin dissociation curve, oxygen content is not related to oxygen tension in a linear manner (as is the case with carbon dioxide tension and content). It is clear from the shape of the curve relating oxygen tension to oxygen content that decreases in content caused by low oxygen tension cannot be compensated for by simply increasing oxygen tension.

tant in determining the P_aO_2 and P_aCO_2 when the lung is abnormal. Since PCO_2 and carbon dioxide are related in a linear fashion, high and low PCO_2 values in blood leaving areas of lung with low and high V/Q ratios can balance each other and result in a normal carbon dioxide content in "mixed" arterial blood resulting in a normal P_aCO_2. Thus, as long as the overall V/Q ratio for the entire lung approximates 1, the P_aCO_2 will remain normal. This relationship is not true for oxygen. Although low and high V/Q areas result in correspondingly low and high values for PO_2 in blood leaving these areas, the oxygen content is not increased proportionately in the blood with a high PO_2 (Fig. 22-6). Thus blood with a high PO_2 leaving areas of lung with high V/Q ratios cannot compensate for blood with low oxygen content caused by low V/Q areas. Therefore hypoxemia will be present even if the overall V/Q ratio for the lung approximates 1 (Fig. 22-7).

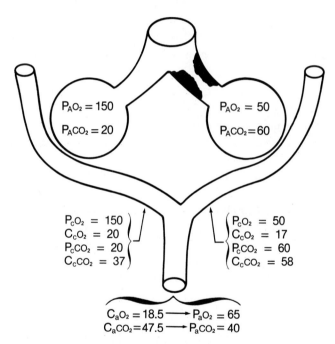

Fig. 22-7. Two-compartment lung with the compartments having equal blood flow but markedly different V/Q ratios. The different relationships between partial pressure and content for oxygen and carbon dioxide influence arterial blood gases under this circumstance. Since the relationship between content and partial pressure is essentially linear for carbon dioxide, a normal arterial carbon dioxide tension can be maintained despite marked abnormalities in regional V/Q ratios. In contrast, increasing oxygen tension does not cause a proportional increase in oxygen content, thus resulting in a low arterial oxygen tension under identical circumstances. Representative values for alveolar gas tensions (*Pa*), pulmonary-capillary gas tensions (*Pc*), contents (*Cc*), arterial gas tensions (*Pa*), and contents (*Ca*) are given.

Abnormalities in arterial blood gases

Various physiologic states produce abnormalities in arterial oxygen and carbon dioxide tensions. It is simplest to begin by considering the basis for alterations in the P_aCO_2. Since the P_aCO_2 is directly proportional to alveolar ventilation, abnormalities in the P_aCO_2 are caused only by abnormalities in alveolar ventilation.

Hypocapnia. If alveolar ventilation exceeds that required for a given level of carbon dioxide production, the P_aCO_2 will be lower than normal. Alveolar hyperventilation may occur as a result of either acute or chronic lung disease. In addition, hyperventilation may be observed in patients with a variety of metabolic or central nervous system diseases that directly stimulate ventilation through central nervous system mechanisms. Hyperventilation may also occur in patients with metabolic acidosis. In this condition alveolar hyperventilation serves as a mechanism for lowering the P_aCO_2 to compensate for the decrease in HCO_3^- caused by the metabolic derangement and thus protect to some degree the systemic arterial pH.

Hypercapnia. Inadequate alveolar ventilation results in an increase in the P_aCO_2. Hypoventilation is in almost all cases a manifestation of lung disease or an abnormality in central respiratory control mechanism or ineffective ventilatory action of the chest cage. Because of a marked increase in the physiologic dead space, total minute ventilation is often greater than normal in patients with alveolar hypoventilation caused by lung disease. However, in some cases central or peripheral obstruction to airflow may simply prevent inadequate ventilation of a large number of alveoli resulting in a fall in total alveolar ventilation without an increase in total minute ventilation.

Neuromuscular diseases that affect the respiratory muscles may also produce hypoventilation if the respiratory muscles are unable to generate the mechanical forces required for effective bellows-like function of the chest cage.

Similarly, abnormalities in respiratory control mechanisms may also produce alveolar hypoventilation. If the brainstem is damaged by drugs, trauma, or disease, appropriate neural impulses may not be transmitted to the respiratory muscles in response to either hypoxemia or hypercapnia. As a result of inadequate respiratory muscle activity, alveolar ventilation may become deficient, resulting in an increase in the P_aCO_2.

In contrast to the efficient compensatory hyperventilation response to acidosis, alveolar ventilation does not decrease in most situations when metabolic alkalosis is present. Thus an elevated P_aCO_2 is almost always indicative of disease of the respiratory system and only occasionally occurs as compensation for metabolic alkalosis.

Hypoxemia. Several pathophysiologic states alter gas exchange across the lung and produce hypoxemia. First, it is important to reemphasize that an isolated abnormality causing impairment of diffusion of oxygen across the alveolar-capillary membrane does not produce hypoxemia under normal conditions. However, impaired diffusion may accentuate the severity of hypoxemia caused by other mechanisms. *Alveolar hypoventilation, ventilation-perfusion mismatching,* and an *increase in the intrapulmonary shunt volume* are the three pathophysiologic mechanisms that produce hypoxemia.

The alveolar-arterial oxygen gradient A-aDO$_2$ is a useful index of oxygen exchange across the lung. Under normal circumstances it is less than 20 mm Hg. The difference that is measured in normal individuals is not truly caused by a difference in oxygen tensions across the alveolar-capillary membrane. Blood leaving the pulmonary capillary has a PO$_2$ that is equal to the alveolar PO$_2$. The difference that is measured is caused by the fact that the PO$_2$ of systemic arterial blood is lower than the PO$_2$ of oxygenated blood leaving the pulmonary capillaries. The drop that occurs in the PO$_2$ in the systemic circulation results from the fact that approximately 5% of the cardiac output shunts across the lung without being oxygenated. As a result, this blood has a low arterial oxygen content. Mixing of this blood with fully oxygenated blood leaving the pulmonary capillaries results in a small fall in the mean oxygen content of arterial blood and thus a drop in the PO$_2$ below that of the blood leaving the pulmonary capillaries.

Despite the fact that alveolar hypoventilation causes hypoxemia, this condition does not produce an abnormality in oxygen exchange across the lung. The decrease in P$_a$O$_2$ is directly caused by a decrease in P$_A$O$_2$. When alveolar ventilation decreases relative to perfusion, the partial pressure of oxygen in the alveolus decreases, since oxygen is removed from the alveolus more rapidly than it is supplied by ventilation. As discussed previously, the partial pressure of oxygen in blood leaving the alveolar capillary is identical to the partial pressure in the alveolus. Thus, if the P$_A$O$_2$ is low, the P$_a$O$_2$ must also be low. However, the difference between the P$_A$O$_2$ and P$_a$O$_2$ (A-aDO$_2$) will be normal in this situation.

If V/Q mismatching is present in the lung so that blood is not fully oxygenated during its course through the pulmonary capillaries, the P$_a$O$_2$ will reflect both this defect in oxygen exchange and the drop in PO$_2$ resulting from the normal shunt fraction. Thus the A-aDO$_2$ will be greater than normal. Similarly, if there is an increase in the fraction of the cardiac output shunting across the lung because of intrapulmonary shunting, the A-aDO$_2$ will also increase. Thus measurement of the A-aDO$_2$ can be useful in determining whether in the presence of alveolar hypoventilation the degree of hypoxemia is totally caused by hypoventilation or whether an abnormality in oxygen exchange is also present. In the former situation, the A-aDO$_2$ will be normal, but in the latter it will be increased.

The most common cause of hypoxemia is V/Q mismatching. In this pathophysiologic state, a larger percentage of pulmonary blood flow is distributed to gas-exchanging units with V/Q ratios of less than 1. As a result, blood leaving some pulmonary capillaries is not fully oxygenated and thus has a low oxygen content. Since the oxygen content does not increase proportionately when the PO$_2$ exceeds

100 mm Hg, the low oxygen content of blood leaving low V/Q regions cannot be compensated for by blood leaving high V/Q regions, despite the fact that the PO_2 is increased in this blood. Thus V/Q mismatching must result in hypoxemia.

It is important to understand that, in contrast to the physiology of an intrapulmonary shunt lesion, with V/Q mismatching all blood perfusing the lung is being distributed to alveoli that are being ventilated. As a result, increasing the P_AO_2 by having a patient breathe a gas mixture enriched with oxygen should produce an increase in the PO_2 of blood leaving all capillaries, even those which are associated with gas-exchanging units with low V/Q ratios. Since the oxygen content in the blood leaving these areas will be increased under these circumstances, the oxygen content of arterial blood will be more nearly normal, and therefore the P_aO_2 will increase. In fact, even when marked V/Q mismatching is present, it may be possible to completely normalize the P_aO_2 by increasing the inspired oxygen concentration (F_IO_2).

An increase in the intrapulmonary shunt fraction occurs when blood perfuses capillary beds of alveoli that are not ventilated. In this situation, there is no potential for gas exchange across the alveolar-capillary membrane. As a result, the partial pressure of oxygen and carbon dioxide in blood leaving these capillaries is identical to the partial pressure of these gases in blood as it enters the capillaries (mixed venous values). Since these units have no potential for gas exchange, increasing the F_IO_2 can have no effect on the PO_2 of blood leaving these capillaries, and the oxygen content of this blood will not increase, regardless of the F_IO_2. Therefore hypoxemia will persist despite oxygen therapy provided that the shunt volume is large enough so that the low oxygen content of this blood cannot be compensated for by mixing with blood containing maximum amounts of dissolved oxygen. As the shunt fraction increases, it has a progressively more adverse effect on the P_aO_2. In fact, when the shunt fraction exceeds 30%, the P_aO_2 changes very little even when the F_IO_2 is increased from 0.2 (room air) to 1.

When hypoxemia is documented, a logical approach may determine which of three pathophysiologic abnormalities of gas exchange are responsible. Hypoventilation can be excluded if the P_aCO_2 is not elevated. If the P_aCO_2 is elevated, measurement of the A-aDO_2 will determine whether the hypoxemia is totally caused by hypoventilation or whether the gas-exchange function across the lung is abnormal. If the A-aDO_2 is less than 20 mm Hg, pure hypoventilation is responsible. If the A-aDO_2 is greater than 20 mm Hg, V/Q mismatching or an increase in the intrapulmonary shunt must also be present.

Measurement of the P_aO_2 after an adequate period of oxygen breathing (100% oxygen for 20 min) will determine whether an intrapulmonary shunt lesion is present. If the shunt volume is normal, the P_aO_2 should exceed 500 mm Hg. At an F_IO_2 of 1, a P_aO_2 in excess of 500 mm Hg means that the A-aDO_2 at this F_IO_2 is normal. In effect this means that breathing 100% oxygen eliminates any gas-exchange abnormality caused by V/Q mismatching. This occurs because all perfused alveoli are ventilated to some degree. Regardless of the relative ventilation, nitrogen will eventually be washed out of all alveoli, leaving a $P_{A}O_2$ in all alveoli that is nearly identical. Therefore the blood leaving all capillaries will be identical to that in the alveoli, and there will be no decrease in the P_aO_2 when these various blood samples mix in the arterial system. Thus any abnormality in gas exchange across the lung during inspiration of 100% oxygen must be caused by the presence of some blood with a low oxygen content. This situation can only occur if blood is shunted through nonventilated alveoli. Thus a P_aO_2 of less than 500 mm Hg during inspiration of 100% oxygen indicates the presence of a shunt lesion. This does not mean that V/Q mismatching is not also present. If there is no shunt, the hypoxemia can be totally attributed to V/Q mismatching. If there is a shunt, it is likely that there is also V/Q mismatching, but this can only be determined by rather sophisticated techniques.

With a technique based on the relative solubility of six inert gases, it is possible to actually measure the relative distribution of ventilation and perfusion of lung zones that contain different V/Q ratios. The presence of V/Q mismatching and true shunts can be determined by this technique. However, this measurement is truly a research procedure and may not be applied for routine clinical evaluation of gas exchange across the lungs. Similarly, it is possible to partition V/Q mismatching and shunt lesions by measuring alveolar-to-arterial gradients at varying values for F_IO_2. This procedure also requires careful attention to technical detail and careful analysis of data and is not directly applicable or particularly useful for the clinical evaluation of gas-exchange abnormalities.

Chapter 23

RESPIRATORY FAILURE WITH NORMAL LUNGS

Respiratory failure may occur in patients with normal lungs if either the ventilatory function of the chest cage or ventilatory control mechanisms are impaired. A number of different conditions may produce this form of respiratory failure. For the purpose of discussion, these conditions will be classified by the mechanism that interferes with effective ventilation.

PATHOPHYSIOLOGY

Alveolar hypoventilation is the primary physiologic abnormality in this form of respiratory failure. As a result, hypercapnia is always present in this condition. Hypoxemia is also regularly present. In cases in which pure hypoventilation is present, oxygen exchange across the lung is normal; that is, the alveolar-arterial oxygen gradient (A-aDo$_2$) is normal. In these cases the degree of arterial hypoxemia is directly proportional to the degree of alveolar hypoventilation. However, in most cases ineffective ventilation leads to atelectasis or other pulmonary complications. As a result of these conditions, ventilation-perfusion (V/Q) mismatching develops, causing abnormal oxygen exchange across the lungs. Thus in the majority of patients, the A-aDo$_2$ is increased. Patients with conditions causing acute alveolar hypoventilation are most likely to have pure hypoventilation with no associated abnormality in oxygen exchange.

CLINICAL MANIFESTATIONS

The majority of the clinical manifestations that occur in patients with respiratory failure and normal lungs are caused by the condition responsible for the development of the respiratory failure. A description of the varied manifestations of these conditions is beyond the scope of this discussion. However, it is important to recognize that in some patients cor pulmonale with right ventricular failure may be the only manifestation of this form of respiratory failure. The presence of respiratory failure will be recognized in these patients only if hypercapnia is detected by arterial blood gas analysis. These patients do not have pulmonary symptoms unless they have an unrelated form of lung disease.

DIAGNOSIS

In most cases recognition of this form of respiratory failure is not difficult. The diagnosis is clear in patients with no clinical, roentgenographic, or physiologic manifestations of lung disease in whom hypoxemia and hypercapnia are demonstrated by arterial blood gas analysis.

It is far more difficult to recognize this form of respiratory failure in patients who also have lung disease. The major diagnostic difficulty occurs in patients with chronic bronchitis and emphysema, since chronic hypercapnia is most likely to occur in these diseases. In this situation, a decision must be made as to whether the hypercapnia is caused by the lung disease or whether it results from one of the conditions that lead to nonpulmonary respiratory failure. This distinction can only be made on the basis of the results of clinical pulmonary function tests. A marked decrease in expiratory flow rates is uniformly present in patients with chronic bronchitis and emphysema who develop hypercapnia. As a general rule, hypoventilation does not occur in these diseases unless the forced expired volume is less than 1300 cc.

Hypercapnia rarely develops in patients with diffuse diseases of the lung parenchyma and then only when a severe, restrictive ventilatory defect is present. Although no specific values define the limits of the total lung capacity that are compatible with the development of hypercapnia in these diseases, the restrictive defect should be severe before attributing hypoventilation to these diseases.

The ventilatory response to hypoxemia and hypercapnia can be evaluated in the physiology laboratory. On occasions these tests may be useful in patients suspected of having hypoventilation resulting from disease of the brainstem involving the respiratory control center. Patients with a disease of the respiratory control center do not augment ventilation appropriately in response to inhalation of gas mixtures that induce either hypoxemia or hypercapnia. However, these tests are not specific for an abnormality in central chemoreceptor activity. The neuromuscular function of the chest cage must be normal for ventilation to increase appropriately in response to increased neural output from central nervous system centers. Thus diseases that interfere with effective ventilatory activity of the chest cage will also produce abnormal ventilatory responses to the gas mixtures. Furthermore, patients with lung disease may also have abnormal responses. Therefore these tests are not particularly useful in clinical practice.

ETIOLOGIC FACTORS

All cases of nonpulmonary respiratory failure can be classified into one of two major categories: those which suppress central ventilatory control mechanisms and those which interfere with effective ventilatory function of the chest cage. The following conditions cause alveolar hypoventilation by interfering with the effective ventilatory function of the chest cage:

Chest wall abnormalities
    Trauma
    Kyphoscoliosis
    Obesity
Neuromuscular conditions
    Guillain-Barré syndrome
    Myasthenia gravis
    Drug-induced neuromuscular blockade
    Bilateral diaphragmatic paralysis
    Myxedema
    Hypophosphatemia

The relationship between these conditions and ventilatory failure are fairly straightforward and warrant little further discussion. A description of the clinical manifestations of these conditions is beyond the scope of this chapter.

Various conditions may suppress central ventilatory control mechanisms:

Idiopathic hypoventilation
Sleep apnea syndrome
Pickwickian syndrome
Drugs (central nervous system suppressants)
Central nervous system trauma
Cerebrovascular events
Central nervous system infection

Trauma and drug overdose usually produce a completely reversible form of respiratory failure, provided that the patient recovers from the catastrophic event. The clinical presentation of these conditions is usually dominated by other evidence of brain dysfunction, and thus the cause of the respiratory failure is evident. Because these conditions are fairly clear, they will not be discussed in any detail.

Idiopathic hypoventilation, the sleep apnea syndromes, and the pickwickian syndrome are the three conditions that are most likely to cause diagnostic confusion. In recent years a great deal has been learned about these disorders, and, although it is now clear that they are not totally distinct entities, it is useful to consider them individually.

Idiopathic hypoventilation

Idiopathic hypoventilation appears to be caused by an abnormality in the respiratory control center of the brainstem. The ventilatory response to carbon dioxide inhalation is markedly blunted or absent in patients with this condition. Although the condition appears to be acquired postnatally, there is not clear history of trauma or infection of the brainstem in patients with the idiopathic form of this disease.

Some evidence suggests that genetic factors may play a role in the development of the condition. Patients are usually asymptomatic unless they have cor pulmonale. Idiopathic hypoventilation has no other distinguishing features.

Sleep apnea syndromes

The sleep apnea syndromes encompass a group of abnormalities of ventilation that occur during sleep. In most patients the apneic episodes are primarily obstructive. The episodes are caused by obstruction to airflow through the pharynx caused by incoordination and relaxation of various pharyngeal muscles during sleep. It has been suggested that an abnormality in the function of the reticular substance of the brainstem is primarily responsible for the obstructive phenomenon.

In some patients the apneic episodes result primarily from a lack of central stimulation of respiratory muscle activity during rapid eye movement (REM) sleep. The basis of this abnormality is unclear. Hypoxemia appears to be the predominant stimulus for ventilation during REM sleep. Thus it is possible that these patients may have an abnormality in chemoreceptor responsiveness to hypoxemia.

Regardless of the type of sleep apnea, hypersomnolence is the primary complaint in the majority of patients. Patients with obstructive sleep apnea are often noted by close relatives to have loud snoring. The severity of these complaints is extremely varied. The physical examination is normal in most patients. However, some patients have evidence of cor pulmonale.

During apneic episodes the arterial oxygen tension drops, and the arterial carbon dioxide tension increases. The apneic episodes generally last from 30 to 60 seconds each. In some patients the majority of sleep time will be apneic as a result of multiple episodes. Thus the arterial oxygen tension may be dangerously low for most of the sleeping hours. This degree of hypoxia may be a potent stimulus to pulmonary vasospasm in some individuals and is probably responsible for the development of cor pulmonale. It is likely that this sequence of events is much more common in patients who are obese or who have underlying lung disease and thus have some degree of hypoxemia while awake. There is no good evidence that patients with sleep apnea eventually develop hypoventilation while awake. The majority of patients have nearly normal arterial blood gases while awake. Thus the presence of resting hypercapnia in the awake state in patients who are documented to have sleep apnea probably reflects the fact that several different abnormalities in ventilatory function are present.

Drug therapy may be beneficial in some patients with sleep apnea. Patients with central episodes may benefit from medroxyprogesterone, a drug known to be a central respiratory stimulant. Patients with obstructive episodes may benefit from protriptyline, a tricyclic antidepressant. The mechanism by which this drug works in this form of sleep apnea is unknown. If obstructive episodes are extremely severe, or if a patient has right ventricular failure, a tracheostomy may be required to provide rapid relief from airway obstruction and reversal of respiratory failure while drug therapy is initiated. The condition of patients with sleep apnea is extremely complex and must be thoroughly evaluated. This syndrome has been associated with a number of other neurologic conditions.

Pickwickian syndrome

Classically the pickwickian syndrome is characterized by alveolar hypoventilation, obesity, and hypersomnolence. This syndrome is perhaps the most difficult to clearly define at this point because it seems likely that many patients have a combination of several abnormalities in ventilatory control. For instance, it is clear that many patients but not all have both central and obstructive sleep apneic episodes. However, as previously mentioned, the great majority of patients with sleep apnea are not obese and do not have hypercapnia while awake. Thus the relationship between these conditions is unclear. Furthermore, a characteristic of the pickwickian syndrome is that the alveolar hypoventilation may resolve with weight loss. In addition, some patients appear to have reasonably normal carbon dioxide response curves when tested in the laboratory. Thus a complex interrelationship clearly exists between central respiratory control mechanisms and ventilation during both wake and sleep states in many of these patients.

Nonetheless, patients with the pickwickian syndrome have characteristic clinical manifestations. They are usually markedly obese and have a ruddy, plethoric appearance. They fall asleep frequently, even during conversations and while being examined. Peripheral edema and other manifestations of cor pulmonale with right ventricular failure are often present. Arterial blood gas analysis reveals hypercapnia and hypoxemia. The degree of hypoxemia is always caused by both hypoventilation and V/Q mismatching associated with obesity. Erythrocytosis is often present.

Weight loss is the primary approach to the management of this syndrome. During the period of weight loss, progesterone may be of value in stimulating ventilation. Obstructive sleep apnea may occur in these patients; thus appropriate therapy for these episodes can be initiated if necessary. Diuretics and oxygen administration may be of value during periods of acute cardiac decompensation.

Chapter 24

ACUTE RESPIRATORY FAILURE

Acute, diffuse alveolar wall injury on occasion may be so severe that it leads to the development of respiratory failure even in individuals with normal lungs. This form of acute respiratory failure is characterized by the presence of diffuse, bilateral, alveolar infiltrates on the chest roentgenogram and severe refractory hypoxemia. The descriptive term "adult respiratory distress syndrome" (ARDS) is employed to describe this clinical entity. This term does not define a specific disease but simply indicates the presence of certain clinical, roentgenographic, and physiologic manifestations that are common to this form of respiratory failure.

PATHOLOGIC CHANGES

Although certain diseases that produce lung injury may cause distinctive pathologic changes, the changes observed in the lung in most cases of ARDS are nonspecific and simply reflect the limited way in which lung tissue may respond to acute injury. It is obviously impossible to completely reconstruct the sequence of changes that occurs in the severely injured lung without examining serial biopsy specimens. Nevertheless, it is possible to describe the sequence of pathologic changes that probably occur in this syndrome based on the spectrum of changes observed in different lungs examined at varying intervals from the onset of the injury. Thus the pathologic changes observed in individual cases are primarily determined by the interval between the onset of lung injury and the time at which a specimen of lung is obtained for examination.

The alveolar wall is the site of the injury in this syndrome. (The normal structure and function of the alveolar wall is described in Chapter 7.) One of the earliest changes that occurs in the alveolar wall in response to acute injury appears to be the development of edema in the interstitial space. Since both the capillary endothelial cell and the type I epithelial cell are important in limiting the permeability of the alveolar-capillary membrane, damage to either of these cells may result in increased filtration of fluid into the alveolar wall interstitial space. It should be recalled that an increase in alveolar-capillary membrane permeability may occur despite the absence of pathologic changes that can be observed by light microscopy. Shortly after the development of edema, the alveolar wall and intra-alveolar space are infiltrated by inflammatory cells. Type I pneumocytes slough from the epithelial surface early in the course of injury and type II pneumocytes proliferate to line the epithelial surface.

As the process evolves, several important changes occur that dramatically alter the alveolar wall and lung structure. First, proteins contained in the intra-alveolar edematous fluid precipitate as hyaline membranes along the epithelial surface of the alveolar wall. These hyaline membranes are characteristic findings in acute lung injury. Second, connective tissue proteins begin to accumulate in the alveolar wall, producing diffuse fibrosis of the lung that on occasion may be marked. Third, individual alveoli throughout the lung become atelectatic. As a result, the total number of ventilated alveoli in the lung may be markedly decreased. During this stage of the syndrome inflammatory cells persist, but edema formation is pronounced.

If the patient survives, diffuse alveolar wall fibrosis is the most prominent pathologic change observed. Both the edema fluid and active inflammatory cell infiltration gradually resolve during the chronic stage. The long-term pathologic sequelae of this form of acute lung injury have not been adequately documented. However, based on physiologic studies, it seems likely that minimum changes consisting of persistent thickening of the alveolar wall caused by the accumulation of alveolar wall connective tissue proteins persist in the lung several months after the acute injury.

PATHOGENESIS AND ETIOLOGIC FACTORS

Two major pathogenetic mechanisms may produce acute alveolar wall injury. First, the alveolar wall may be directly injured by external agents. Microorganisms or noxious gases inhaled into the lung, certain drugs, or direct physical agents such as radiation may cause direct alveolar wall injury. Second, certain naturally occurring substances in blood may on occasion cause alveolar wall injury primarily by their effect on the lung microvasculature, particularly the capillary endothelial cell. At present it is possible only to speculate on the nature of these substances. However, it has been suggested that certain of the prostaglandins, clotting factors, and complement components may produce this type of acute lung injury by altering the permeability of the alveolar-capillary membrane and by provoking an acute inflammatory reaction in the lung. This mechanism is thought to be responsible for the acute lung injury that occurs in acute pancreatitis, sepsis, and shock.

CLINICAL MANIFESTATIONS

The clinical manifestations of acute lung injury are entirely nonspecific. Patients usually have rapidly progressive dyspnea, and the entire syndrome evolves within 1 or 2 days and frequently within hours. Patients often complain of cough but usually have scanty sputum production. However, on occasion copious amounts of frothy edema fluid, frequently blood tinged and occasionally grossly bloody, will be expectorated during the acute stage of ARDS.

During physical examination patients usually appear anxious and are markedly tachypneic. Characteristically diffuse rales are present over all lung fields but on occasion may be absent. Cyanosis is often evident, even in patients receiving oxygen. Other physical findings that can be attributed to a specific disease causing ARDS may be present in individual cases. A description of the clinical manifestations of each of the diseases that may be associated with this syndrome is clearly beyond the scope of this discussion.

ROENTGENOGRAPHIC MANIFESTATIONS

Diffuse, bilateral, alveolar infiltrates are the characteristic roentgenographic manifestation of ARDS (Fig. 24-1). Although in most cases the infiltrates are bilaterally symmetric, there may be marked unilateral predominance in some cases. Occasionally the chest roentgenogram is entirely normal during the early stage of the syndrome. However, roentgenographic abnormalities usually develop rapidly

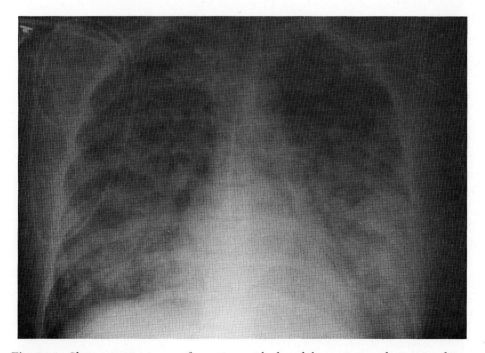

Fig. 24-1. Chest roentgenogram of a patient with the adult respiratory distress syndrome (acute respiratory failure). Diffuse bilateral alveolar infiltrates are present, and heart size is normal.

in these cases. No distinguishing features of the roentgenographic changes suggest the diagnosis of a specific disease associated with ARDS.

As the disease progresses, the roentgenographic manifestations tend to mirror the clinical course. If the patient does not recover, the infiltrates persist without change. If the patient survives, diffuse linear infiltrates may persist for a variable period of time; however, the chest roentgenogram eventually becomes normal in the majority of survivors.

PHYSIOLOGIC MANIFESTATIONS

A marked increase in the intrapulmonary shunt fraction is the characteristic physiologic abnormality affecting gas exchange in ARDS. The presence of refractory hypoxemia caused by the increased shunt fraction is the critical determinant of this form of respiratory failure. A diagnosis of ARDS should not be made in patients with clinical and roentgenographic abnormalities who do not have refractory hypoxemia.

The marked increase in the intrapulmonary shunt fraction can be attributed to the presence of both fluid-filled and collapsed alveoli. In either condition gas exchange between capillary blood and the alveolar air space cannot occur, since the alveoli are not ventilated. As a result the partial pressures of carbon dioxide and oxygen are identical in blood entering and leaving the capillaries of these alveoli. Individual "shunts" of this nature occur diffusely throughout the lung. The sum of the individual capillary shunts represents the total intrapulmonary shunt fraction. In ARDS the shunt fraction usually represents 25% to 50% of the cardiac output.

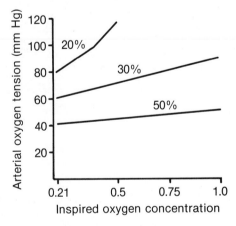

Fig. 24-2. Relationship between the inspired oxygen concentration and the arterial oxygen tension is plotted and compared under circumstances in which the intrapulmonary shunt fraction is 20%, 30%, or 50% of the cardiac output. As the shunt fraction increases, raising the inspired oxygen concentration has less and less effect on the arterial oxygen tension.

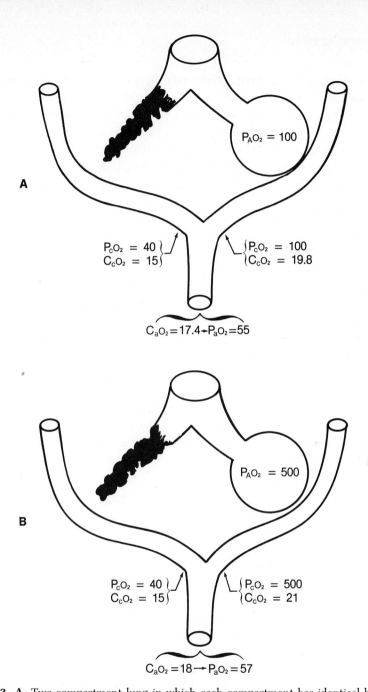

Fig. 24-3. A, Two-compartment lung in which each compartment has identical blood flow. One compartment is normal, whereas the other represents shunt physiology. In the situation depicted, the intrapulmonary shunt fraction would be 50% of the cardiac output. Under this circumstance the arterial oxygen tension during inspiration of room air would be 55 mm Hg. **B,** Identical two-compartment lung is depicted, but the alveolar oxygen tension in the normal lung compartment is 500 mm Hg. This value would be equivalent to breathing a gas mixture containing almost 80% oxygen. Despite the marked increment in the inspired oxygen concentration and alveolar oxygen tension in the normal lung compartment, the arterial oxygen tension increased only to 57 mm Hg. The reason for the minimum increase in arterial oxygen tension is apparent by comparing the arterial oxygen contents under the two circumstances illustrated in **A** and **B.**

Large shunt fractions have an adverse effect on gas exchange and produce severe hypoxemia. In the presence of a large shunt fraction, the arterial oxygen tension (P_aO_2) may be influenced little by increases in the inspired oxygen concentration (F_IO_2). In fact, if the shunt fraction is large enough, the P_aO_2 may remain almost constant despite increasing the F_IO_2 from 0.2 to 1. The relationship between the size of the shunt fraction, the P_aO_2, and the F_IO_2 is depicted in Fig. 24-2. The characteristics of the binding of oxygen by hemoglobin that limit the oxygen content of blood with a high oxygen tension (PO_2) is responsible for this relationship.

The PO_2 of blood in a systemic artery is determined by the proportional mean of the oxygen content of blood leaving all pulmonary capillary beds. Since this is a difficult concept to grasp, it is useful simply to consider how the P_aO_2 is determined under various circumstances when the lung functions as if only two sources of pulmonary venous blood contribute to the arterial system. (Fig. 24-3). It is critical to understand that the P_aO_2 is not determined by the proportional mean of the PO_2 in blood leaving different lung compartments, since, because of the characteristics of hemoglobin, the relationship between oxygen content and PO_2 in blood is not linear. As a result, blood with a high PO_2 cannot adequately compensate in terms of oxygen content for blood with a low PO_2.

DIAGNOSIS

The diagnosis of ARDS is based on the presence of clinical, physiologic, and roentgenographic manifestations consistent with this form of respiratory failure. When diagnosing ARDS, two important aspects must be emphasized.

First, the clinical, roentgenographic, and physiologic manifestations of ARDS may be indistinguishable from those caused by cardiogenic pulmonary edema. ARDS and cardiogenic pulmonary edema can only be accurately distinguished by hemodynamic measurements. Thus it is essential that a Swan-Ganz catheter be inserted for diagnostic purposes in all patients considered to have ARDS. If the pulmonary-capillary wedge pressure is elevated, the diagnosis of cardiogenic pulmonary edema must be made and appropriate therapy instituted. If the pulmonary-capillary wedge pressure is not elevated, the diagnosis of ARDS is confirmed.

Occasionally vigorous therapy for cardiac failure (diuretics, inotropic agents, and vasodilators) is instituted before hemodynamic measurements are obtained. In this situation a normal pulmonary-capillary wedge pressure may not exclude cardiogenic pulmonary edema, since the hemodynamic alterations of left ventricular decompensation resolve much more rapidly than the other manifestations of the condition. In this setting measurement of the protein concentration of edema fluid aspirated from the lung may prove useful. The protein concentration of pulmonary edema fluid caused by increased hydrostatic pressure usually aproximates half that of plasma. A protein concentration nearly equal to that of plasma indicates an increase in pulmonary-capillary permeability consistent with diffuse lung injury. This diagnostic approach is infrequently used and obviously is of little value in patients with little edema fluid.

Second, an attempt should be made to identify a specific, treatable disease causing the syndrome. The most common conditions associated with ARDS follow:

Direct lung injury	Indirect lung injury
Infection	Sepsis
Toxic gas inhalation	Shock
Drug poisoning	Trauma
Near drowning	Pancreatitis
Aspiration	

Identification of a cause is often a frustrating experience, since diagnostic tests used to identify many of the diseases associated with ARDS are not clinically available. All too frequently a diagnosis is made too late to influence the course of the lung injury by specific therapy. Thus empiric therapy for certain treatable diseases must be initiated when the patient is first examined.

TREATMENT

As a general rule the treatment of ARDS is supportive, since specific treatment exists for only a few of the diseases associated with this syndrome. Furthermore, no specific therapy can be used to reverse the nonspecific pathologic response of the lung to injury. Regardless, corticosteroids are often used empirically for this purpose as part of the initial therapy of patients with this syndrome. The rationale for the use of these agents is based on the assumption that circulating substances produce lung injury primarily by altering the permeability of the alveolar-capillary membrane and by provoking an inflammatory reaction in the lung. These agents are employed because of their anti-inflammatory activity and their theoretic role in stabilizing cell membranes. There is no clear evidence that this therapy is beneficial.

Mechanical ventilation is the most important aspect of the supportive management of patients with ARDS. Mechanical ventilation is employed in this form of respiratory failure primarily to improve oxygenation and not to maintain adequate alveolar ventilation. Although high concentrations of oxygen may be administered by other techniques, these are usually of limited value in correcting hypoxemia in patients with ARDS and thus will not be discussed. Mechanical ventilation employing positive end expiratory pressure (PEEP) is often required to oxygenate patients with this form of respiratory failure. Since this form of ventilator management is unique to ARDS, the indications for PEEP and some of the fundamental concepts governing its use will be described in some detail.

As discussed previously, the major determinant of the hypoxemia observed in patients with ARDS is the size of the intrapulmonary shunt fraction. Because of the adverse effect of a shunt lesion on pulmonary gas exchange, oxygenation can be improved only if the shunt fraction can be decreased. Mechanical ventilation with PEEP is an effective way of decreasing the shunt fraction in many patients with ARDS.

PEEP is thought to be effective in improving oxygenation primarily by preventing closure of airways and collapse of gas-exchanging alveolar units. The mechanical events producing airway closure and collapse of gas-exchanging units in ARDS are not completely understood. Nevertheless, as previously atelectatic alveoli become ventilated, they once again participate in gas exchange, and the total shunt fraction decreases by an amount that can roughly be attributed to the volume of perfusion of these units.

In addition to reexpanding collapsed alveoli, PEEP may also decrease fluid filtration across the alveolar-capillary membrane. Although this cannot be quantitated, it is reasonable to assume that PEEP may increase the tissue hydrostatic pressure and thus decrease the hydrostatic gradient for fluid filtration into the interstitial space of the alveolar wall. As a result, oxygen exchange is expected to improve somewhat, since fluid already in the lung was removed by clearance mechanisms. This hypothesis is consistent with the observation that oxygen exchange may continue to improve slowly for hours after institution of optimum levels of PEEP. It appears that PEEP decreases the intrapulmonary shunt fraction and thus improves oxygenation by two mechanisms. There is an almost immediate effect caused by the recruitment of collapsed alveoli for gas exchange and a delayed effect resulting from the inhibition of further filtration of fluid into the lung.

The improvment in oxygen exchange across the lung manifest by an increase in the P_aO_2 must be balanced against the adverse hemodynamic effects of PEEP. To understand the way in which PEEP affects hemodynamics, a brief review of the hemodynamic effects of mechanical ventilation is necessary. During spontaneous ventilation, mean intrathoracic pressure is negative to atmosphere. It has been clearly shown that venous return to the heart is maximum during inspiration, since the pressure gradient for blood flow into the thorax is greatest when the intrathoracic pressure is most negative. In contrast, mechanical ventilation produces a positive intrathoracic pressure during inspiration. Furthermore, the lowest intrathoracic pressure occurs at the end of expiration when airway pressure only equals atmospheric pressure. Therefore, during mechanical ventilation, venous return is greatest during the expiratory phase of the respiratory cycle. However, since the mean intrathoracic pressure after expiration is not as low as that which occurs during inspiration with spontaneous breathing, expiratory time must be prolonged when a patient is undergoing mechanical ventilation to optimize venous return. If the expiratory time is too short, venous return and thus cardiac output decrease resulting in hypoperfusion of vital organs.

Mechanical ventilation with PEEP exaggerates these hemodynamic alterations by further increasing the mean intrathoracic pressure during the end expiratory period. If, as a result, cardiac output falls, delivery of oxygen to tissue may actually decrease, even though the P_aO_2 increases substantially because of the decrease in the intrapulmonary shunt fraction. Thus, to evaluate the effect of PEEP, it is not adequate to simply monitor changes in P_aO_2. Oxygen delivery (oxygen content times cardiac output) must be calculated, and the level of PEEP adjusted to provide maximum oxygen delivery.

Indications for the use of PEEP in patients with ARDS are generally well accepted. If a P_aO_2 of 60 mm Hg cannot be attained by mechanical ventilation with an F_IO_2 of 0.6, PEEP should be instituted. The amount of end expiratory pressure should be increased in gradual increments while the effect of PEEP on oxygen delivery is monitored. Since cardiac output must be measured to calculate oxygen delivery, a Swan-Ganz catheter must be inserted. Placement of a Swan-Ganz catheter also allows the pulmonary-capillary wedge pressure to be directly measured. This is extremely important during initial treatment of ARDS, since fluid and electrolyte balance may be severely deranged. Since increased fluid filtration into the lung occurs in most cases of ARDS, the pulmonary-capillary wedge pressure should be kept low to minimize this phenomenon. Within this context fluid therapy can be managed intelligently only if the pulmonary-capillary wedge pressure can be measured.

• • •

ARDS is a condition that is associated with high mortality even with optimum management. Although oxygenation can usually be maintained by mechanical ventilation with PEEP, patients often die as a result of complications of therapy, bleeding, infection, or progression of the primary disease. Some evidence suggests that the response to PEEP may have prognostic value. If the response to PEEP is rapid, it appears that edema is the major pathologic abnormality in the lung, and the prognosis is favorable. If the response is delayed or there is no response, varying degrees of fibrosis and gross distortion of the lung architecture are present, and the prognosis is less favorable. These are only general guidelines and obviously are of limited value in individual cases. Patients who recover may eventually regain near normal lung function regardless of the severity of their disease.

Chapter 25

CHRONIC RESPIRATORY FAILURE

Chronic respiratory failure occurs most often in patients with chronic bronchitis and/or emphysema. It is characterized by chronic hypoxemia primarily caused by ventilation-perfusion (V/Q) mismatching. Chronic hypercapnia is also present in some patients. The clinical course of this form of respiratory failure is punctuated by intermittent episodes of clinical deterioration during which gas exchange becomes more abnormal resulting in life-threatening hypoxemia in most patients and progressive hypercapnia in some. This discussion will focus primarily on the episodes of acute respiratory decompensation.

PATHOLOGIC CHANGES

The pathologic manifestations of chronic bronchitis and emphysema have been discussed in previous chapters. Other than the extent and severity of both emphysema and pathologic changes in small airways, no distinguishing pathologic changes are observed in the lungs of patients with these diseases who develop respiratory failure. The majority of patients with chronic respiratory failure also have cor pulmonale. Thus pathologic changes consistent with this condition may also be observed in the right ventricle and pulmonary arterial system.

PATHOGENESIS

A number of conditions may precipitate acute respiratory decompensation in patients with chronic bronchitis and emphysema:

Exacerbation of bronchitis	Left ventricular failure
Pneumonia	Drugs
Pneumothorax	Oxygen administration
Pulmonary emboli	Sepsis
Chest trauma	Severe anemia

An exacerbation of bronchitis, pneumonia, left ventricular decompensation, oxygen administration, and administration of certain drugs are probably the most important precipating events. An exacerbation of bronchitis is probably the most common of these conditions. As discussed in Chapter 5, careful studies have demonstrated that these episodes are not necessarily related to infection. Thus the cause of these exacerbations of bronchitis is not clear.

The role of left ventricular decompensation in precipitating acute respiratory decompensation is controversial. There is no question that pulmonary edema caused by left ventricular failure alone can produce hypoxemic, hypercapnic respiratory failure in patients with no underlying lung disease. Therefore it seems reasonable to assume that even mild left ventricular decompensation might precipitate respiratory decompensation in patients with chronic bronchitis and/or emphysema. Clearly this sequence of events must occur in some patients. However, since physical findings of left ventricular failure are difficult if not impossible to detect in patients with severe lung disease, it is impossible to accurately determine how frequently this sequence of events occurs.

In some patients the administration of oxygen is responsible for precipitating respiratory decompensation. This phenomenon has been explained by the fact that under certain circumstances oxygen may suppress ventilatory drive. The arterial carbon dioxide tension (P_aCO_2) is the primary determinant of ventilation in normal humans, and the arterial oxygen tension (P_aO_2) is of relatively little importance. To attribute the suppression of ventilation to an increase in the P_aO_2 caused by oxygen administration, the assumption must be made that, in some patients with chronic respiratory failure, ventilation is primarily controlled by a hypoxic stimulus. If this is the case, administration of oxygen by raising the P_aO_2 may remove the primary stimulus for ventilation and cause hypoventilation. Although this sequence of events is observed clinically, recent studies have raised doubts about the validity of this explanation. These studies have shown that patients who experience suppression of ventilation by oxygen administration during respiratory decompensation do not demonstrate this phenomenon when tested in a laboratory after recovery. Regardless, oxygen must be administered cautiously to patients with chronic bronchitis and emphysema to avoid precipitation or aggravating respiratory decompensation.

A number of drugs may directly suppress respiratory drive. For the most part these drugs act centrally on the ventilatory control center. However, some drugs may induce partial neuromuscular blockade and precipitate respiratory decompensation in this manner. Finally, it seems likely that certain systemic disorders which increase metabolism may also precipitate respiratory decompensation by increasing ventilatory requirements. This is probably an unusual cause of respiratory decompensation in patients with chronic bronchitis and emphysema.

CLINICAL MANIFESTATIONS

The clinical features that develop in patients during an episode of decompensation may be caused by severe hypoxemia or hypercapnia or by the condition precipitating the episode. A complete description of the various manifestations of the conditions that may precipitate respiratory decompensation is beyond the scope of this discussion. These features are usually fairly straightforward and do not require detailed description.

Cyanosis, tachycardia, and hypertension are frequently present in patients with hypoxemia. However, as the hypoxemia becomes more severe, bradycardia and hypotension may develop. Mental status changes and headache may be caused by either severe hypoxemia or hypercapnia. These changes are usually greatest in patients with progressive hypercapnia. At times hypercapnia may produce somnolence or coma.

Cor pulmonale is present in the majority of patients with chronic respiratory failure. Right ventricular failure frequently develops when respiratory decompensation occurs. Thus hepatomegaly and peripheral edema may develop during an episode of respiratory decompensation.

PATHOPHYSIOLOGY

A deterioration in pulmonary gas exchange is the major physiologic abnormality that accompanies episodes of respiratory decompensation. Since routine pulmonary function tests are usually not obtained during an episode of acute respiratory decompensation, the spectrum of abnormalities that may occur in these tests has not been described. Certainly expiratory flow rates will be expected to decrease in patients with an exacerbation of bronchitis.

Two major abnormalities in pulmonary gas exchange may occur during these episodes. First, V/Q mismatching becomes more abnormal with a shift of blood flow to gas-exchange units with low V/Q ratios. As a result, the alveolar-arterial oxygen gradient increases, and the P_aO_2 decreases. In the majority of patients the P_aO_2 ranges from 40 to 50 mm Hg at the time of hospitalization. It is important to recognize that the intrapulmonary shunt fraction is usually not increased in this form of respiratory failure. This contrasts dramatically with the form of acute respiratory failure associated with diffuse lung injury.

Alveolar hypoventilation is the second major gas-exchange abnormality that may develop or become more severe during respiratory decompensation. Alveolar hypoventilation may be caused by progressive maldistribution of ventilation as a result of increasing airways obstruction or by suppression of ventilation by the administration of oxygen or drugs. However, it is worth reemphasizing that hypercapnia does not necessarily occur during respiratory decompensation and in fact is probably present in a minority of patients. In contrast, severe hypoxemia is uniformly present.

In addition to the gas-exchange abnormalities, two other major pathophysiologic conditions develop during episodes of respiratory decompensation. First, right ventricular failure frequently occurs during these episodes. Presumably alveolar hypoxia stimulates an increase in pulmonary vascular resistance and increases right ventricular work. As a result, the right ventricle may eventually decompensate, leading to systemic venous hypertension and retention of salt and water. Second, respiratory acidosis may develop if alveolar hypoventilation results in carbon dioxide retention. At times life-threatening acidemia may occur during these episodes.

These pathophysiologic conditions are entirely reversible if appropriate therapy is instituted and the patient survives the episode of respiratory decompensation. Obviously, however, the physiologic abnormalities directly related to the presence of chronic bronchitis or emphysema do not disappear. Thus the goal of therapy is to return the patient's physiologic state to a baseline status that existed before the episode of respiratory decompensation. There should be no attempt to normalize gas exchange or lung mechanics.

TREATMENT

Several extremely important principles guide the therapy of acute respiratory decompensation in a patient with chronic respiratory failure associated with chronic bronchitis and/or emphysema. These principles differ from those which should be followed in the management of other forms of respiratory failure. First and most important are the principles that must be observed in correcting life-threatening hypoxemia by oxygen administration. Since a real threat exists that oxygen administration may suppress respiratiory drive, oxygen must be administered in a judicious, controlled manner. As a general rule, life-threatening complications of hypoxemia do not occur if the P_aO_2 is greater than 50 mm Hg. Similarly, suppression of ventilatory drive is unlikely to occur if the P_aO_2 remains below 60 mm Hg. Thus the goal of oxygen therapy during episodes of respiratory decompensation is to maintain the P_aO_2 between 50 and 60 mm Hg. Raising the P_aO_2 from less than 50 mm Hg into this therapeutic range may at first seem almost inconsequential. However, it is important to recall that the oxyhemoglobin dissociation curve is steep in this range; thus small increments in P_aO_2 result in proportionately larger increments in the oxygen content of arterial blood. Since tissue oxygenation is directly influenced by arterial oxygen content, the small increment in P_aO_2 that occurs with therapy results in substantial improvement in cell function.

As mentioned previously, the hypoxemia of chronic bronchitis and emphysema is caused by V/Q mismatching. As a result, relatively small increases in the concentration of oxygen in inspired air (F_IO_2) will usually boost the P_aO_2 into the desirable therapeutic range. In clinical practice an F_IO_2 of 0.24 to 0.30 will usually raise the P_aO_2 into the 50 to 60 mm Hg range. Oxygen may be administered in these low concentrations either by using a Venturi type of face mask that delivers a fixed F_IO_2 or by delivering oxygen at low rates (1 to 2 l/minute) through nasal prongs. Both techniques have advantages. Regardless of the technique used, changes in the P_aO_2 should be closely monitored by serial arterial blood gas measurements.

Occasionally even small increments in the P_aO_2 may be associated with progressive hypoventilation. When this situation occurs, the usual course of action is to decrease the F_IO_2 in the hope that a fall in the P_aO_2 will restore an appropriate stimulus to ventilation. However, if the P_aO_2 is not in the desirable therapeutic range, the F_IO_2 must not be decreased, since to do so would perpetuate the duration of life-threatening hypoxemia. Thus it is essential to understand that an increase in the P_aCO_2 is not an indication to decrease the F_IO_2 when the P_aO_2 is appropriate. Under no circumstances should the concern over an increase in the P_aCO_2 be considered an indication for allowing the P_aO_2 to fall below 50 mm Hg by decreasing the F_IO_2.

Another important principle that guides the management of respiratory decompensation in patients with chronic respiratory failure is that mechanical ventilation should be used only after a trial of conservative management has failed. As a general rule, only two indications for mechanical ventilation exist in this situation. If an increase in the P_aCO_2 produces life-threatening acidemia (pH less than 7.1) or carbon dioxide narcosis, mechanical ventilation is clearly indicated. Under almost all other circumstances, mechanical ventilation should not be employed. It is essential to recognize that no absolute level of P_aCO_2 indicates institution of mechanical ventilation. The majority of patients with respiratory decompensation associated with chronic bronchitis and/or emphysema do not require mechanical ventilation.

In addition to adhering to the therapeutic principles that guide oxygen therapy and mechanical ventilation, other therapeutic measures directed at specific conditions which may be responsible for precipating respiratory decompensation should be employed when indicated. In a large percentage of patients with acute respiratory decompensation, a specific precipitating event cannot be identified. Thus it is common practice to initiate empiric forms of therapy. Since an exacerbation of broncitis is often responsible for these episodes, a broad-spectrum antibiotic is usually prescribed. In addition, ultrasonic nebulization, chest physical therapy, and postural drainage are beneficial in some patients. Parenteral administration of theophylline may also be beneficial in promoting bronchodilation. Sympathomimetics should be employed with caution because of the inherent risks associated with the use of these drugs in hypoxemic, adult patients. Occasionally corticosteroids may be beneficial. These agents probably improve V/Q relationships and gas exchange by decreasing bronchiolar inflammation. Finally, since right ventricular decompensation is present in most patients with respiratory decompensation, diuretics may be of value by decreasing both total body and extravascular lung water. There is no evidence that respiratory stimulants are of any value in the treatment of patients with chronic respiratory failure.

INFECTIONS OF THE LUNG

Chapter 26

PATHOGENESIS AND EPIDEMIOLOGIC CLASSIFICATION

Infections of the lung are among the most common pulmonary diseases encountered in clinical medicine. Despite the fact that many different organisms with varied biologic characteristics may infect the lung, there is a great deal of similarity in the clinical and roentgenographic manifestations of these infections. In this chapter factors that are important in the pathogenesis of pulmonary infection will be discussed, and a classification scheme that is useful in guiding a general approach to the diagnosis and treatment of these infections will be described. The specific features of the major pulmonary infectious diseases will be discussed in subsequent chapters.

PATHOGENESIS

For pulmonary infection to occur, pathogenic organisms must first reach the parenchyma of the lung and then proliferate in the local alveolar environment. Therefore, to gain a general understanding of the pathogenesis of these infections, one must be aware of the routes by which pathogenic organisms may reach the lung parenchyma and the intricate defense mechanisms that prevent organisms from reaching the alveolar environment or multiplying at this site.

Routes of infection

Inhalation of airborne organisms is probably the most common mechanism by which pathogens gain access to the lung. This route of infection is particularly important in human-to-human transmission of certain organisms, since coughing is an effective way of aerosolizing organisms into the environment. Organisms that are not spread by human-to-human transmission may also gain access to the lung by the inhalation route. Organisms that normally reside in soil and water may be aerosolized by wind turbulence, digging, or construction work and thus inhaled by individuals in the immediate area. Similarly, organisms that may be in animal furs or hides may be aerosolized during the processing of these materials and inhaled by individuals working with them.

The secretions of the pharynx and mouth contain a large number of organisms that may reach the lung parenchyma if oropharyngeal secretions are aspirated. Normally coordinating mechanisms of the upper respiratory tract prevent aspiration of pharyngeal contents into the trachea during swallowing. These mechanisms are impaired to some degree during sleep in normal individuals and appear to be impaired to a much greater extent during periods of altered consciousness. Thus anesthetized patients or patients with brain damage, seizures, or drug- or alcohol-induced unconsciousness are particularly susceptible to aspiration of oropharyngeal secretions. The nature of the pulmonary infection that results is determined by the composition of the microbial flora of the oropharynx.

Organisms may be hematogenously disseminated to the lung from localized sites of infection elsewhere in the body. The urinary tract is probably the most common source for organisms that produce hematogenous pulmonary infection. Hematogenous pulmonary infection may also occur if contaminated intravenous solutions are inadvertently infused into a patient or if indwelling vascular devices become infected.

Finally, organisms on occasion may be directly introduced into the lung during performance of a diagnostic or therapeutic procedure, as a result of trauma, or as a result of contiguous spread of infection from a neighboring intrathoracic structure. This is the least common route by which organisms reach the lung parenchyma.

Pulmonary defenses

By virtue of being in direct contact with the environment, the lung is vulnerable to infection by a host of organisms. In reality environmental organisms produce pulmonary infection only infrequently because the complex defense mechanisms of the respiratory tract that prevent infection by organisms which gain access to the lung are effective. Components of the pulmonary defense system have been described in previous chapters. In this discussion the complex defense mechanisms of the lung that specifically limit pulmonary infection will be emphasized:

> Airways
>> Mucociliary blanket
>>> Mechanical clearance
>> Secretory IgA
>>> Inactivation of viruses
>>> Aggregation of bacteria
>>> Lysis of bacteria, activation of alternate complement pathway
> Alveolar environment
>> B-lymphocytes (IgG and IgM synthesis)
>>> Opsonization of bacteria
>>> Lysis of bacteria, activation of classic complement pathway

T-lymphocytes (lymphokine synthesis)
    Chemotaxis of mononuclear phagocytes
    Activation of inflammatory effector cells
Alveolar macrophages
    Phagocytosis of organisms
    Chemotaxis of polymorphonuclear leukocytes

Both immunologic and nonimmunologic mechanisms prevent pulmonary infection by microorganisms that gain access to the tracheobronchial tree. To begin with, these organisms may sediment onto the mucociliary blanket of the airways and be removed mechanically. In addition, sedimented organisms may be rendered harmless by local immunologic mechanisms. Secretory IgA, the most abundant immunoglobulin in airway secretions, is the predominant immunologic defense against organisms that sediment on the mucociliary blanket. This immunoglobulin appears to play an important role in preventing viruses that sediment on the surface of the airways from becoming locally invasive. The specific mechanism by which IgA accomplishes this is unknown. Secretory IgA may also play an important role in preventing some bacterial infections. Although secretory IgA does not function as an opsonizing antibody by promoting ingestion and killing of bacteria by phagocytic cells, this immunoglobulin may agglutinate bacteria on the surface of the airways and in this manner prevent tissue invasion and promote mechanical clearance of the organisms. In addition, once bound to organisms, secretory IgA may activate the alternate complement pathway and cause lysis of the organisms in this manner. Experimental evidence also suggests that nonantibody components of airway secretions have the ability to promote ingestion and killing of bacteria by phagocytic cells and thus contribute to the immunologic defense of the tracheobronchial tree.

Once microorganisms reach the alveolar milieu, more complex immunologic mechanisms are required to prevent multiplication of the organisms. The nature of the immunologic response depends to a great extent on the infecting organism. The immunologic response of the host may be primarily humoral (antibody mediated) or cellular (lymphocyte-macrophage mediated). Bacteria generally elicit a humoral immune response, whereas viruses, fungi, and mycobacteria elicit a cellular immune response. An immune response may occur in the lung without evidence of a systemic immune response. Thus the lung appears to have an intact immune system that, although dependent on systemic support, can function somewhat autonomously.

The major humoral immune response to most bacteria is the production of IgG. The major function of IgG is to bind to the surface of organisms, thus making them susceptible either to lysis by complement activation or to ingestion by phagocytic cells. IgG is the predominant immunoglobulin in the alveolar environment and is presumably produced within the lung by plasma cells located in the interstitium of the alveolar wall. Since the components of the classic complement pathway are present in only trace amounts in the alveolar environment, it is unlikely that complement-mediated lysis of bacteria is of any significance in the defense of the lung against bacterial infection. Phagocytosis of opsonized microorganisms is thus particularly important.

The alveolar macrophage is the primary, resident phagocytic cell in the lung and thus provides the first line of alveolar defense against bacterial infection. Although a number of experimental studies have clearly demonstrated the importance of macrophages in the initial defense against bacterial infection, migration of polymorphonuclear leukocytes (PMNs) into the lung from the peripheral circulation is essential for the resolution of most bacterial infections. PMNs are active phagocytes and contain more efficient metabolic mechanisms for killing ingested organisms than alveolar macrophages. Thus, despite the important role for alveolar macrophages in the initial defense of the lung against some bacteria, PMNs are more important once a critical number of organisms reach the lung.

Shortly after an inoculum of bacteria reaches the lung parenchyma, PMNs begin to migrate into the lung. These cells are presumably attracted by humoral chemotactic factors. Although the origin of the chemotactic factors produced in the lung is unknown, alveolar macrophages have been shown to produce these factors under certain conditions.

Cellular immune responses are important in the defense of the lung against a variety of pathogens. Cell-mediated immunity is the primary defense against tuberculous and fungal organism. The initiation of cellular immune responses against infecting organisms depends on recognition of the antigenic determinants of the organism by T-lymphocytes. The T-lymphocytes are present in the lymphocyte population of the lung in approximately the same proportion that they are present in the peripheral blood; these cells possess all of the functional characteristics of T-lymphocytes elsewhere in the body. T-lymphocytes mediate the immune response by the synthesis and release of a number of proteins (lymphokines) that possess a variety of biologic activities. Within the context of this discussion, the most important lymphokines are those which stimulate effector cells to ingest and kill certain pathogenic organisms.

In contrast to humoral immune responses, mononuclear cells are the most important cells involved in cellular immune responses. In response to certain lymphokines, alveolar macrophages rapidly accumulate at the site of infection. In addition, peripheral blood monocytes, precursors of alveolar macrophages, migrate into the lung to participate in the immune response. In fact, after several days monocytes recently released from the bone marrow can be shown to be the predominant cell in the inflammatory response.

Based on an awareness of these fundamentals of the pulmonary immune responses, certain clinical and pathologic observations made in patients with pulmonary infection can be better understood. First, it should be readily apparent that acute bacterial pneumonia is characterized by the presence of large numbers of

PMNs. In contrast, infection by organisms that evoke a cellular immune response is characterized pathologically by the presence of lymphocytes, monocytes, and macrophages.

In addition, it should be apparent that the organisms which are likely to cause pulmonary infection in an immunocompromised patient are predictable on the basis of the defect in the patient's immune system. Individuals with a deficiency of PMNs or abnormalities in leukocyte function or immunoglobulin production are prone to develop bacterial pneumonias. In contrast, individuals with abnormalities in T-lymphocytes or monocyte-macrophage function are expected to have a higher incidence of infection with organisms that depend on the cellular immune mechanisms for killing. Thus tuberculous and fungal infection is expected to occur more frequently in individuals with diseases that result in impaired cell-mediated immunity or individuals receiving drugs that suppress these immune mechanisms.

EPIDEMIOLOGIC CLASSIFICATION OF LUNG INFECTIONS

Since the organisms that may produce pulmonary infection are extremely varied in their biologic characteristics, a number of different diagnostic techniques may have to be performed to identify in the laboratory the pathogen responsible for a given case of pneumonia. Although some pathogenic organisms can be easily identified by routine smears and cultures of expectorated sputum, others may be identified only by performing more complex bacteriologic or histopathologic studies on secretions or tissue specimens obtained by invasive techniques. It is clearly not feasible to perform routinely all possible diagnostic tests on all patients with pulmonary infection. Thus it is extremely important that an organized approach be used to evaluate patients with lung infection so that diagnostic techiques can be logically employed on a selective basis. In this discussion, the infections of the lung will be classified on the basis of certain epidemiologic characteristics. Based on this classification scheme, it is possible to organize a logical approach to the diagnosis of pulmonary infections.

Pulmonary infections can be classified into five major categories. Category I consists of the usual community-acquired pneumonias. The true incidence of infection by various pathogenic organisms in this clinical setting is unknown. However, at least half of the community-acquired pneumonias appear to be nonbacterial in origin, and the balance are caused by a relatively small number of bacteria. The majority of community-acquired bacterial pneumonias are caused by *Streptococcus pneumoniae*. *Staphylococcus aureus*, *Streptococcus pyogenes*, *Hemophilus influenzae*, and *Klebsiella pneumoniae* each cause a small percentage of these infections. Since routine Gram stains of sputum suggest the correct diagnosis in the great majority of these cases, appropriate therapy can usually be selected on the basis of the Gram stain examination. It is important to realize that a specific diagnosis cannot be made by these routine bacteriologic studies in patients with community-acquired, nonbacterial pneumonias. However, since pathogens that can be identified only by invasive diagnostic techniques or complex bacteriologic studies rarely produce community-acquired pneumonias in normal individuals, there is no necessity to undertake a more vigorous diagnostic evaluation in patients in whom routine bacteriologic studies are nondiagnostic unless suspicious clinical features suggest the presence of an unusual pathogen.

Category II consists of aspiration pneumonias caused by anaerobic organisms. Most patients with these infections have a "community-acquired" pneumonia. Thus it is only the role of aspiration in the pathogenesis of the infection that distinguishes these patients from those in category I. Furthermore, since anaerobic organisms can be cultured only with special bacteriologic techniques, these infections cannot be distinguished from other community-acquired pneumonias by routine bacteriologic studies.

Aspiration, anaerobic pulmonary infection may also be acquired in the hospital. However, in contrast to community-acquired aspiration pneumonias that are uniformly caused by anaerobic organisms, approximately a third of hospital-acquired, aspiration pneumonias will be caused by gram-negative, aerobic organisms. It is important to be aware of this fact when evaluating a patient with a hospital-acquired, aspiration pneumonia, since the treatment of anaerobic pulmonary infection differs from that of aerobic, gram-negative pulmonary infection.

Category III consists of hospital-acquired (nosocomial) pneumonias. The lung is the second most common site of nosocomial infection. These pneumonias are usually caused by gram-negative, aerobic organisms. The most common organisms that cause hospital-acquired lung infections are *Escherichia coli, Pseudomonas aeruginosa, Aerobacter* species, and *K. pneumoniae*. Although aspiration is important in the pathogenesis of many hospital-acquired pneumonias, many are caused by hematogenous dissemination of organisms to the lung from extrathoracic sites. Occasionally these infections can be caused by exposure to contaminated inhalation therapy equipment or inadvertent infusion of contaminated parenteral fluids. The mortality of nosocomial pneumonias is extremely high because of the inherent virulence of the organisms that cause these infections and the fact that they often occur in seriously ill patients.

Category IV consists of chronic infections of the lung. At the time of initial examination, it is often impossible to know whether a patient has a chronic pneumonia unless a series of chest roentgenograms is available for review. In the absence of previous roentgenograms, the physician may suspect that a patient has a chronic pneumonia only on the basis of the duration and nature of the symptoms or certain roentgenographic manifestations of the infection. The nature of the infection ultimately becomes apparent when the patient's condition fails to resolve with standard treatment.

Most chronic lung infections are caused by mycobacteria or fungi. These organisms can be identified in sputum and other secretions only by special staining techniques. In addition, special bacteriologic techniques are required to grow the organisms in culture. On occasion, invasive techniques may be required to obtain tissue specimens for culture or histopathologic identification of the organism. Thus recognition that a patient has a chronic infection of the lung dictates a totally different diagnostic approach from that required in patients with acute pneumonias.

On occasion certain bacteria may produce chronic pulmonary infection. These chronic bacterial infections usually occur as chronic lung abscess and are most often caused by anaerobic organisms. However, *K. pneumoniae, P. aeruginosa,* or *S. aureus* may on occasion be responsible. In addition, *Brucella* species, *Bacillus anthracis,* and several other less frequently encountered organisms may also cause chronic pneumonias. When mycobacteria or fungi cannot be isolated from a patient with a chronic pneumonia, a specific epidemiologic history consistent with exposure to one of these pathogens should be sought.

Category V consists of infection caused by opportunistic organisms. For many reasons, immunocompromised patients with pulmonary infection are the most difficult patients to evaluate, since they may have an acute, community-acquired pneumonia or pneumonia caused by such diverse organisms as *Pneumocystis carinii, Aspergillus* species, cytomegalovirus, and a host of other organisms that are rarely pathogenic in the normal host. The value of negative routine smears and cultures of sputum is limited in these patients, since many of the organisms that produce opportunistic infections can be diagnosed only by invasive techniques to obtain specimens for special analysis. Thus, when routine diagnostic studies are negative, the physician must determine the extent of invasion necessary to make a specific diagnosis.

The evaluation of immunocompromised patients is further complicated by the fact that noninfectious pulmonary diseases somewhat unique to their underlying disease may mimic certain opportunistic pulmonary infections. In addition, these patients are often ill or have complications of their underlying disease that limit the diagnostic evaluation. Nevertheless, there are several points to bear in mind. First, the most common pneumonias in these patients are the usual acute, community-acquired pneumonias observed in normal individuals. Thus *S. pneumoniae* is the most common treatable cause of pneumonia in these patients. Second, the clinical and roentgenographic manifestations of the infection frequently provide important clues such as the presence of bilateral pulmonary infiltrates, to the fact that the infection may be caused by an unusual pathogen. There is no substitute for sound clinical judgment and experience in making decisions about the diagnostic evaluation of immunosuppressed hosts with pulmonary infection.

Chapter 27

COMMUNITY-ACQUIRED PNEUMONIAS

It has been estimated that approximately half of acute, community-acquired pneumonias are bacterial in origin and half nonbacterial:

Nonbacterial infections
  Viruses
  Mycoplasma pneumoniae
Bacterial infections
  Streptococcus pneumoniae
  Legionella pneumophila
  Staphylococcus aureus
  Streptococcus pyogenes
  Hemophilus influenzae
  Klebsiella pneumoniae

Despite the fact that certain clinical manifestations of pneumonia are more characteristic of either bacterial or nonbacterial infection (Table 8), such overlap exists that it is often impossible to make a clear distinction between these kinds of infection on clinical grounds alone. In this chapter the most important of the community-acquired pneumonias will be discussed.

BACTERIAL PNEUMONIAS
Streptococcus pneumoniae infection

Most community-acquired, bacterial pneumonias are caused by *Streptococcus pneumoniae*. This organism usually appears in sputum as a gram-positive, lancet-shaped diplococcus. However, it grows in culture as short chains of cocci, thus explaining its classification as a streptococcus.

Pulmonary infection is acquired by inhalation of the organism from the environment. Although the organism spreads within the community by human-to-human transmission, major epidemics do not occur, since the organism is not highly

TABLE 8

Characteristics of community-acquired bacterial and nonbacterial pneumonias

Characteristic	Bacterial	Nonbacterial
Fever	Often high (>101° F)	Low-grade
Chills	Common	Uncommon
Sputum production	Usually abundant	Scanty
Gram stain	Many organisms; predominant pathogen	Few organisms; pleomorphic population
Leukocyte count	Elevated	Normal
Chest roentgenogram	Usually unilobar	Varied, often bilateral; diffuse interstitial infiltrates on occasion

virulent. Nevertheless, many cases may be observed in conditions in which over-crowding of a large number of highly susceptible individuals exists. This infection may occur at any age and is generally more serious in the very young or elderly.

The major immune response to this infection is production of antibody directed against specific antigenic determinants of the organism, primarily capsular polysaccharides. Based on differences in these capsular antigens, eighty-three different types of pneumococci are known to exist. It appears that fourteen types are responsible for 75% of pneumococcal pulmonary infections. Individuals who are unable to mount an effective antibody response against the organism are at greater risk of developing serious pneumococcal infection. Patients with hereditary or acquired immunoglobulin deficiency states or individuals who have undergone splenectomy fall into this category.

Clinical and roentgenographic manifestations. Pneumococcal pneumonia is characterized by the abrupt onset of fever and shaking chills (rigor). Cough with production of mucoid and frequently reddish-brown sputum, chest pain, and generalized symptoms of anorexia and malaise follow within hours. Since pneumococcal pneumonia occurs in many patients after a viral, upper respiratory tract infection, prodromal symptoms of low-grade fever, sore throat, arthralgia, and myalgia may be present. During physical examination the major findings are localized to the involved hemithorax. Physical findings of lobar consolidation are often present. However, it is important to recognize that examination of the lungs may be entirely normal in some patients.

If a patient with pneumococcal pneumonia is treated appropriately, clinical improvement manifest by defervescence of fever and a marked improvement in the patient's sense of well-being usually occurs within 48 to 72 hours. Despite clinical improvement, abnormal physical findings may persist over the area of involved lung for many days and even several weeks. If the patient does not receive an appropriate antibiotic or does not respond to therapy, signs and symptoms attributable to complications of the infection may develop. An increase in chest pain, shortness of breath, and persistent fever may occur in patients who develop a parapneumonic pleural effusion or empyema. These complications usually do not appear until 5 to 7 days after the onset of the pneumonia. Occasionally meningitis or endocarditis may develop. These complications may be manifest by seizures, obtundation, coma, or heart failure. Before the availability of antibiotic therapy, more than 30% of patients with pneumococcal pneumonia died. At present approximately 10% of patients die, usually early in the course of the disease rather than as a result of late complications of the infection.

The roentgenographic manifestations of pneumococcal pneumonia are entirely nonspecific. Involvement of the lung is usually unilobar, but two or more lobes may be involved in some cases (Fig. 27-1). Patchy alveolar infiltrates or complete lobar consolidation may be present. Cavitation of pulmonary infiltrates is extremely uncommon but may occur with infection caused by type III organisms. Pleural effusions may be observed but, as mentioned previously, usually do not appear

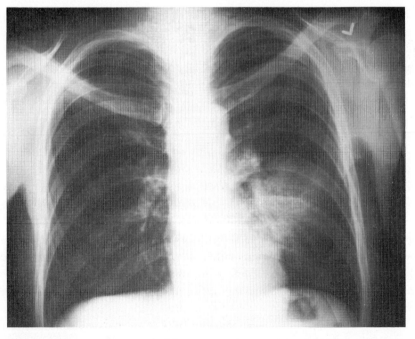

Fig. 27-1. Lingular pneumonia caused by *Streptococcus pneumoniae:* an example of a unilobar, consolidating process characteristic of pneumococcal pneumonia.

until infection has been present for 5 to 7 days. Massive fluid accumulation may be observed in some cases.

With appropriate treatment, the roentgenographic abnormalities resolve almost completely. However, the rate of resolution may be slow. In patients less than 50 years of age who do not have underlying systemic disease, the chest roentgenogram will almost always return to baseline within 6 weeks. However, roentgenographic abnormalities may persist for months in patients over 50 years of age who are alcoholics or who have chronic lung disease. Lobar consolidation may still be present after a month in as many as a third of patients. Because of the slow and varied rate of roentgenographic resolution, the therapeutic response must be assessed by evaluating clinical manifestations of the infection. Furthermore, it should be apparent that serial films to assess roentgenographic clearing need not be obtained more often than every 4 to 6 weeks.

Diagnosis. A tentative diagnosis of pneumococcal pneumonia can usually be made by examination of a suitably prepared, gram-stained sputum specimen. Identification of abundant, gram-positive diplococci in areas of the smear containing polymorphonuclear leukocytes (PMNs) and alveolar macrophages is sufficient evidence for making a diagnosis and instituting therapy. Bacteriologic confirmation of the diagnosis does not occur in many cases. Culture of the sputum is positive in only about half of patients who have positive sputum smears and are proved to have *S. pneumoniae* infection on the basis of positive blood cultures. The reason for this discrepancy is not entirely clear. However, it emphasizes the fact that negative sputum cultures are not a sufficient reason for changing a diagnosis that was based on examination of a gram-stained sputum specimen or for altering therapy.

Since bacteremia occurs in some patients with pneumococcal disease, blood cultures are useful for substantiating the diagnosis. Blood cultures may be positive in as many as a third of patients with lobar consolidation. Although capsular polysaccharide antigen and type-specific, human agglutinating antibody can be detected in the serum of patients with pneumococcal infection, these serologic tests have not proved to be clinically useful for the routine diagnosis of this infection.

Treatment and prevention. Penicillin is the drug of choice for the treatment of seriously ill patients with pneumococcal pneumonia. Isolates of *S. pneumoniae* are almost always exquisitely sensitive to the drug. Standard treatment of hospitalized patients in most medical centers consists of parenteral administration of 1 to 2 million units of penicillin per day. In recent years, isolates of *S. pneumoniae* displaying relative resistance to penicillin have been identified. These organisms still respond to large doses of penicillin. Since these relatively resistant strains have yet to become clinically important, standard doses of penicillin should continue to be employed for the routine treatment of patients with pneumococcal pneumonia. Although patients with multilobar infection are frequently given higher doses of penicillin, no evidence suggests that this treatment is necessary. Patients with serious infection seem to do well whether they receive standard or high-dose treatment.

Although a number of other antibiotics are effective in treating *S. pneumoniae* infection, there is little indication for their use except in patients who are allergic to penicillin. One exception is the use of erythromycin in ambulatory patients who are not very sick. In this clinical situation it is often not possible to determine whether a patient has pneumococcal pneumonia or a nonbacterial infection. Thus use of erythromycin, an effective drug for treating pneumococcal infection, has two potential advantages in this clinical setting: the patients are not exposed to the risk of a serious penicillin reaction as a result of prior sensitization to the drug, and patients who have *Mycoplasma pneumoniae* infection or Legionnaires disease will benefit whereas they would not with penicillin.

A commercially produced, pneumococcal vaccine has been available for clinical use for several years. This vaccine contains capsular antigenic material from fourteen of the eighty-three known types of *S. pneumoniae*. These fourteen types are estimated to be responsible for approximately 75% of the cases of pneumococcal pneumonia. The vaccine is generally recommended for use in individuals who are at high risk for increased morbidity or mortality from pneumococcal infection. The true efficacy of the vaccine in these patients is unknown.

Failure of the vaccine to protect susceptible individuals may occur because the individual becomes infected with an organism that is not one of the types contained in the vaccine or because the individual does not develop an adequate antibody response to the vaccine. In normal, healthy individuals, an inadequate antibody response occurs approximately 20% of the time. Recent evidence suggests that this occurs much more often in high-risk patient populations who most need protection. Infants and some patients with Hodgkin disease, sickle cell disease, and primary or acquired immunoglobulin deficiency states have poor antibody responses to the vaccine. Furthermore, some patients with these diseases do not receive adequate protection, despite what appears to be a good antibody response to the vaccine. The reason for vaccine failure in this situation is unknown.

Legionnaires disease

The clinical and roentgenographic manifestations of *Legionella pneumophila* pulmonary infection and the approach to diagnosis and treatment of this disease have only recently been described. Since this organism was identified as a result of a dramatic outbreak of respiratory infections in individuals attending an American Legion convention in Philadelphia, the disease has become popularly known as Legionnaires disease.

Epidemiologic studies have shown that the etiologic agent of this infection is a gram-negative bacillus. Respiratory tract infection occurs in a person who inhales the organism from the environment. The organism appears to be present in soil or water and may be aerosolized into the environment by mechanical means. Several studies strongly suggest that the organism may be distributed throughout a building by way of the fresh air vents. The organism is a major cause of hospital-acquired, pulmonary infections in some institutions. Although clustering of hospital-acquired cases has received a great deal of publicity, the majority of cases of Legionnaires disease are sporadic in nature. Human-to-human transmission of the organism does not appear to occur.

The results of epidemiologic studies have clearly shown that a wide range exists in the severity of respiratory infection caused by *L. pneumophila*. In some epidemics the majority of patients have had relatively mild upper respiratory tract infections, whereas in others serious pneumonias, leading to the development of the adult respiratory distress syndrome (ARDS) in many patients, have been prominent. Although the organism may be cultured from blood and has been identified in lymph nodes and other extrathoracic organs, extrathoracic dissemination of the organism is rare.

Clinical manifestations. The clinical manifestations of Legionnaires disease obviously overlap with those observed in other pulmonary infections. However, mental confusion and diarrhea are prominent symptoms in many patients with this infection. Although the chest roentgenogram usually shows localized unilateral pulmonary infiltrates, bilateral or diffuse infiltrates may occur in some patients. Necrosis of lung tissue and pleural effusions are distinctly uncommon. With prompt institution of therapy the great majority of patients survive. Although infection with this organism has been shown to evoke a marked fibrotic response in the lungs, patients who survive, even those who develop ARDS, do not have persistent impairment of lung function.

Diagnosis. It may be extremely difficult to make an accurate diagnosis of acute Legionnaires disease. Since the organism resides intracellularly, it is not seen in gram-stained sputum preparations. Thus use of Gram stain, which is so valuable in other bacterial infections of the lung, is not helpful. The best technique for early diagnosis is direct immunofluorescent staining of lung secretions or lung tissue by fluorescent-tagged antibody raised against antigenic determinants of the organism. Although this diagnostic technique is valuable, it is not widely available at this time.

Serologic diagnosis can be made by demonstrating a fourfold rise in serum antibody titer to at least 1:128. Although this technique is useful, it has practical limitations, since serologic conversion is not usually apparent until several weeks after the onset of the acute illness. Thus this technique has virtually no value in the diagnosis of acutely ill patients at the time that therapeutic decisions must be made. Diagnosis by culture also has great limitations because of the delay in obtaining positive information and the unknown sensitivity of culture techniques for isolating the organism from pulmonary secretions or blood.

Treatment. Erythromycin is the drug of choice for the treatment of Legionnaires disease. In mild cases the drug can be given orally. However, in patients who are seriously ill, the drug should be given intravenously (2 gm/day). The efficacy of other antibiotics in the treatment of this infection is unknown.

NONBACTERIAL PNEUMONIAS

At least half of community-acquired, pulmonary infections are nonbacterial in origin. As mentioned previously, it may be impossible to differentiate nonbacterial from bacterial infection on the basis of the clinical and laboratory features of the illness. However, sputum examination can be helpful. The absence of sputum production or scant sputum that contains few pathogenic bacteria favors the presence of nonbacterial infection. However, it must be remembered that Legionnaires disease is characterized by similar findings and that early in the course of other bacterial infections sputum production may be minimum.

The presence of diffuse interstitial infiltrates on the chest roentgenogram favors nonbacterial infection. Although bacterial infection may cause bilateral infiltrates, the disease is usually distributed in a patchy or lobar manner. The character of these infiltrates contrasts with the linear and nodular infiltrates that may occur with nonbacterial infections. There are several exceptions to this rule. *Hemophilus influenzae* infection may occasionally produce diffuse nodular infiltrates on the chest roentgenogram, whereas *Legionella pneumophila* infection may cause diffuse interstitial infiltrates. For practical purposes, other bacterial infections do not cause similar roentgenographic abnormalities.

VIRAL PNEUMONIAS

In adults the majority of nonbacterial pneumonias are caused by viruses. Following are the causes and hosts of the various pneumonias:

Adenoviruses	Adults
Influenza viruses	Adults
Rhinovirus	Children and adults (rare)
Coxsackievirus	Children and young adults (rare)
Echovirus	Children and young adults (rare)
Parainfluenza viruses	Children (rare)
Respiratory syncytial virus	Infants (rare)
Herpesviruses	Immunocompromised hosts

Most viral pneumonias are characterized by rather mild clinical symptoms and localized infiltrates on the chest roentgenogram. However, some viral pneumonias may cause severe symptoms and even death. These cases are almost always characterized by diffuse infiltrates on the chest roentgenogram (Fig. 27-2).

Since there is such similarity in the clinical manifestations of the various viral infections, these diseases will not be discussed individually. At present, there is no way of making an absolute diagnosis during the acute stage of viral pneumonia short

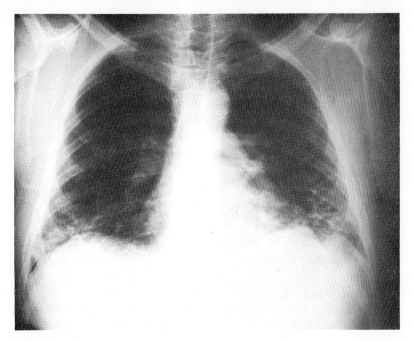

Fig. 27-2. Bibasilar interstitial infiltrates caused by adenovirus infection. This roentgeno-graphic pattern is rarely caused by bacterial infection.

of performing a lung biopsy to demonstrate intracellular inclusion bodies in the respiratory epithelial cells. Viral culture and serologic studies are of value only in retrospect, since the acute course of the disease will have resolved before the results of these studies are available. Finally, no effective therapy for these infections exists. Thus identification of the specific virus producing pulmonary infection cannot be translated into a specific therapeutic decision.

MYCOPLASMA PNEUMONIAE INFECTION

Mycoplasma pneumoniae is a common cause of upper respiratory tract infection. Approximately 5% to 10% of individuals with upper respiratory tract infection develop clinical evidence of pneumonia. The organism can be isolated from individuals with respiratory tract infection throughout the year; however, outbreaks of infection tend to begin in late summer and early fall. Since the organism is apparently spread within the community by human-to-human transmission, a large number of cases may occur when susceptible individuals cluster. Although the organism is not highly contagious in that it does not spread rapidly among a group of susceptible individuals, it appears that high percentages of susceptible contacts eventually become infected. This organism is responsible for 10% to 30% of all pneumonias in adults. Although it is responsible for a larger percentage of pneumonias in older children and teenagers, it is an uncommon cause of pneumonia in children under 5 years of age.

M. pneumoniae primarily infects the respiratory epithelium of both the upper and lower respiratory tracts. The organism has been isolated from extrapulmonary sites in several instances; however, it is not clear how often extensive systemic dissemination of the organism occurs. This fact is of interest, since, based on the results of experimental studies in animals, a number of extrapulmonary manifestations of *M. pneumoniae* infection are probably caused by immunologic reactions and not direct tissue invasion by the organism.

Clinical and roentgenographic manifestations

The clinical manifestations of *M. pneumoniae* infection are nonspecific. Fever, chills, headache, malaise, and cough occur in the majority of patients. The cough is frequently nonproductive, but some patients expectorate purulent sputum. Nausea, vomiting, myalgia, arthralgia, sore throat, and rhinorrhea occur in some patients. Physical examination reveals rales over involved areas of lung in the majority of patients. Pharyngitis, conjunctivitis, skin rash, and cervical adenopathy are present in a small number of patients.

Ocasionally a patient may have symptoms and physical findings consistent with extrapulmonary disease. Hepatitis, polyarthritis, pericarditis, myocarditis, splenomegaly, and various neurologic disorders have been described in patients with *M. pneumoniae* infection. Detailed description of the findings that may be associated with these complications is beyond the scope of this discussion.

A number of roentgenographic patterns have been observed in patients with this infection. Pulmonary infiltrates are characteristically unilateral and focal in nature. The lower lobes are involved most frequently. Bilateral infiltrates occur in many patients. In some these appear as diffuse reticulonodular infiltrates. Small pleural effusions occur in 10% to 20% of patients. Despite appropriate antibiotic therapy, the disease may progress and involve new areas of lung in some patients. In the majority of patients the infiltrates resolve within 3 weeks. Occasionally infiltrates appear after the patient's condition has responded to therapy and the intial infiltrates have resolved.

Diagnosis

M. pneumoniae may be cultured from sputum, pharyngeal washing, or pharyngeal swabs. Isolation of the organism requires special culture media. Growth does not usually appear until 7 to 10 days after inoculation. For these reasons, culture of the organism is not a useful diagnostic technique during the acute stage of the disease.

Measurement of the serum antibody response to the organism is the most useful technique for the diagnosis of mycoplasma infection. A fourfold rise in the titer of complement-fixing antibody in paired sera (acute and convalescent) or a titer of 1:64 or greater in convalescent serum is virtually diagnostic of recent *M. pneumoniae* infection. Since antibody titers usually increase only 7 to 10 days after the onset of infection, serologic studies are of limited value during the acute stage of the illness when diagnosis is most important.

Cold hemagglutinins, which can be detected rather easily in the laboratory or at the bedside, develop in many patients with *M. pneumoniae* infection. These agglutinins usually appear about 7 days after the onset of infection and increase in titer for a period of several weeks. Cold agglutinins also develop during other infections, particularly viral pneumonias. However, the higher the titer, the more likely that the patient has *M. pneumoniae* infection.

Routine laboratory studies are of little value in the diagnosis of this disease; even sputum examination has limited value. If the patient has a productive cough, the sputum characteristically contains PMNs but no organisms.

Treatment

Clinical trials in young adults have shown that the morbidity associated with *M. pneumoniae* infection can be reduced by treatment with either erythromycin or tetracycline. In vitro studies have also shown the organism to be sensitive to these drugs. Not only is the duration of fever and symptoms shortened by treatment with these drugs, pulmonary infiltrates also appear to resolve sooner in treated patients. Despite these observations, the organism can be cultured for many days from the respiratory secretions of patients receiving these antimicrobial agents. The significance of this observation is unknown.

Although both erythromycin and tetracycline are effective, erythromycin should be employed as the drug of choice, since it is also effective in treating *Streptococcus pneumoniae* or *Legionella pneumophila* infection. It may be difficult to distinguish between these infections on clinical grounds alone. Thus it is best to use an antimicrobial agent that will be effective in each of these infections. Tetracycline is a poor choice, since many strains of *S. pneumoniae* are resistant to it, and its efficacy in treating Legionnaires disease is unknown.

Chapter 28

ASPIRATION PNEUMONIAS

Anaerobic bacteria are important causes of pleuropulmonary infections. Since multiple anaerobic organisms can be cultured from most patients with anaerobic pneumonia, these organisms will be considered as a group rather than individually. Most anaerobic pulmonary infections result from aspiration of these organisms into the lung. Anaerobic bacteria are the predominant organisms in the flora of the mouth and pharynx of normal individuals. As a result, aspiration of oropharyngeal secretions results primarily in anaerobic infection. A history of an aspiration episode or a period of unconsciousness that indicates predisposition to aspiration can be obtained from most but not all patients who have anaerobic pulmonary infection. Aspiration of oropharyngeal secretions probably occurs during sleep in perfectly normal adults. Therefore it is reasonable to conclude that anaerobic infections of the lung are almost always caused by aspiration of the organisms, regardless of whether a clear history of an aspiration episode exists. Aspiration is also important in the pathogenesis of many nosocomial, aerobic, gram-negative bacterial pneumonias (Chapter 29). However, for the purpose of this discussion, aspiration pneumonia will be used interchangeably with anaerobic pulmonary infection.

As mentioned previously, it is uncommon for a single organism to be isolated from patients with anaerobic pulmonary infection. This fact is not surprising, since a large number of different organisms are present in the pharyngeal flora. An average of almost three different anaerobic organisms can be isolated from each patient. In almost half the cases, both aerobic and anaerobic organisms can be isolated. Since these infections respond clinically to treatment for the anaerobic organisms alone, it appears that the aerobic organisms are of little pathogenic importance. Because virtually all anaerobic organisms are sensitive to the same antibiotics, a single antimicrobial agent can be used for treatment of these infections, regardless of the number of different organisms isolated. Following are the most common anaerobic organisms isolated from patients with anaerobic pulmonary infection:

Gram-negative bacilli
  Fusobacterium nucleatum
  Bacteroides fragilis
  Bacteroides melaninogenicus
Gram-positive cocci
  Peptostreptococcus species
  Peptococcus species
  Microaerophilic streptococcus

Anaerobic organisms may also be important pathogens in some extrathoracic infections. On occasion these organisms may be hematogenously disseminated to the lungs and produce anaerobic pulmonary infection in this way. The clinical features of this form of anaerobic pneumonia are often different from those associated with aspiration, anaerobic pneumonia. It is important to make this distinction, since the pattern of antibiotic sensitivity of hematogenously spread anaerobic organisms may be different from those associated with anaerobic organisms of the nasopharynx. This is particularly true of *Bacteroides fragilis*, which is likely to respond to penicillin if the organism originates in the upper respiratory tract but is unlikely to be penicillin responsive if it originates from the pelvis or abdomen.

CLINICAL MANIFESTATIONS

Infection of the lung by anaerobic bacteria may result in one of several distinct clinical entities—nonnecrotizing pneumonia, necrotizing pneumonia, lung abscess, and empyema. These distinct clinical entities simply represent different end points in the evolution of anaerobic pulmonary infection. Several of these manifestations of anaerobic infection may be present in a single patient. The following summarizes the relative frequency* with which each of these entities is observed:

Nonnecrotizing pneumonitis	35%
Lung abscess	20%
Empyema	15%
Necrotizing pneumonitis	14%
Lung abscess and empyema	10%
Necrotizing pneumonitis and empyema	6%

Nonnecrotizing pneumonia, clinically indistinguishable for the most part from other bacterial pneumonias, is the most common manifestation of anaerobic pulmonary infection. Although the area of pneumonia is usually limited to one lung, multilobar infiltrates may occur (Fig. 28-1). Since aspiration is the pathogenetic mechanism involved in the development of these pneumonias the infiltrates are usually located in dependent regions of the lung. Fever, productive cough, and systemic symptoms are usually present. In some patients the sputum may have a

---

*Approximate incidence reported in various published series.

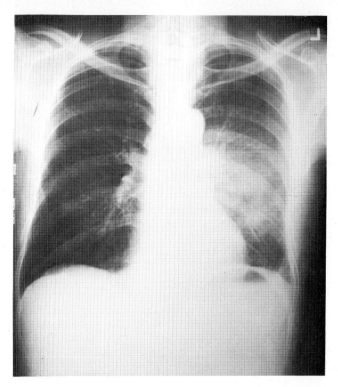

Fig. 28-1. Left lower lobe pneumonia caused by anaerobic organisms. Pleural involvement is evident.

putrid odor, which should strongly suggest anaerobic infection. In contrast to infection by *Streptococcus pneumoniae* and other bacteria, shaking chills are extremely uncommon.

Tissue necrosis, a characteristic feature of pulmonary infection caused by anaerobic bacteria, is responsible for the other pathologic and roentgenographic manifestations of aspiration pneumonia. Necrotizing pneumonia is characterized by the development of multiple areas of necrosis within an area of infection. Necrosis usually becomes roentgenographically apparent 7 or more days after the onset of the infection and may develop despite adequate antibiotic therapy (Fig. 28-2). The areas of necrosis may coalesce to form a single, large abscess cavity. Patients with necrotizing pneumonia tend to be more seriously ill than are patients without tissue necrosis. If massive necrosis of lung tissue occurs, the mortality is higher than that observed in patients with a nonnecrotizing process.

Lung abscesses may become apparent to the physician in several different ways. If an abscess develops during the acute stage of anaerobic infection, the clinical manifestations tend to be similar to those observed with any necrotizing pneu-

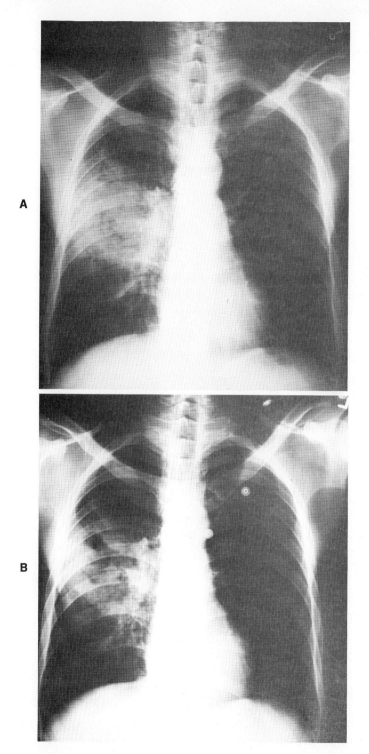

Fig. 28-2. A, Necrotizing pneumonia in the superior segment of the right lower lobe. **B,** The necrotic areas have undergone progressive enlargement and coalescence.

monia. However, many patients with a lung abscess have a more subacute or chronic illness characterized by cough, recurrent fever, weight loss, anorexia, and malaise. Lung abscesses usually respond well to appropriate antibiotic therapy. On occasion surgical resection may be required if the abscess fails to resolve after an appropriate period of treatment. Since abscess cavities less than 4 cm in diameter uniformly close, the need for surgical resection can be anticipated only when large abscess cavities are present. Bleeding within an abscess cavity is also an important indication for considering surgical resection, since without it life-threatening hemorrhage may occur. Bleeding is usually manifest by the onset of hemoptysis and filling of the cavity on the chest roentgenogram.

Patients with empyema may have acute or chronic symptoms such as chest pain and increasing shortness of breath. The diagnosis of empyema is often suspected on the basis of the roentgenographic abnormality and confirmed by thoracentesis (Fig. 28-3). In addition to appropriate antibiotic therapy, drainage of the pleural space is required for optimum management.

The mortality for anaerobic pulmonary infection is in the range of 10% to

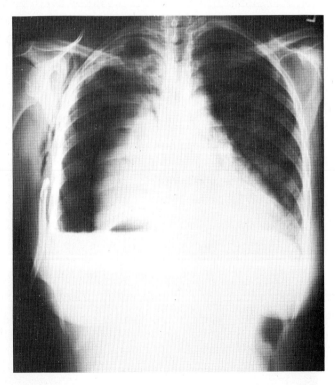

Fig. 28-3. Acute bronchopleural fistula. Several cavities are evident in the opacified, atelectatic lung. A thoracentesis yielded pus containing numerous anaerobic organisms.

15%. With appropriate antibiotic therapy the acute infection resolves in the majority of patients; however, there are several serious chronic complications of anaerobic pulmonary infection. One of the most serious is the development of a chronic bronchopleural fistula. Patients with this complication usually have chronic cough, weight loss, and generalized malaise. Recurrent episodes of chest pain and fever should alert the physician to the possibility that this complication has occurred. A chronic fibrothorax may persist in patients with empyema after the pleural space infection has resolved. These patients may have persistent exertional dyspnea but usually do not have systemic symptoms or continued evidence of intrathoracic infection. In some patients localized bronchiectasis or chronic lung abscess may occur as a result of a necrotizing parenchymal process. These patients may have recurrent episodes of pulmonary infection and recurrent hemoptysis. As mentioned previously, life-threatening hemorrhage may occur on occasion.

DIAGNOSIS

A definitive diagnosis of anaerobic pulmonary infection may be extremely difficult to make, since there are stringent requirements for handling appropriate specimens to grow anaerobic organisms in the routine clinical bacteriology laboratory. Since anaerobic organisms are present in the normal oropharyngeal flora, any specimens that are contaminated by oropharyngeal secretions will grow anaerobes if cultured properly. Thus expectorated sputum or respiratory secretions aspirated through a bronchoscope cannot be used for diagnostic purposes when anaerobic infection is suspected. Two methods for obtaining respiratory tract secretions for anaerobic culture are acceptable. Transtracheal aspiration is the most frequently employed technique for this purpose. More recently catheter systems that can be passed through a fiberoptic bronchoscope and obtain noncontaminated respiratory secretions have become available for clinical use.

It should be emphasized that it is often not necessary to undertake these techniques to confirm a diagnosis of anaerobic infection. In many patients a tentative diagnosis can be made on the basis of the roentgenographic manifestations of the infection, examination of a gram-stained sputum specimen demonstrating a pleomorphic bacterial population, and the clinical setting in which the infection occurred (i.e., a history of aspiration episode or altered consciousness).

Pleural fluid cultures can be useful for confirming the diagnosis of anaerobic pleuropulmonary infection, provided that proper attention is paid to obtaining the fluid anaerobically and assuring that it is handled and cultured under anaerobic conditions. Blood cultures are usually not helpful, since they are positive in only a few patients with this type of infection. Percutaneous aspiration of a lung abscess may be of value in selected patients. However, there are few indications for performing this procedure, since life-threatening bleeding is a potential complication of the procedure.

TREATMENT

Penicillin is the drug of choice for the treatment of anaerobic pleuropulmonary infections. The exact dose of penicillin and duration of therapy are not known. However, it is standard practice to initially administer approximately 10 million units of penicillin per day intravenously. The duration of intravenous therapy is generally guided by the clinical response of the disease. In patients with uncomplicated pneumonia, 7 to 10 days of therapy is adequate. Patients with a lung abscess or empyema usually require a much longer period of treatment. There are no clearly defined guidelines for determining the optimum treatment of these diseases.

Penicillin is the preferred drug for treatment of aspiration anaerobic infections of the lung regardless of the apparent in vitro sensitivity of the infecting organisms. *Bacteroides fragilis* is usually resistant to penicillin in vitro. Nevertheless, the condition of patients infected with this organism usually responds well to penicillin therapy. This response is not true if the organism arises from a nonrespiratory source. Patients with *B. fragilis* infection arising from the abdomen or pelvis usually do not respond well to penicillin and require treatment with an alternate antibiotic.

Clindamycin and chloramphenicol are excellent antibiotics for treating anaerobic infections. As a general rule all anaerobic organisms respond well to either of these agents. These drugs are limited in use only by their relative toxicity when compared with penicillin. Nevertheless, either drug will be effective in patients who are unable to receive penicillin because of drug hypersensitivity or in patients who do not respond appropriately to penicillin.

As mentioned previously, both aerobic and anaerobic organisms are isolated from the respiratory secretions of many patients with aspiration pneumonias. In a great majority of these patients, antibiotic treatment directed against the anaerobic organism is all that is required for treatment. The reason for this is unclear, but it suggests that the aerobic organisms are only colonizing organisms, whereas the anaerobic organisms are truly important in the pathogenesis of the infection.

Chapter 29

NOSOCOMIAL PNEUMONIAS

The lung is the second most common organ involved in hospital-acquired infections. The majority of nosocomial (hospital-acquired) pulmonary infections are caused by gram-negative, aerobic bacteria. Aspiration of oropharyngeal secretions contaminated with aerobic, gram-negative bacteria or hematogenous dissemination of these organisms from extrathoracic sites of infection are the most important mechanisms involved in the pathogenesis of nosocomial pneumonias.

It is unusual for normal individuals to develop gram-negative, aerobic pulmonary infection in the community because gram-negative, aerobic bacteria are usually not present in substantial numbers in their oropharyngeal secretions. Thus aspiration of upper respiratory secretions in this setting does not lead to gram-negative, bacillary pneumonia. Although gram-negative, aerobic bacteria only rarely colonize the oropharynx in normal individuals, colonization occurs with some regularity in persons with serious underlying disease. Epidemiologic studies of hospitalized patients have shown that gram-negative, aerobic organisms tend to colonize the upper respiratory tract in direct relationship to the severity of the illness for which the patient is hospitalized. Careful studies of patients admitted directly to medical intensive care units have shown that the rate of colonization of the oropharynx by gram-negative, aerobic bacteria increases substantially after the patient has been hospitalized for 48 to 72 hours. Colonization occurs more slowly and less often in patients with less serious disease and only occasionally in "well patients" such as young persons hospitalized with fractures.

Hematogenous gram-negative, aerobic pulmonary infections also occur most often in hospitalized patients. Urinary tract or intra-abdominal infections are the most common sources for the organisms that produce hematogenous pneumonias. However, infection of indwelling vascular catheters and monitoring devices and on occasion infusion of contaminated parenteral fluids may also be responsible for bacteremia and the development of hematogenous pneumonia.

In the past, gram-negative pulmonary infections occasionally developed as a result of aerosolization of organisms into the lung from contaminated respiratory therapy equipment. Since most gram-negative, aerobic organisms proliferate well in tap water, a heavy concentration of organisms can develop in humidifiers and nebulizers containing contaminated water and be inhaled into the lung. This hazard has been well recognized, and appropriate procedures are now employed to prevent this from happening.

CLINICAL AND ROENTGENOGRAPHIC MANIFESTATIONS

Since the clinical and roentgenographic manifestations of the various gram-negative, bacillary pneumonias are similar, a detailed discussion of each of these infections is not warranted. Following is the incidence* of these nosocomial pneumonias:

Organism	Incidence (percent)
Escherichia coli	5-25
Pseudomonas aeruginosa	10-60
Proteus species	5-25
Klebsiella pneumoniae	0-15
Enterobacter species	0-10
Serratia marcescens	0-20

As with most pulmonary infections, fever, cough, shortness of breath, and chest pain are usually present. Physical findings on examination of the lungs vary widely but generally reflect the distribution and extent of pulmonary involvement.

All these infections may be characterized roentgenographically by focal infiltrates in single or multiple lobes. Hematogenous infection is particularly likely to cause multilobar, focal infiltrates. Necrosis of involved lung tissue and rapid development of a pleural effusion are also frequently observed during infections caused by all these organisms (Figs. 29-1 to 29-3).

DIAGNOSIS

A tentative diagnosis of gram-negative, aerobic pneumonia must be based on examination of gram-stained sputum preparations. The presence of abundant gram-negative organisms is suggestive enough of gram-negative, aerobic infection to warrant empiric antibiotic therapy to combat these organisms. Since colonization of upper respiratory tract by gram-negative organisms occurs regularly in seriously ill patients, examination of expectorated sputum specimens in these patients may be misleading. In this clinical situation, it may be necessary to obtain respiratory se-

---

*Approximate range of incidence in various published series. Incidence varies widely because of fluctuation in predominant pathogens causing infection in different institutions.

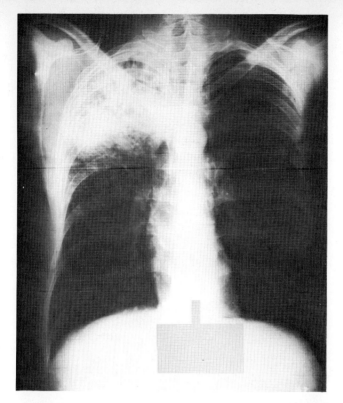

Fig. 29-1. Necrotizing pneumonia in the right upper lobe caused by *Klebsiella pneumoniae*.

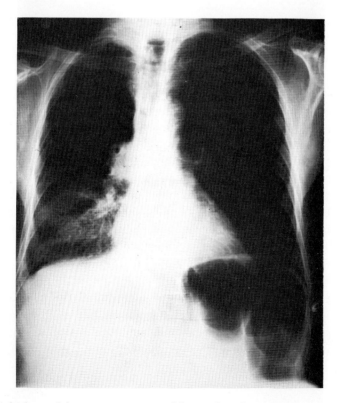

Fig. 29-2. Right lower lobe pneumonia caused by *Escherichia coli*. Pleural involvement is evident.

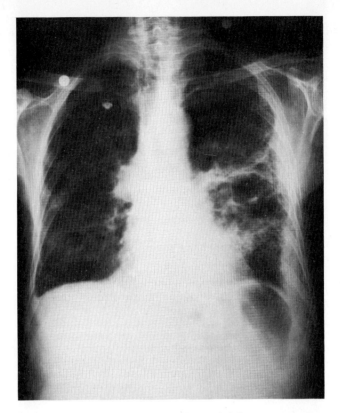

Fig. 29-3. *Pseudomonas aeruginosa* infection. The multilobar pneumonia is extensive and complicated by empyema of the left pleural space.

cretions by transtracheal aspiration, since this technique prevents contamination of the specimen by upper respiratory tract secretions. Furthermore, patients with chronic lung disease may have colonization of the major airways by gram-negative organisms, thus invalidating to some degree interpretation of the sputum smear in these individuals. Ultimate diagnosis requires isolation of the organism in culture from appropriately obtained respiratory secretions, blood, or pleural fluid. Positive blood or pleural fluid cultures are extremely valuable, since these specimens are rarely contaminated by gram-negative, aerobic bacteria. Other laboratory studies are of no value for making a definitive diagnosis.

TREATMENT

Antibiotics that provide a broad spectrum of antimicrobial coverage should be instituted empirically once the diagnosis of gram-negative, aerobic bacillary pneumonia is considered. In most institutions the antibiotic regimen consists of an aminoglycoside and a cephalosporin. The specific antibiotics employed in the regimen vary from institution to institution based on the sensitivity pattern of gram-negative, aerobic organisms in each institution. After the organism has been isolated in culture and antibiotic sensitivity tests have been performed on the isolate, therapy can be altered appropriately. Because of the high mortality associated with these infections, a combination of two antibiotics to which the organism is sensitive is usually employed. Despite the availability of effective antibiotics, the overall mortality of gram-negative, aerobic infection is probably 50%. To a great extent this reflects the pathogenicity of the organism but also the fact that patients who develop gram-negative, bacillary infections tend to have serious underlying chronic disease or to be acutely ill from other diseases.

Chapter 30

CHRONIC PNEUMONIAS
tuberculous and fungal infections

At one time pulmonary infection caused by *Mycobacterium tuberculosis* was one of the major causes of morbidity and mortality in the United States. The introduction of effective drug therapy in the early 1950s revolutionized the approach to the management of this disease and had a dramatic impact on the morbidity and mortality of this infection. At present, tuberculosis has become a relatively uncommon disease in the United States. Approximately 30,000 new cases are reported annually across the entire country. Nevertheless, it is extremely important to understand the principles of diagnosis and treatment of this infection.

PATHOGENESIS
With rare exceptions, infection by *M. tuberculosis* is caused by inhalation of viable organisms into the lung as a result of contact with an infected individual who is aerosolizing organisms into the environment by coughing. In most susceptible individuals the initial site of infection occurs in the lower lobe. The pleura and hilar lymph nodes are frequently involved during this stage of the infection.

In the great majority of patients the primary infection resolves spontaneously. However, during this period, organisms are probably hematogenously disseminated throughout the lungs and remainder of the body. As a result, foci of viable organisms are established in the lungs and many extrathoracic organs.

Infection by *M. tuberculosis* elicits a classic cellular immune response. This response is characterized by an influx of lymphocytes, monocytes, and macrophages into the areas of infection. This inflammatory response ultimately leads to the formation of granulomas. Although the host's immune response usually controls the primary infection, the disease is progressive (progressive primary infection) in a small percentage of patients. It is not entirely clear why this progression occurs in some individuals; however, impaired cellular immune function predisposes individuals to this clinical course.

In most individuals the foci of viable organisms located in the lungs and extrathoracic organs remain dormant after resolution of the primary infection. However, in a small percentage of patients these foci ultimately reactivate and produce clinical manifestations of disease. In most patients the site of reactivation is in the lungs. However, extrathoracic foci may reactivate and produce clinical manifestations of extrathoracic disease without evidence of active pulmonary infection. It is not known why these quiescent foci of organisms activate after many years. However, some factors are known to predispose to this. Any condition that impairs the host's immune response, such as malignancy, malnutrition, chronic renal failure, diabetes mellitus, or prolonged administration of immunosuppressive drugs, predisposes to reactivation of these foci.

CLINICAL MANIFESTATIONS

The clinical manifestations of tuberculosis are extremely varied. During the stage of primary infection, the majority of patients are asymptomatic or have only mild symptoms consistent with a virus-like syndrome. Patients who develop a pleural effusion may have pleuritic chest pain and more severe constitutional symptoms. Regardless of the nature of the symptoms, spontaneous resolution of primary infection is the rule.

The clinical manifestations of reactivation tuberculosis depend on the extent of the disease and the site of reactivation. Cough with sputum production, hemoptysis, fever, night sweats, anorexia, malaise, and weight loss are characteristic symptoms of reactivation pulmonary tuberculosis. However, some patients with rather extensive pulmonary tuberculosis may be asymptomatic or have surprisingly few symptoms. As the disease progresses, the symptoms increase in severity, and evidence of severe malnutrition may become apparent.

Since infection with *M. tuberculosis* may involve almost any organ, the symptoms of extrathoracic tuberculosis are varied. A detailed description of the manifestations of extrathoracic tuberculosis is beyond the scope of this discussion.

With effective treatment, patients often notice improvement in their systemic condition and a decrease in frequency of cough in days to weeks. In patients with pulmonary tuberculosis, symptomatic improvement generally occurs long before there is any evidence of roentgenographic clearing of the disease.

ROENTGENOGRAPHIC MANIFESTATIONS

There are many different roentgenographic manifestations of pulmonary tuberculosis. From a diagnostic standpoint it is important to recognize the roentgenographic abnormalities that correlate with the various stages of tuberculous infection. The three characteristic roentgenographic manifestations of primary tuberculous infection are a lower lung field infiltrate, pleural effusion, and hilar adenopathy. These abnormalities may be observed alone or in any combination. The most

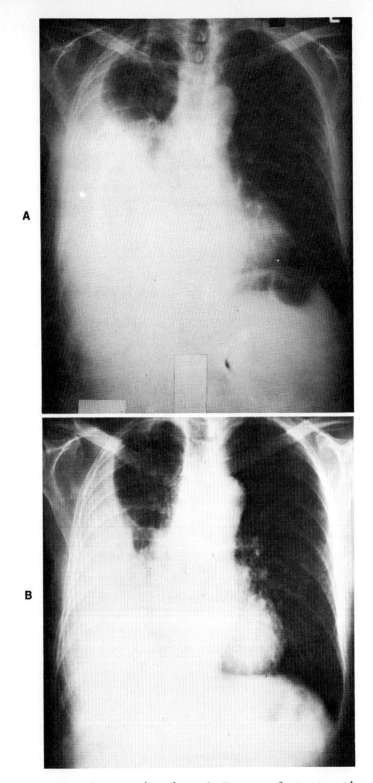

Fig. 30-1. Progressive primary tuberculosis. **A,** Primary infection is evident by a right pleural effusion. **B,** Progressive disease is manifest by the development of diffuse miliary infiltrates in a subsequent film.

frequently observed abnormality is an isolated pleural effusion. These manifestations of primary infection usually resolve spontaneously. However, with progressive primary disease new infiltrates may develop in any part of the lung and may ultimately cavitate. In some patients, diffuse micronodular, or miliary, infiltrates may develop during this stage of the disease (Fig. 30-1).

During the quiescent stage of the disease, the chest roentgenogram may be entirely normal. However, subtle abnormalities representing healed primary infection may be observed. A small, calcified granuloma may be present at the site of initial infection. Similarly, lymph nodes involved in the primary infection may also calcify. The combination of both a calcified parenchymal focus and calcified lymph nodes is known as a Ghon complex (Fig. 30-2). Small nodular lesions may also be observed in the upper lobes. There, lesions may contain viable organisms and serve as the foci for reactivation pulmonary tuberculosis.

Reactivation tuberculosis is characterized by the presence of extensive upper lobe infiltrates that often undergo cavitation. These infiltrates are usually located in the apical or posterior segments of the upper lobe; isolated anterior segment involvement is unusual. As the disease progresses, infiltrates may develop in the

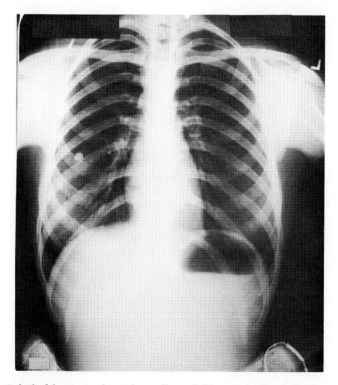

Fig. 30-2. Calcified lesion in the right midlung field typical of healed primary infection.

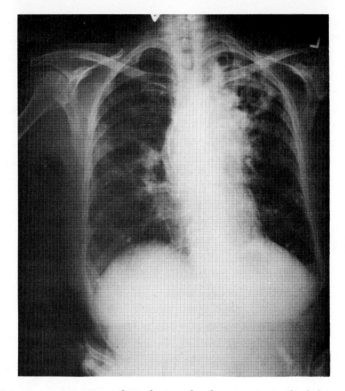

Fig. 30-3. Extensive reactivation tuberculosis with a large cavity in the left upper lobe and evidence of bronchogenic spread of disease to the lower lobes.

lower lung fields as a result of bronchogenic spread of secretions containing viable organisms into these areas (Fig. 30-3). Miliary infiltrates may also occur during the stage of reactivation tuberculosis. Hilar lymph node enlargement does not occur during this stage of the disease.

Pleural effusions or tuberculous empyemas may be observed during reactivation tuberculosis. Pleural involvement tends to occur in patients with extensive disease. Occasionally extensive cavitary tuberculosis will rupture into the pleural space, resulting in the formation of a bronchopleural fistula.

As tuberculosis heals, particularly in cases with cavitary disease, extensive fibrosis and volume loss occurs in the affected lobes. Since the upper lobes are most often affected by extensive infection, healing results in a shift of the superior mediastinum toward the side of involvement and retraction of the ipsilateral hilum toward the apex. When present on a chest roentgenogram, these abnormalities may indicate that a patient has had previous tuberculosis regardless of whether the diagnosis was made in the past.

DIAGNOSIS
Tuberculin skin test

The tuberculin skin test is an extremely valuable technique for documenting that an individual has been infected with *M. tuberculosis*. However, since skin test reactivity is present from the time of primary infection for the duration of life, the skin test is of no value in documenting active infection in patients suspected of having the disease. Nevertheless, it is important to understand the rationale for performing the skin test and the basis for its interpretation.

As mentioned previously, a classic cellular immune response develops during the stage of primary infection. As an integral part of the response, a population of T-lymphocytes with memory for antigenic determinants of *M. tuberculosis* become established in the body. When the sensitized individual is subsequently challenged with an appropriate antigen, these lymphocytes will be stimulated to provoke a cellular immune response. If the antigen is deposited intradermally, mononuclear cells will migrate to the area of antigen deposition and produce visible intradermal infiltration within 48 to 72 hours. This reaction is the basis for the intradermal skin test used to detect prior infection with *M. tuberculosis*.

A purified protein derivative from cultures of *M. tuberculosis* is used as the stimulating antigen in this skin test. Since the dose of antigen to be injected intradermally can be quantitated, it has been possible to define diagnostic criteria based on the skin test response. Three concentrations of protein are commercially available for intradermal skin testing. First-strength material contains 1 tuberculin unit; intermediate-strength, 5 tuberculin units (TU); and second-strength, 250 TU. The cutaneous response to the intermediate-strength dose is used for documenting previous *M. tuberculosis* infection. Induration at 48 hours of less than 5 mm is considered a negative result. A reaction of 5 to 9 mm is positive but not necessarily indicative of previous infection with *M. tuberculosis*, whereas a reaction of 10 mm or greater generally indicates previous *M. tuberculosis* infection.

Many variables may influence the skin test response. Under certain circumstances, the response may be boosted by a previous skin test, resulting in an exaggerated or false positive test. Although this may influence certain epidemiologic considerations, it rarely causes confusion in the evaluation of a patient suspected of having active disease. Conversely many factors may suppress skin test reactivity and produce false negative tests. Drugs or diseases that specifically affect the cellular immune response or conditions such as malnutrition, uremia, or severe illness that nonspecifically alter immune responses may affect skin test reactivity. Obviously, technical errors in application or interpretation of the skin test may also lead to false negative results. A false negative skin test is more important than a false positive test, since it may stop the physician from further consideration of tuberculosis in a patient with the disease. In some series as many as 20% to 30% of patients with active tuberculosis have had a negative skin test during initial testing.

The greatest value of the skin test is its ability to identify patients who have had recent primary infection. Since most patients with primary infection are asymptomatic or have only minimum symptoms, *M. tuberculosis* infection is usually not documented during this stage of the disease. However, documentation that an individual has converted the skin test from negative to positive is evidence that infection has occurred during the interval. If the interval between the tests is short, recent infection can be inferred. As will be discussed later, this is useful information when considering attempts to prevent the development of reactivation tuberculosis.

Acid-fast smears

Unlike most organisms, mycobacteria that have been stained by certain dyes and fluorescent compounds retain the dye when washed with acid alcohol (acid-fast). The Ziehl-Neelsen stain is used for identifying acid-fast organisms under light microscopy, whereas the auromine-O stain is used for fluorescence microscopy. When acid-fast organisms are identified by these staining techniques, the diagnosis of *M. tuberculosis* is strongly suggested. However, since other organisms are also acid-fast, the results of the stains are not unequivocally diagnostic. It is important to confirm the diagnosis by identification of the organisms in culture when positive smears are obtained.

Furthermore, organisms may be present in respiratory secretions but not identified by these staining techniques. Because of the inherent sensitivity of these techniques, a large number of organisms must be present before smears are positive. Thus negative smears do not exclude the diagnosis. Appropriate specimens must be cultured in suspected cases. The smear techniques are far less valuable when body fluids or tissue is employed. Therefore negative smears of these specimens are of little importance in the overall diagnostic evaluation of a patient suspected of having tuberculosis.

Culture

A definitive diagnosis of active pulmonary tuberculosis is made by culturing the organism from either expectorated sputum, secretions obtained at bronchoscopy, or biopsy specimens obtained from the lung. It is extremely important that the organism be accurately identified in culture so that there will be no confusion with other diseases that can cause similar clinical and roentgenographic manifestations. In patients with extrathoracic tuberculosis, the organism may be cultured from body fluids and tissue. On occasion a definitive diagnosis can be made in a patient with pulmonary tuberculosis who does not cough and expectorate secretions for culture by isolating the organism from an extrathoracic site. Pleural, peritoneal, or cerebrospinal fluid may yield positive cultures in some patients, whereas liver, bone marrow, pericardial, pleural, or peritoneal biopsies may be positive in others. Samples for culture should be introduced into Löwenstein-Jensen medium or Middlebrook agar. *M. tuberculosis* produces smooth, buff-colored colonies that can usually be detected within 2 to 3 weeks after inoculation. However, cultures should not be considered negative until 4 to 6 weeks have elapsed without growth.

Miscellaneous diagnostic studies

Infection with *M. tuberculosis* is characterized by granulomatous inflammation; thus demonstration of granulomas in involved tissue can be useful in suggesting the correct diagnosis in some clinical situations. However, since granulomatous inflammation occurs in a number of diseases, this finding cannot be considered diagnostic of tuberculosis. If caseation necrosis is present within the areas of inflammation, tuberculosis is more likely, since this form of necrosis does not occur in most other diseases that cause granulomatous inflammation.

Finally, several comments should be made about the nature of the inflammatory response detected in body fluids in extrapulmonary tuberculosis. Since pleural involvement is the most common clinically recognized form of primary tuberculous infection, pleural fluid is the most common body fluid studied in patients suspected of having tuberculosis. Tuberculous pleural effusions are generally exudates, and the cells obtained from the fluid in most but not all cases are predominantly lymphocytes. Since many other causes of lymphocytic pleural exudates exist, routine pleural fluid analysis is of limited value in the diagnosis of pleural tuberculosis. Pleural biopsies demonstrating pleural granulomas and identification of the organisms by culture of the biopsy specimen or pleural fluid is required for definitive diagnosis. Similar comments can be made about peritoneal or joint fluid in cases of tuberculous peritonitis and arthritis.

Although a number of studies may suggest the diagnosis of tuberculosis, definitive diagnosis requires identification of the organism in culture. In some cases this is not accomplished for one reason or another. Nevertheless, the physician should strive for this goal in evaluating a patient suspected of having active tuberculosis. An additional reason for isolating the organism in culture is that the sensitivity of the organism to various drugs which may be employed in treating the infection can only be assessed once this has been accomplished. Although not common, primary drug resistance can only be recognized by performing in vitro drug sensitivity tests on organisms subcultured from the original isolates. Thus every attempt should be made to isolate the organism from patients with active disease.

TREATMENT

Chemoprophylaxis is an important concept in the overall approach to the therapy for tuberculosis. The rationale for chemoprophylaxis is that reactivation of quiescent foci of viable organisms can be prevented by appropriate drug therapy. At present, 300 mg of isoniazid daily for a year is the only form of chemoprophylaxis that has been documented to be effective. Only patients who are known to have had previous tuberculous infection based on skin test reactivity are candidates for chemoprophylaxis. Although isoniazid is effective in decreasing the incidence of reactivation of tuberculosis in persons with positive skin tests, some controversy remains regarding the indications for its use. For chemoprophylaxis to be justified, the decrease in the incidence of reactivation disease has to be balanced against the toxicity of the drug.

In recent years the indications for isoniazid chemoprophylaxis have been better defined:

1. Household members and other close contacts of patients with recently diagnosed tuberculosis
2. Patients with recent infection documented by skin test conversion
3. Tuberculin-positive individuals with roentgenographic abnormalities consistent with nonprogressive tuberculosis who also have negative smears and cultures and have never received adequate chemotherapy
4. Tuberculin-positive individuals with associated conditions that are known to predispose to reactivation tuberculosis, for example, diabetics or patients receiving immunosuppressive drugs
5. Tuberculin-positive individuals between 6 and 35 years of age

Since only a small percentage of these patients actually develop active tuberculosis, the potential toxicity of the drug must still be considered before instituting therapy.

At least 10% of patients who receive isoniazid as chemoprophylaxis develop minor liver toxicity manifested by an increase in liver enzymes within the first month or two of treatment. However, the drug may also produce serious hepatotoxicity, occasionally leading to fatal liver failure. Severe liver toxicity may occur at any time during the period that the drug is being administered. Although drug toxicity should be closely monitored, when isoniazid is employed, it is not always possible to anticipate the development of life-threatening toxicity by monitoring symptoms or obtaining serial liver enzyme studies. The likelihood of serious hepatotoxicity appears to be increased in older individuals, particularly women over 45 years of age. Thus routine chemoprophylaxis should not be used in these individuals.

A number of drugs are effective for treating active infection caused by *M. tuberculosis* (Table 9). With a complete course of therapy, at least 95% of patients will be cured. This contrasts dramatically with the course of the disease in the preantibiotic era when approximately a third of patients ultimately died of tuberculosis and only a third improved spontaneously. With effective therapy, sputum conversion occurs roughly at a rate of 20% to 30% each month. Thus by 5 months essentially all patients should have negative smears and cultures. Continued therapy beyond this point prevents clinical and roentgenographic relapse. Relapse after completion of treatment occurs in only a small percentage of patients and usually within the first year after stopping therapy. Thus there is no reason to evaluate patients on a regular basis with chest roentgenograms or sputum bacteriologic studies beyond this period.

TABLE 9
Antituberculous drugs

Drug	Standard daily dose	Major toxicity
Primary drugs		
Isoniazid	5-10 mg/kg (300 mg maximum)	Hepatitis, peripheral neuritis
Rifampin	10-20 mg/kg (600 mg maximum)	Hepatitis
Secondary drugs		
Ethambutol	15-25 mg/kg	Optic neuritis
Para-aminosalicylic acid (PAS)	12-15 gm	Hepatotoxic, gastrointestinal intolerance
Pyrazinamide	20-35 mg/kg (3 gm maximum)	Hepatotoxic
Streptomycin	1 gm (intramuscularly)	Eighth cranial nerve damage, nephrotoxic
Tertiary drugs		
Capreomycin	*	Eighth cranial nerve damage, nephrotoxic
Cycloserine	*	Convulsions, psychosis
Ethionamide	*	Hepatotoxic
Kanamycin	*	Eighth cranial nerve damage, nephrotoxic

*Tertiary drugs are rarely used except in treatment of drug-resistant tuberculosis.

The treatment of active pulmonary tuberculosis has undergone continuous modifications since the introduction of effective drugs approximately 30 years ago. The combination of isoniazid and rifampin, 300 mg and 600 mg respectively, daily for 9 months is the regimen recommended for routine use at present. Regimens using combinations of isoniazid, ethambutal, and streptomycin for 18 to 24 months may also achieve comparable therapeutic results. Since using short courses of therapy has many obvious advantages, the 9-month regimen of isoniazid and rifampin is preferred.

Several effective antituberculous regimens require that drugs be administered only two or three times each week. This approach to therapy is particularly valuable for treating individuals with active disease who are unlikely to comply with a prescribed regimen. Since these regimens can be administered by a health care worker, accepabable therapeutic results can be guaranteed. This approach to therapy has gained acceptance in programs administered by some intercity health departments.

A description of the treatment of drug-resistant tuberculosis is beyond the scope of this discussion. However, several general principles are important in preventing the development of drug resistance. The most important principle is that patients should never be treated in such a way that their organisms will be exposed to only one effective drug. If single-drug therapy is employed, strains of *M. tuber-*

culosis resistant to the drug will selectively emerge as the predominant population of organisms causing disease. Since this population of organisms will be unresponsive to the drug being administered, the disease may progress unless therapy is altered.

Most drug-resistant tuberculosis develops when a noncompliant patient takes only one of the drugs included in the therapeutic regimen. If a patient stops taking all the drugs, resistant organisms do not emerge, and progressive disease is caused by organisms that are sensitive to the original drug regimen. Whenever patients do not respond appropriately to treatment or have evidence of clinical or roentgenographic relapse while receiving therapy, poor drug compliance should be suspected.

Unfortunately, resistant tuberculosis develops in some patients because inappropriate treatment is prescribed by a physician. A physician may inadvertently prescribe only a single effective drug for a patient with active tuberculosis: because of negative smears, the physician may believe that a patient does not have active disease and prescribe only isoniazid prophylaxis, or the physician may prescribe a two-drug regimen containing a drug to which the patient's organisms are resistant, and thus, in effect, the patient is receiving only single drug treatment. Under both circumstances, strains of *M. tuberculosis* resistant to the single drug may emerge. When drug resistance is suspected during the course of therapy, it is absolutely essential that therapy be altered by adding to the regimen two new drugs that the patient has not previously received. If only a single drug is prescribed, strains resistant to this drug may also emerge, and the patient may ultimately be infected with organisms that display multiple drug resistance.

NONTUBERCULOUS MYCOBACTERIA

A number of other mycobacteria may produce disease in humans. These organisms are referred to as "nontuberculous mycobacteria" and are classified on the basis of their growth characteristic in culture. Since these organisms are "acid fast," they cannot be clearly distinguished from *M. tuberculosis* by standarad staining techniques. Thus the organisms must be identified in culture.

Only a small number of nontuberculous mycobacteria have been documented to cause pulmonary infection:

Slowly growing organisms
  M. kansasii (photochromogen)
  M. simiae (photochromogen)
  M. scrofulaceum (scotochromogen)
  M. xenopi (scotochromogen)
  M. szulgai (scotochromogen)
  M. avium–intracellulare (nonchromogen)
Rapidly growing organisms
  M. fortuitium
  M. cheloni

Most of these infections are caused by *M. kansasii* or the *avium-intracellulare* group. The clinical and roentgenographic manifestations of pulmonary infection caused by these organisms are indistinguishable from those caused by *M. tuberculosis* and will not be described any further. Although these organisms may produce lung disease, they also may occur as colonizing organisms. Thus sporadic isolation of any one of these organisms cannot be interpreted as evidence of infection. The physician can diagnose an infection caused by one of these organisms when the patient has lung disease compatible with mycobacterial infection and multiple isolates of the organisms from sputum.

Other nontuberculous mycobacteria may on occasion be isolated from the sputum of patients with lung disease. These isolates are almost always caused by colonization of the lung and not true infection. The diagnosis of pulmonary infection caused by these organisms should be made only after due consideration has been paid to other possible explanations for the patient's lung disease.

In contrast to *M. tuberculosis*, the nontuberculous mycobacteria are not contracted by human-to-human transmission. These organisms are found in water and soil. Humans are infected by contact with these organisms in their environment. *M. kansasii* and the *avium-intracellulare* group of organisms tend to be distributed on a regional basis in the United States. Infection is far more prevalent in the southeast and central United States than in the Northeast or far West.

The pathogenesis of infection in humans, although not as well defined, is probably similar to that of *M. tuberculosis*. However, extrathoracic disease is distinctly less common and generally is observed only in seriously immunocompromised hosts. In addition, the pulmonary infection tends to be less progressive in nature even in the absence of effective chemotherapy. In many patients, generally those without underlying lung disease, the disease may undergo spontaneous resolution.

As mentioned previously, the diagnosis of pulmonary infection caused by these organisms is based on repetitive isolation of the organism from sputum in a patient with compatible manifestations of lung disease. Because these organisms cannot be specifically distinguished by smear techniques, culture identification is absolutely essential.

The same antituberculous agents that are used to treat *M. tuberculosis* are used for the treatment of infections caused by the nontuberculous mycobacteria. However, the therapeutic principles employed in selecting appropriate drug regimens are less well defined, and the response of these infections to treatment is less predictable. In general, infections with *M. kansasii* respond to therapy with regimens containing at least three drugs. This tends to be the case even if the organisms display in vitro resistance to one or more of the drugs in the regimen. Infections caused by the *avium-intracellulare* group of organisms respond less well to treatment. Some investigators have proposed that four or five drug regimens should be routinely employed in treating infections caused by these organisms. In addition, it has been proposed that these infections should be treated by surgical excision of the involved area of lung after a period of drug therapy. This approach has been proposed because of the unsatisfactory results of medical treatment alone in some patients.

FUNGAL INFECTIONS

Three dimorphic fungi, *Histoplasma capsulatum, Blastomyces dermatitides,* and *Coccidioides immitis,* are responsible for the majority of pulmonary fungal infections. Since the clinical and roentgenographic manifestations of these infections are similar, they will be discussed together.

Pathogenesis and epidemiologic factors

Although the epidemiologic factors of these infections differ markedly, each of these organisms resides in soil and produces pulmonary infection when virulent spores are inhaled into the lungs. Human-to-human transmission of these organisms does not occur. Coccidioidomycosis occurs primarily in southern California and the Southwest, histoplasmosis in the Ohio and Mississippi river valley regions, and blastomycosis in the north and central regions of the United States.

C. immitis resides primarily in arid regions of California, Nevada, New Mexico, Utah, Arizona, and western Texas. The mycelial form of the organism exists in soil and forms highly virulent arthrospores. The virulence of the arthrospores is evident by the fact that the majority of individuals who move into an endemic region become infected within a year. A number of small epidemics of coccidioidomycosis have occurred in groups of individuals involved in anthropologic or archaeologic exploration in endemic areas. Although infection usually occurs in a rural setting, arthrospores may be borne long distances by windstorms and thus produce infection in urban dwellers. *C. immitis* also produces highly virulent arthrospores when cultured in the bacteriology laboratory. Thus, when attempts are made to grow the organism in a laboratory, precautions must be taken to prevent infection of laboratory personnel.

H. capsulatum exists in mycelial form in nature. Infection is produced by inhalation of airborne spores. The organism is most often isolated from areas highly contaminated by bird droppings. Old farm buildings and chicken houses are a common source of infection in endemic regions of the United States. Similarly, soil around trees in which starlings and pigeons roost may be heavily contaminated with the organism. Although histoplasmosis occurs most often in rural settings, wind-borne spores may cause infection in urban dwellers. The epidemiologic factors of histoplasmosis are not as well documented as those of coccidioidomycosis. Nevertheless, it is known that a high percentage of individuals who reside in endemic regions become infected with *H. capsulatum* at some time during their lifetimes.

The epidemiologic factors of blastomycosis are less well defined than those of coccidioidomycosis or histoplasmosis. It is presumed that *B. dermatitides* resides in soil in a mycelial form and that inhalation of airborne spores causes infection. However, with few exceptions it has not been possible to isolate the organism from the soil in regions known to be endemic for infection. Since there is no satisfactory skin test for epidemiologic surveys, the prevalence of infection in endemic areas cannot be clearly ascertained. However, small clusters of infection may occur among groups of individuals with a common source of exposure.

As with mycobacterial infection, a cellular immune response is the primary immunologic response to these organisms. The initial infection of the lung resolves spontaneously in the great majority of infected persons. However, to some extent hematogenous spread of organisms to extrathoracic organs probably occurs during this period. In the great majority of patients, hematogenous dissemination of the organisms does not result in clinical manifestation of disease. However, some patients have prominent clinical manifestations of disseminated disease. Any condition that alters cellular immunity is likely to promote widespread dissemination of the organism. Genetic factors also appear to play a role in the ability of the host to contain these infections. Dissemination seems to occur must more frequently in dark-skinned ethnic groups than in whites. This occurrence has been best documented with *C. immitis* infection.

Clinical manifestations

In general the clinical manifestations of these three infections are similar. Certain distinguishing clinical features are listed in Table 10. In the great majority of patients, lung involvement is responsible for the predominant clinical manifestations of the disease. During the stage of primary infection patients usually develop a nonproductive cough, fever, myalgia, arthralgia, and generalized malaise. With diffuse lung involvement extreme shortness of breath may also be present. These symptoms typically last for a period of several days to several weeks and resolve spontaneously. If disseminated infection occurs at this stage, varied clinical manifestations attributable to extrathoracic organ involvement develop, and systemic symptoms of high fever and progressive weight loss are usually prominent.

Reactivation of pulmonary infection may mimic pulmonary tuberculosis in every respect. Chronic cough, hemoptysis, weight loss, and fever are the most common symptoms. Clinical evidence of dissemination may also occur during this stage of the infection, and manifestations of specific organ involvement may be prominent features of the disease. The usual pattern of extrathoracic involvement with each organism is summarized in Table 10.

Complete resolution of the disease occurs with appropriate therapy in many patients. However, chronic infection with frequent clinical relapses characterize the course of others. Some patients may suffer severe organ damage and be left with disabling respiratory or extrathoracic disease despite ultimate cure of the infection.

TABLE 10

Comparison of the pulmonary mycoses

	Blastomycosis	Coccidioidomycosis	Histoplasmosis
Chest roentgenogram			
Acute disease	Focal alveolar infiltrates	Focal alveolar infiltrates Pleural effusions Hilar adenopathy	Focal alveolar infiltrates Diffuse nodules Hilar adenopathy
Chronic disease	Cavities Masses	Thin-walled cavities	Cavities Parenchymal calcifications Fibrosing mediastinitis
Sites of dissemination	Skin Bone Male genital tract	Skin Bone Meninges	Liver and spleen Mucosal surfaces Adrenal glands
Diagnostic studies			
Skin test	No value	Excellent epidemiologic tool	Limited value
Serologic tests	No value	Diagnostic and prognostic value	Limited value

Roentgenographic manifestations

The roentgenographic manifestations of these infections are also similar. During the stage of primary infection, localized alveolar infiltrates or diffuse micronodular infiltrates may be observed (Fig. 30-4). Hilar adenopathy may also be present. As these infiltrates heal, they may calcify and thus be visible on the roentgenogram. Healing of histoplasmosis is particularly likely to produce multiple parenchymal calcifications (Figs. 30-5 and 30-6). Each of these infections may also produce chronic cavitary upper lobe infiltrates identical to those observed with mycobacterial infection. However, infection by *C. immitis* regularly produces thin-walled cavitary lesions, infrequently observed in other infections (Fig. 30-7). These lesions are usually located in the periphery of the lung and thus may rupture spontaneously into the pleural space, producing a pneumothorax. Pleural effusions may be observed during these infections, most frequently those caused by *C. immitis*. Chronic empyemas and bronchopleural fistulas may occur rarely during each disease.

Diagnosis

The diagnosis of these diseases is based on histopathologic identification of the organisms in tissue specimens or bacteriologic isolation of the organisms from

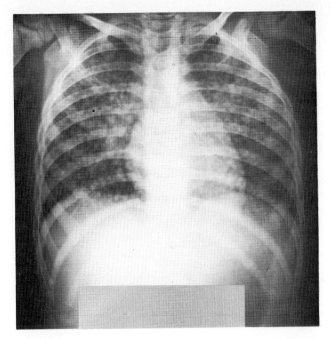

Fig. 30-4. Acute inhalational histoplasmosis in a child. The diffuse nodular lesions are characteristic of this type of infection.

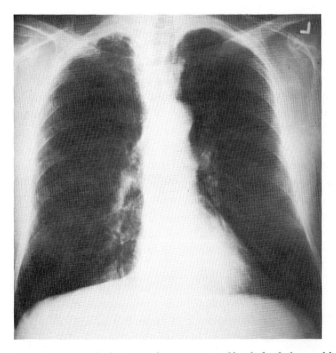

Fig. 30-5. Diffuse pulmonary calcifications characteristic of healed inhalational histoplasmosis as depicted in Fig. 30-4.

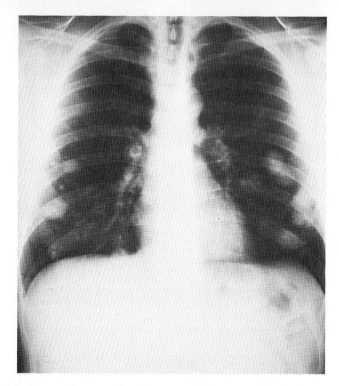

Fig. 30-6. Multiple granulomas and pulmonary calcifications. These changes may be seen with any of the pulmonary mycoses but are most often caused by *Histoplasma capsulatum*.

appropriately cultured specimens. The organisms can be identified in respiratory secretions and tissue with methenamine silver or periodic acid–Schiff stains. The organisms grow well on Sabouraud agar. Colonies may appear 2 to 3 days after inoculation, but occasionally 7 to 21 days may be required before growth is apparent. The source of material submitted for bacteriologic or histopathologic study depends on the clinical manifestations that are present in a given case. The organisms can be isolated from sputum in most patients with cavitary pulmonary disease. However, in patients with systemic disease, cultures of other body fluids or tissues may be required for diagnosis. The organisms may be identified in liver, bone, skin, or mucosal lesions or cultured from bone marrow, blood, urine, or cerebrospinal fluid.

Skin tests and serologic tests have variable reliability. Although these studies may be very useful in coccidioidomycosis, they are essentially of no value in blastomycosis. For absolute diagnosis, it is important to identify these organisms by histopathologic or bacteriologic techniques.

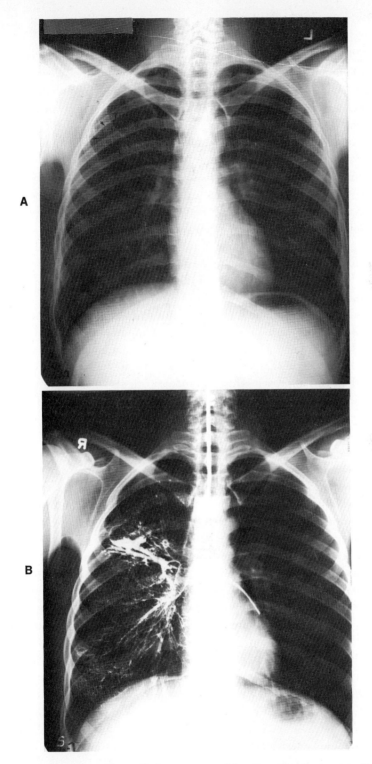

Fig. 30-7. A, Characteristic thin-walled cavity caused by *Coccidioides immitis*. **B,** Cavity is better outlined by bronchographic contrast material.

Treatment

Amphotericin B is currently the drug of choice for treatment of these infections. Toxicity is a limiting factor in using this drug. Fever, chills, nausea, arthralgia, myalgia, and generalized malaise may occur during intravenous infusion of the drug. During the course of therapy, anemia, azotemia, and hypocalcemia may develop. These complications usually resolve when the daily dose of the drug is decreased or the drug is discontinued.

During the primary stage of infection, treatment is generally unnecessary. However, if clinical manifestations of extrathoracic dissemination become evident during this stage of the disease, therapy should be instituted. The optimum dose of the drug under this circumstance is not known. Some patients with systemic symptoms respond well to relatively small doses of the drug and continue to do well when the drug is discontinued. Other patients with obvious extrathoracic involvement may have progressive disease and ultimately die despite amphotericin B administration.

Chronic cavitary infection caused by these fungi is also treated with amphotericin B. At present the goal of therapy is to administer the drug in daily or intermittent doses of approximately 0.5 to 1 mg/kg of body weight until the patient has received a total dose in the range of 2.0 to 2.5 gm. The majority of patients appear to be cured by this approach. However, some patients relapse and require retreatment. Several courses of therapy may have to be administered to some patients before they are cured.

It has been suggested that patients with coccidioidomycosis whose clinical course is characterized by chronic infection and poor response to amphotericin B have impaired immune response to the organism. Some of these patients have been treated with transfer factor with good results. This therapeutic approach has not been used widely in treating either chronic blastomycosis or histoplasmosis.

Fungal meningitis is extremely difficult to treat. Since parenteral administration of amphotericin B results in subtherapeutic cerebrospinal fluid levels of the drug, intrathecal therapy is required. In some patients with chronic meningitis, an Ommaya reservoir has been placed in a lateral ventricle to administer the drug on a long-term, chronic basis.

Other antifungal agents (miconazole and ketoconazole) have undergone clinical trials to determine their efficacy in treating these fungal infections. The role for these drugs in the treatment of the pulmonary mycoses has yet to be defined. Although these drugs appear to be less toxic than amphotericin B, it is not known whether they are more or less efficacious than amphotericin B for treating these three fungal diseases.

Chapter 31

OPPORTUNISTIC PNEUMONIAS

Pulmonary infection is a serious problem in immunocompromised individuals. Most infections in these patients are caused by the same organisms that usually cause infection in individuals with intact immunologic defenses. However, a number of organisms usually do not infect normal individuals but produce serious pulmonary infection in the immunocompromised host:

Bacteria
  Nocardia asteroides
Fungi
  Aspergillus species
  Candida albicans
  Cryptococcus neoformans
  Phycomycetes
  Torulopsis glabrata
Viruses
  Cytomegalovirus
  Herpes simplex virus
  Varicella-zoster
Protozoa
  Pneumocystis carinii
  Toxoplasma gondii
Helminths
  Strongyloides stercoralis

In this chapter the most common of these opportunistic infections will be discussed, particularly those which are potentially treatable:

Organism	Treatment
Apergillus species	Amphotericin B
Candida albicans	Amphotericin B and 5-fluorocytosine
Cryptococcus neoformans	Amphotericin B and 5-fluorocytosine
Nocardia asteroides	Sulfonamides
Pneumocystis carinii	Trimethoprim and sulfamethoxazole

PNEUMOCYSTIS CARINII

In many institutions *Pneumocystis carinii* infection is the most common, treatable opportunistic infection observed in patients with compromised immunologic defenses. Although usually classified as a protozoan, the taxonomy of this organism is somewhat unclear. Since the organism cannot be cultured in the routine clinical laboratory, infection must be documented by histopathologic identification of the organism in pulmonary secretions or living tissues. The organism is generally present in these specimens in the form of a cyst containing a number of merozoites.

Epidemiologic factors and pathogenesis

P. carinii can cause two distinct clinical syndromes. The organism was first identified as a cause of epidemic pulmonary infection in malnourished infants in Europe. This entity is now of little significance and will not be discussed further. Approximately 15 years ago the organism was recognized as a cause of pulmonary infection in immunocompromised patients. This form of infection has achieved major clinical significance, since an increasing number of patients with a variety of diseases have undergone immunosuppression during the course of modern therapy.

The epidemiologic factors of the infection are unclear. Some observations suggest that human-to-human transmission of the organism may occur. It is also clear that the organism may reside in the lung without causing clinical manifestations of infection. Impairment of cellular immunity appears to be important in the activation of latent infection and the development of clinical manifestations of disease. As will be pointed out in the following paragraphs, activation of latent infection can be prevented with appropriate therapy.

Clinical and roentgenographic manifestations

P. carinii infection is characterized by the development of fever, dyspnea, and nonproductive cough. In some patients the disease progresses rapidly in only a few days, but in others it evolves gradually over a period of 5 to 7 days. Physical findings are often not impressive. However, tachypnea and cyanosis are usually present, and rales may be audible during auscultation of the lungs. With prompt institution of therapy, many patients recover, the disease may progress despite therapy. If the disease is not treated, all patients eventually develop progressive respiratory disease and die within days.

At the onset of the disease the chest roentgenogram may reveal only a localized alveolar filling process. However, a characteristic diffuse, bilateral, ground-glass, alveolar filling pattern usually evolves over several days (Fig. 31-1). Nodular densities and pleural effusion have been identified in some cases but are extremely uncommon. With successful treatment the chest roentgenogram usually returns to normal.

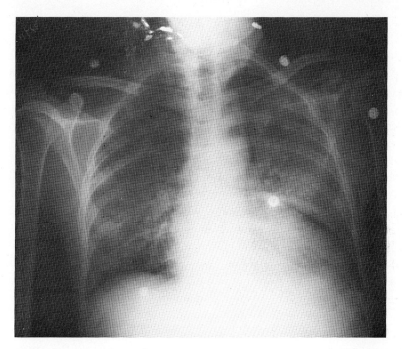

Fig. 31-1. *Pneumocystis carinii* infection with a diffuse, gound-glass, alveolar filling pattern.

Diagnosis

The diagnosis of *P. carinii* infection is made by demonstrating the organism in respiratory secretions or lung tissue. No other diagnostic studies are of value. If a patient is suspected of having *P. carinii* infection, a variety of techniques can be employed to obtain material for histopathologic examination.

Examination of tissue obtained by open lung biopsy is the most sensitive and specific method for diagnosis. Although open lung biopsy has the disadvantage of being a major surgical procedure that requires general anesthesia, seriously ill patients tolerate the procedure surprisingly well. Open lung biopsy should be performed in the majority of patients who are suspected of having this infection when the diagnosis cannot be substantiated by other methods.

Transbronchial lung biopsy through the fiberoptic bronchoscope is also an excellent diagnostic technique. False negative results appear to occur infrequently when adequate tissue is obtained for examination. Unfortunately, the more serious the patient's respiratory distress, the less applicable the technique, since patient cooperation and breath holding are required to perform the biopsy. Severe hypoxemia despite oxygen therapy should be considered a relative contraindication to transbronchial biopsy, since the development of a pneumothorax may further compromise gas exchange and produce life-threatening hypoxemia. The procedure is absolutely contraindicated in patients who are undergoing mechanical ventilation.

The pathologic features of *P. carinii* infection are characteristic. Routine hematoxylin and eosin stains reveal hyperplasia of the type II alveolar pneumocytes and the presence of foamy, eosinophilic material in the alveolar space. Inflammatory cell infiltration is usually minimum. Using silver stains, the cystic form of the organism can usually be easily identified in the alveolar spaces. The cysts appear oval or crescentic and are often present in groups.

The organism may also be identified in various respiratory secretions. In a small percentage of cases the organism can be identified in sputum. Although organisms may be identified in material obtained by brushing areas of involved lung at the time of bronchoscopy, the sensitivity of this technique is not high. Recent studies suggest that in a high percentage of cases, organisms may be observed in the pellet of the effluent obtained by subsegmental bronchoalveolar lavage. If further studies confirm that the yield of this procedure is high, it will be extremely valuable, since the procedure can be easily performed under almost all conditions.

Treatment

A combination of trimethoprim and sulfamethoxazole is the treatment of choice for *P. carinii* infection. The results of therapy are at least in part related to the interval between the onset of clinical manifestations of infection and institution of the drugs. As a general rule, the shorter the interval, the more likely that the patient will survive. When given orally once a day, this drug combination also appears to be effective in preventing infection in high-risk patients. Since this drug combination is relatively nontoxic, it is almost an ideal form of treatment for this infection.

Pentamidine isothionate is an effective drug for treating *P. carinii* infection and was extensively employed in the past. In contrast to the combination of trimethoprim and sulfamethoxazole, this drug has a number of serious side effects; thus it is now used only in patients who do not appear to be responding to trimethoprim-sulfamethoxazole therapy.

CRYPTOCOCCOSIS

Cryptococcus neoformans exists in nature as an unencapsulated yeast form. The organism that is frequently isolated from soil contaminated by pigeon and chicken droppings may cause pulmonary infection when inhaled into the lung from environmental sources. Human-to-human transmission of the organism does not seem to occur. Although the organism may produce infection in normal individuals, it appears that the incidence of infection is increased in some immunocompromised individuals, particularly patients with Hodgkin disease and those receiving corticosteroids.

Clinical manifestations

Cough, with or without sputum production; weight loss; fever; and chest pain are the most common symptoms observed in patients with pulmonary cryptococcosis. However, almost a third of patients are asymptomatic despite roentgenographic evidence of infection. In immunocompetent individuals, infection is usually localized to the lung. In contrast, immunocompromised hosts almost always have disseminated disease. Meningitis is the most common manifestation of disseminated disease in these patients. In this situation manifestations of meningeal disease usually dominate the clinical picture, and there may be few if any pulmonary symptoms.

The roentgenographic manifestations of pulmonary crytococcosis are varied. Localized segmental or lobar infiltrates are the most common abnormalities observed. Cavitation may occur in some areas of localized infiltrative disease. Single or multiple nodules, or mass lesions, are also frequently present. These lesions also cavitate on occasion (Fig. 31-2). Diffuse infiltrates occur primarily in immunocompromised hosts and may be observed in approximately 20% of such patients. Hilar adenopathy and pleural effusions are present in a small percentage of patients.

Diagnosis

The diagnosis of cryptococcosis is based on identification of the organism in culture or histopathologic identification of the organism in tissue. *C. neoformans* may be identified in smears of sputum and cerebrospinal fluid in patients with pulmonary or meningeal involvement respectively. Since the organism may on occasion colonize the respiratory tract, sputum isolates are not necessarily indicative of pulmonary infection. However, identification of the organism in sputum from hosts with compromised immunologic defenses should not be treated lightly. If pulmonary infiltrates are present, treatment should be instituted immediately. The organism may be isolated from blood, urine, prostatic secretions, and skin lesions in patients with disseminated disease.

Both cryptococcal antigen and antibody can be measured by serologic tests. Detection of antigen in serum or cerebrospinal fluid is diagnostic of the disease. Although false positive tests do not occur, these tests lack sensitivity. Antigen cannot be detected in the sera of as many as a third of patients with disease. Tests for cryptococcal antibody are of less value, since the false positive rate is significant. Both tests are limited in their clinical use by the inherent delay in obtaining the test results.

Treatment

The most effective treatment for cryptococcosis is not known. The organism is clearly susceptible to amphotericin B, but the toxicity of the drug often limits its use in infected patients. Furthermore, the total dose and duration of therapy with this drug is unknown. Therapy can be guided only by the clinical and roentgeno-

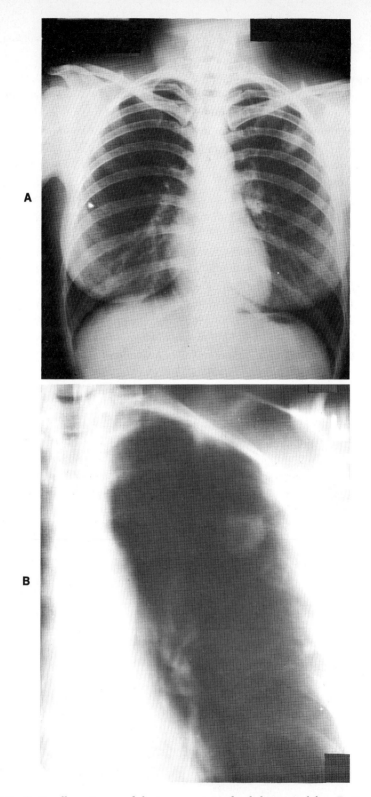

Fig. 31-2. A, Small cavitary nodule is present in the left upper lobe. **B,** Lesion is well defined by tomography. *Cryptococcus neoformans* was grown from a bronchial brush specimen.

graphic response of the patient's condition during treatment. Since spontaneous resolution of pulmonary infection may occur in patients who are not immunocompromised, it is unclear whether these patients need to be treated. Patients with impaired immunologic defenses should be treated for pulmonary cryptococcosis to prevent dissemination of the infection.

5-Fluorocytosine (5-FC) has also been employed successfully in treating cryptococcosis. This drug cannot be used alone, since drug resistance frequently develops during therapy. A combination of 5-FC and low-dose amphotericin B may be the most effective form of therapy for immunocompromised hosts.

ASPERGILLOSIS

Pulmonary infection by various *Aspergillus* species, usually *A. fumigatus,* is believed to result primarily from inhalation of spores into the respiratory tract from the environment. In some patients pulmonary infection may occur as a result of hematogenous spread of the organism from a primary site of infection in the gastrointestinal tract or by aspiration of organisms that have colonized the upper respiratory tract. Human-to-human transmission of the organism does not appear to occur.

The *Aspergillus* organism is a common environmental contaminant. Although the organism may be isolated from sputum in a small percentage of both normal individuals and persons with chronic lung disease, invasive pulmonary infection occurs almost exclusively in immunocompromised individuals. The specific immunologic defect that predisposes to tissue invasion by *Aspergillus* species is unknown. A number of factors including serious underlying disease, immunosuppressive drug therapy, antibiotic therapy, and preexistent pulmonary infection appear to contribute to the pathogenesis of this infection.

Clinical and roentgenographic manifestations

The clinical and roentgenographic manifestations of invasive pulmonary aspergillosis are entirely nonspecific. As with any pulmonary infection, dyspnea, nonproductive cough, and fever are usually present. In addition, pleuritic chest pain and hemoptysis occur frequently. Physical findings are varied and tend to conform to what would be expected on the basis of the patient's symptoms and roentgenographic findings.

The roentgenographic manifestations of this infection are extremely varied. Because preexisting pulmonary disease is present in many patients who develop aspergillosis, it is often difficult to correlate roentgenographic abnormalities with the presence of infection. The most common manifestations of *Aspergillus* infection are necrotizing pneumonia and hemorrhagic infarction. The *Aspergillus* organism causes hemorrhagic infarction by invading pulmonary arteries and producing vascular thromboses. Although the roentgenogram may initially be entirely normal in

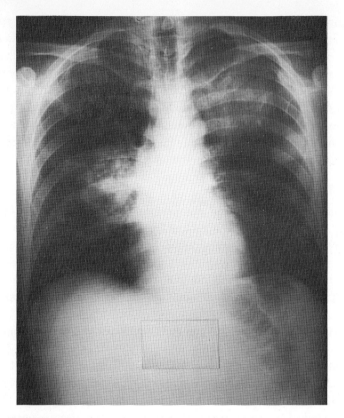

Fig. 31-3. Multilobar necrotizing lesions proven at the postmortem examination to be caused by *Aspergillus fumigatus*.

patients with invasion of pulmonary vessels, parenchymal infiltrates usually develop at some point during the course of the infection. Patchy alveolar infiltrates, lobar consolidation, nodular densities, cavitary densities, and diffuse, nodular, interstitial infiltrates have all been described in patients with aspergillosis (Fig. 31-3). Systemic dissemination of the organism occurs in many patients with invasive pulmonary aspergillosis. A description of the varied manifestations of the systemic dissemination is beyond the scope of this discussion.

Diagnosis

Antemortem diagnosis of invasive aspergillosis is extremely difficult. Since *Aspergillus* species may be a laboratory contaminant or may colonize the respiratory tract, the diagnosis of invasive aspergillosis cannot be based simply on identification of the organism in respiratory secretions. Absolute diagnosis requires both histopathologic identification of hyphae in tissue and bacteriologic identification of the organism in culture.

The pathologic findings of invasive pulmonary aspergillosis are varied. Necrotizing pneumonitis and bronchitis, invasion of small pulmonary vessels, and infarction of lung tissue associated with invasion and occlusion of larger pulmonary vessels are the most common pathologic findings. However, microabscesses, nonnecrotizing pneumonitis, and aspergillomas may also be observed.

Microscopic examination usually reveals invasion of bronchi, bronchioles, and vessels of varying size by hyphae and thrombosis of the involved vessels. Although highly characteristic hyphae may be seen in tissue, absolute diagnosis requires growth of the organism in culture where diagnostic candidiophores may be observed.

From a practical standpoint it is often not possible to obtain lung tissue for definitive diagnosis. Therefore, for a presumptive diagnosis the organism must be identified in respiratory secretions. Unfortunately the majority of patients with invasive pulmonary aspergillosis have negative smears and cultures. Thus the diagnosis is made at autopsy in most immunocompromised hosts who develop this infection.

Precipitating antibody can be detected in the serum of some patients with *Aspergillus* infection. However, serologic tests have not been particularly useful for diagnostic purposes. False negative tests occur in many patients with proven aspergillosis, and a positive test does not necessarily indicate active disease.

Treatment

Amphotericin B is considered the drug of choice for treatment of invasive aspergillosis. However, no convincing data show that amphotericin B has any effect on the course of the disease in patients with malignant diseases, particularly leukemia and lymphoma. Several reports suggest that infection in renal transplant patients may be more responsive to long-term amphotericin B administration.

An aggressive attempt should be undertaken to diagnose *Aspergillus* infection in immunocompromised hosts who may have the disease so that treatment can be instituted as early in the course as possible. It seems reasonable to conclude that the chance of survival is lessened if treatment is delayed until extensive necrotizing pneumonia has developed. No evidence suggests that other antifungal agents have any role in the treatment of this disease.

CANDIDIASIS

Candida albicans and other *Candida* species may cause pulmonary infection in the immunocompromised host. These organisms can be cultured from the oral and gastrointestinal flora of normal individuals and from pulmonary secretions of patients with chronic lung disease and seriously ill patients with other diseases. Thus it is generally assumed that pulmonary infection is caused by aspiration of organisms into the lung or by hematogenous spread of organisms to the lung from extrathoracic sites of infection. Inhalation of the organism from the environment or human-to-human spread of the organism are not considered to play an important role in the pathogenesis of this infection.

Invasive candidiasis is rare in normal individuals. Thus it is clear that impairment of host defenses is critical in the pathogenesis of this infection. Despite a large body of experimental data compiled from animal or in vitro studies, the specific immunologic response that is most critical in protecting against candidal infection is unknown. The use of antibiotics and the presence of indwelling vascular catheters are two factors that seem to predispose to *Candida* pulmonary infection in patients with compromised immunologic defenses. The mechanisms by which these factors predispose to infection is unknown. It is possible that antibiotics, by leading to increased growth of *Candida* organisms on the skin and in the gastrointestinal tract, simply increase the likelihood that tissue invasion will occur. Venous catheters may multiply infection by serving as a route for skin organisms to gain access to the bloodstream or as an intravascular nidus on which the organism may grow.

Clinical and roentgenographic manifestations

The clinical and roentgenographic manifestations of *Candida* pulmonary infection are extremely varied. Shortness of breath, cough, and fever are present in most patients. Although the physical examination may be entirely normal, the physical findings generally reflect the extent of lung involvement visible on the chest roentgenogram. Focal alveolar infiltrates, generally involving multiple lobes, are the most common roentgenographic abnormality observed in candidal infection. Occasionally, multiple small abscesses may be present.

Diagnosis

Pulmonary candidal infection may be extremely difficult to diagnose before death. Definitive diagnosis requires histopathologic identification of the organism invading viable lung tissue. Pathologic examination of involved lung tissue generally reveals focal nodular lesions containing inflammatory cells, predominantly polymorphonuclear leukocytes, and typical budding yeasts and pseudohyphae. Invasion of pulmonary vessels accompanied by thrombosis of the involved vessels is observed in some cases.

Culture of biopsy specimens is not necessarily a reliable way of making a diagnosis, since the organism may be grown from the lung in a small percentage of cases in which no clinical or pathologic evidence of tissue invasion by the organism exists. This observation, plus the fact that colonization of the respiratory tract frequently occurs in seriously ill patients, underscores the difficulty of making a diagnosis by stains or cultures of respiratory secretions. Thus identification of pseudohyphae or yeast forms in respiratory secretions cannot be considered definitive evidence of pulmonary infection.

Identification of *Candida* species in other body fluids is diagnostic of infection. Thus culture of pleural fluid or material aspirated from a lung abscess is useful for making a diagnosis of intrathoracic candidiasis. Since dissemination occurs in most patients with pulmonary infection, identification of the organism in extrathoracic sites is also useful for the diagnosis of pulmonary candidiasis. The kidney is a common site of infection in disseminated candidiasis. Identification of the organism in a clean-catch urine specimen obtained from a patient who has not had an indwelling catheter strongly suggests the presence of renal candidiasis and systemic infection. Similarly, the infection may be diagnosed by identifying the organism in material obtained from other easily accessible sites of infection such as peritoneal or joint fluid or on occasion the aqueous humor of the eye.

Blood cultures are difficult to interpret. Benign candidemia resulting in positive blood cultures may occur in patients who have indwelling venous catheters. Although a positive blood culture is not necessarily indicative of disseminated infection, antifungal therapy should probably be instituted when the organism is isolated from the blood of an immunocompromised patient. Since blood cultures are negative in the majority of patients with disseminated candidal infection, a negative culture does not exclude the diagnosis.

At present, serologic tests have a limited role in the diagnosis of candidal infection. False positive and false negative results occur with the currently available techniques. Thus in the appropriate clinical setting a diagnosis must be based on identification of the organism from appropriate specimens.

Treatment

Amphotericin B is the drug of choice for the treatment of pulmonary candidal infection. The dose and duration of therapy is unknown. Although cure of infection has been documented in some patients, the relative efficacy of this treatment is unknown. In immunocompromised hosts, candidemia should be treated with amphotericin B. However, treatment can be delayed in other patients with positive blood cultures if the patient is clinically stable, has an indwelling venous catheter, and has no evidence of tissue infection. In this setting the catheter should be removed, and serial blood cultures obtained. If positive blood cultures persist for 3 to 4 days, treatment should be instituted. 5-Fluorcytosine, alone or in combination with amphotericin B, has been employed in some patients. There is no evidence that this approach to therapy is any better than amphotericin B alone.

NOCARDIOSIS

Pulmonary infection caused by *Nocardia asteroides* is being increasingly recognized in immunocompromised patients. *N. asteroides* is only one of a number of species of *Nocardia* but by far the most common species associated with pulmonary infection. The organism is a gram-positive, acid-fast bacterium that can be isolated

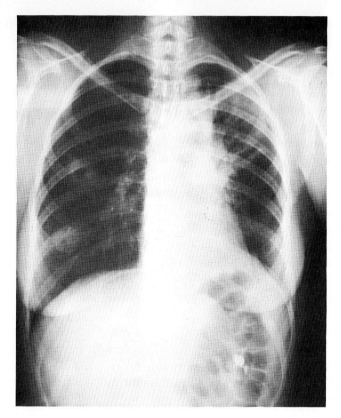

Fig. 31-4. *Nocardia asteroides* infection. Left upper lobe infiltrate and several cavitary nodules in the right lung are evident on the roentgenogram.

from soil. It is generally accepted that pulmonary infection occurs by inhalation of the organism from the environment. Human-to-human transmission of the organism is not thought to be of pathogenetic significance.

Although infection by species of *Nocardia* may occur in perfectly normal individuals, almost half of the cases recorded in the literature have occurred in patients with compromised immunologic defenses, particularly those receiving corticosteroid therapy. The role of both cellular and humeral immunity in the control of nocardial infection has not been established.

Clinical and roentgenographic manifestations

Both the clinical and roentgenographic manifestations of nocardial infection are extremely varied. Some patients are asymptomatic or have only minor symptoms. However, shortness of breath, nonproductive cough, fever, and malaise occur in most patients. Varied pulmonary infiltrates including necrotizing pneumonia, cavitary nodules, mass lesions, and pleural involvement have been observed on chest roentgenograms (Fig. 31-4).

Diagnosis

The diagnosis of pulmonary nocardiosis requires identification of the organism in respiratory secretions or lung tissue obtained by biopsy. Isolation of the organism in culture is usually required, since *Nocardia* organisms cannot be distinguished from actinomycetes by morphologic criteria on stained smears. It is not only difficult to identify the organism in smears of respiratory secretions, but isolation of the organism in culture is often difficult because the plates may be overgrown with other organisms contained in respiratory secretions. Since the *Nocardia* organism is not a common contaminant, its isolation from an immunocompromised host should be considered evidence of infection.

In tissue the organism generally appears in coccobacillary forms or as branching hyphae. Tissue necrosis with polymorphonuclear infiltration is the usual microscopic finding. Areas of chronic inflammation containing lymphocytes and giant cells may be observed on occasion in some regions of lung.

No satisfactory serologic test can detect infection. Other routine laboratory studies are of no diagnostic value.

Treatment

Sulfonamide therapy is the treatment of choice for nocardial infection. The duration of therapy that will produce cure is unknown. In general patients should receive 5 to 10 gm of sulfonamide per day until evidence suggests that the infection has resolved or the disease has become stable. Close observation after cessation of therapy is important to detect clinical relapse. Although other drugs, either alone or in combination with sulfonamides, have been used on occasion to treat nocardial infections, there are no convincing data that this approach is more effective than the use of sulfonamides alone.

INDEX

Italicized page numbers refer to illustrations;
those followed by *T* refer to tables.

Bronchogenic carcinoma
 clinical manifestations of, 67-70
 diagnosis of, 70-71
 epidemiologic factors of, 65-66
 and histopathologic tumor type, 62-63
 mortality rate for, 62
 pathologic features of, 62-65
 prognosis of, 68, 70, 72-73
 staging evaluation of, 71-72
 survival rate in, 72, *72*, 73
 treatment of, 72-73
Bronchogram
 in bronchiectasis, 44-45, 48
 for differential diagnosis of chronic bronchitis, 56
Bronchopleural fistula, chronic, 311
Bronchopulmonary aspergillosis, 155, 156
Bronchoscope, flexible, in diagnosis of bronchogenic carcinoma, 70
Brucella, 295
Bullous emphysema, *120, 121,* 121-122
Busulfan, 181-182
 and direct pulmonary toxicity, 179

C
Calcification, "eggshell," in complicated silicosis, 168, *168*
Candida albicans, 337, 340
Candidiasis
 clinical manifestations of, 346
 diagnosis of, 346-347
 roentgenographic manifestations of, 346
 treatment of, 346
Capillaries
 hydrostatic pressure of, 216
  increased, 217-218
 permeability of, in pulmonary edema, 219
Caplan syndrome
 and coal workers pneumoconiosis, 175, 177
 in silicosis, 168-169
Capreomycin, 327T
Carbon dioxide, 253-255
 content of, in blood, 254
 membrane diffusing capacity for, 96-97
 partial pressure of, 254, 255, 256, 257, 258, 262, 263
 relationship of, to bicarbonate, 257
Carbonic acid, 253
 concentration of, in blood, 254
Carcinogens, environmental, and bronchogenic carcinoma, 66
Carcinoid adenomas, 74-76
Carcinoid syndrome, 76
Carcinoma
 bronchogenic; *see* Bronchogenic carcinoma
 large cell
  in bronchogenic carcinoma, 62, 65
  and ectopic hormone secretion, 69T
 small cell
  in bronchogenic carcinoma, 62, 63, 65, 66

Carcinoma-con't
 small cell-cont'd
  and ectopic hormone secretion, 68, 69T
 squamous cell
  in bronchogenic carcinoma, 62, 63, 65, 66
  and ectopic hormone secretion, 68, 69T
Catheterization, cardiac, in primary pulmonary hypertension, 225
Cellular immune response in pulmonary infections, 292, 293
Central nervous system and sarcoidosis, 147
Centriacinar emphysema, 112, 113, *113, 114,* 115, *116*
Centrilobular emphysema; *see* Centriacinar emphysema
Cephalosporin, 316
Cerebrospinal fluid and ventilation, 257
Chemoprophylaxis for tuberculosis, 325-328
Chemotherapy for bronchogenic carcinoma, 73
Chest, physical examination of
 in bronchiectasis, 42
 in chronic bronchitis, 55
Chloramphenicol, 312
Chronic fibrosing alveolitis; *see* Alveolitis, chronic fibrosing
Ciliated cell, 8, 13
 purpose of, 5
Clara cells, purpose of, 5, 8
Clindamycin, 312
Closing volume, measurement of, 27-28
Coal macule, 174
Coal workers pneumoconiosis; *see* Pneumoconiosis, coal workers
Coccidioides immitis, 330, 331, 332, *335*
Coccidioidomycosis, 330, 336
Colchicine, 186
 and increased alveolar-capillary permeability, 179
Collagen in alveolar wall, 92, 94
Collagen vascular diseases, 232, *233*
Connective tissue diseases and chronic fibrosing alveolitis, 135-140
Cor pulmonale
 in chronic bronchitis, 61
 clinical manifestations of, 213
 definition of, 211
 diagnosis of, 213-214
 in primary pulmonary hypertension, 225
 in respiratory failure, 268-269
 treatment of, 214-215
Corticosteroid therapy, 229, 232, 234, 235, 286
 in acute asthma treatment, 39
 for adult respiratory distress syndrome, 279
 for allergic alveolitis, 161
 for alveolar proteinosis, 195
 for bronchogenic carcinoma, 73
 for chronic bronchitis, 60
 for chronic fibrosing alveolitis, 134-135
 for pulmonary edema, 221
 and radiation pneumonitis, 183
 for sarcoidosis, 151-152